Pharmacogenomics

DRUGS AND THE PHARMACEUTICAL SCIENCES

Executive Editor
James Swarbrick
AAI, Inc.
Wilmington, North Carolina

Advisory Board

DRUGS AND THE PHARMACEUTICAL SCIENCES

A Series of Textbooks and Monographs

1. Pharmacokinetics, *Milo Gibaldi and Donald Perrier*
2. Good Manufacturing Practices for Pharmaceuticals: A Plan for Total Quality Control, *Sidney H. Willig, Murray M. Tuckerman, and William S. Hitchings IV*
3. Microencapsulation, *edited by J. R. Nixon*
4. Drug Metabolism: Chemical and Biochemical Aspects, *Bernard Testa and Peter Jenner*
5. New Drugs: Discovery and Development, *edited by Alan A. Rubin*
6. Sustained and Controlled Release Drug Delivery Systems, *edited by Joseph R. Robinson*
7. Modern Pharmaceutics, *edited by Gilbert S. Banker and Christopher T. Rhodes*
8. Prescription Drugs in Short Supply: Case Histories, *Michael A. Schwartz*
9. Activated Charcoal: Antidotal and Other Medical Uses, *David O. Cooney*
10. Concepts in Drug Metabolism (in two parts), *edited by Peter Jenner and Bernard Testa*
11. Pharmaceutical Analysis: Modern Methods (in two parts), *edited by James W. Munson*
12. Techniques of Solubilization of Drugs, *edited by Samuel H. Yalkowsky*
13. Orphan Drugs, *edited by Fred E. Karch*
14. Novel Drug Delivery Systems: Fundamentals, Developmental Concepts, Biomedical Assessments, *Yie W. Chien*
15. Pharmacokinetics: Second Edition, Revised and Expanded, *Milo Gibaldi and Donald Perrier*
16. Good Manufacturing Practices for Pharmaceuticals: A Plan for Total Quality Control, Second Edition, Revised and Expanded, *Sidney H. Willig, Murray M. Tuckerman, and William S. Hitchings IV*
17. Formulation of Veterinary Dosage Forms, *edited by Jack Blodinger*
18. Dermatological Formulations: Percutaneous Absorption, *Brian W. Barry*
19. The Clinical Research Process in the Pharmaceutical Industry, *edited by Gary M. Matoren*
20. Microencapsulation and Related Drug Processes, *Patrick B. Deasy*
21. Drugs and Nutrients: The Interactive Effects, *edited by Daphne A. Roe and T. Colin Campbell*
22. Biotechnology of Industrial Antibiotics, *Erick J. Vandamme*

23. Pharmaceutical Process Validation, *edited by Bernard T. Loftus and Robert A. Nash*

24. Anticancer and Interferon Agents: Synthesis and Properties, *edited by Raphael M. Ottenbrite and George B. Butler*

25. Pharmaceutical Statistics: Practical and Clinical Applications, *Sanford Bolton*

26. Drug Dynamics for Analytical, Clinical, and Biological Chemists, *Benjamin J. Gudzinowicz, Burrows T. Younkin, Jr., and Michael J. Gudzinowicz*

27. Modern Analysis of Antibiotics, *edited by Adjoran Aszalos*

28. Solubility and Related Properties, *Kenneth C. James*

29. Controlled Drug Delivery: Fundamentals and Applications, Second Edition, Revised and Expanded, *edited by Joseph R. Robinson and Vincent H. Lee*

30. New Drug Approval Process: Clinical and Regulatory Management, *edited by Richard A. Guarino*

31. Transdermal Controlled Systemic Medications, *edited by Yie W. Chien*

32. Drug Delivery Devices: Fundamentals and Applications, *edited by Praveen Tyle*

33. Pharmacokinetics: Regulatory • Industrial • Academic Perspectives, *edited by Peter G. Welling and Francis L. S. Tse*

34. Clinical Drug Trials and Tribulations, *edited by Allen E. Cato*

35. Transdermal Drug Delivery: Developmental Issues and Research Initiatives, *edited by Jonathan Hadgraft and Richard H. Guy*

36. Aqueous Polymeric Coatings for Pharmaceutical Dosage Forms, *edited by James W. McGinity*

37. Pharmaceutical Pelletization Technology, *edited by Isaac Ghebre-Sellassie*

38. Good Laboratory Practice Regulations, *edited by Allen F. Hirsch*

39. Nasal Systemic Drug Delivery, *Yie W. Chien, Kenneth S. E. Su, and Shyi-Feu Chang*

40. Modern Pharmaceutics: Second Edition, Revised and Expanded, *edited by Gilbert S. Banker and Christopher T. Rhodes*

41. Specialized Drug Delivery Systems: Manufacturing and Production Technology, *edited by Praveen Tyle*

42. Topical Drug Delivery Formulations, *edited by David W. Osborne and Anton H. Amann*

43. Drug Stability: Principles and Practices, *Jens T. Carstensen*

44. Pharmaceutical Statistics: Practical and Clinical Applications, Second Edition, Revised and Expanded, *Sanford Bolton*

45. Biodegradable Polymers as Drug Delivery Systems, *edited by Mark Chasin and Robert Langer*

46. Preclinical Drug Disposition: A Laboratory Handbook, *Francis L. S. Tse and James J. Jaffe*

47. HPLC in the Pharmaceutical Industry, *edited by Godwin W. Fong and Stanley K. Lam*

48. Pharmaceutical Bioequivalence, *edited by Peter G. Welling, Francis L. S. Tse, and Shrikant V. Dinghe*

49. Pharmaceutical Dissolution Testing, *Umesh V. Banakar*
50. Novel Drug Delivery Systems: Second Edition, Revised and Expanded, *Yie W. Chien*
51. Managing the Clinical Drug Development Process, *David M. Cocchetto and Ronald V. Nardi*
52. Good Manufacturing Practices for Pharmaceuticals: A Plan for Total Quality Control, Third Edition, *edited by Sidney H. Willig and James R. Stoker*
53. Prodrugs: Topical and Ocular Drug Delivery, *edited by Kenneth B. Sloan*
54. Pharmaceutical Inhalation Aerosol Technology, *edited by Anthony J. Hickey*
55. Radiopharmaceuticals: Chemistry and Pharmacology, *edited by Adrian D. Nunn*
56. New Drug Approval Process: Second Edition, Revised and Expanded, *edited by Richard A. Guarino*
57. Pharmaceutical Process Validation: Second Edition, Revised and Expanded, *edited by Ira R. Berry and Robert A. Nash*
58. Ophthalmic Drug Delivery Systems, *edited by Ashim K. Mitra*
59. Pharmaceutical Skin Penetration Enhancement, *edited by Kenneth A. Walters and Jonathan Hadgraft*
60. Colonic Drug Absorption and Metabolism, *edited by Peter R. Bieck*
61. Pharmaceutical Particulate Carriers: Therapeutic Applications, *edited by Alain Rolland*
62. Drug Permeation Enhancement: Theory and Applications, *edited by Dean S. Hsieh*
63. Glycopeptide Antibiotics, *edited by Ramakrishnan Nagarajan*
64. Achieving Sterility in Medical and Pharmaceutical Products, *Nigel A. Halls*
65. Multiparticulate Oral Drug Delivery, *edited by Isaac Ghebre-Sellassie*
66. Colloidal Drug Delivery Systems, *edited by Jörg Kreuter*
67. Pharmacokinetics: Regulatory • Industrial • Academic Perspectives, Second Edition, *edited by Peter G. Welling and Francis L. S. Tse*
68. Drug Stability: Principles and Practices, Second Edition, Revised and Expanded, *Jens T. Carstensen*
69. Good Laboratory Practice Regulations: Second Edition, Revised and Expanded, *edited by Sandy Weinberg*
70. Physical Characterization of Pharmaceutical Solids, *edited by Harry G. Brittain*
71. Pharmaceutical Powder Compaction Technology, *edited by Göran Alderborn and Christer Nyström*
72. Modern Pharmaceutics: Third Edition, Revised and Expanded, *edited by Gilbert S. Banker and Christopher T. Rhodes*
73. Microencapsulation: Methods and Industrial Applications, *edited by Simon Benita*
74. Oral Mucosal Drug Delivery, *edited by Michael J. Rathbone*
75. Clinical Research in Pharmaceutical Development, *edited by Barry Bleidt and Michael Montagne*

76. The Drug Development Process: Increasing Efficiency and Cost Effectiveness, *edited by Peter G. Welling, Louis Lasagna, and Umesh V. Banakar*

77. Microparticulate Systems for the Delivery of Proteins and Vaccines, *edited by Smadar Cohen and Howard Bernstein*

78. Good Manufacturing Practices for Pharmaceuticals: A Plan for Total Quality Control, Fourth Edition, Revised and Expanded, *Sidney H. Willig and James R. Stoker*

79. Aqueous Polymeric Coatings for Pharmaceutical Dosage Forms: Second Edition, Revised and Expanded, *edited by James W. McGinity*

80. Pharmaceutical Statistics: Practical and Clinical Applications, Third Edition, *Sanford Bolton*

81. Handbook of Pharmaceutical Granulation Technology, *edited by Dilip M. Parikh*

82. Biotechnology of Antibiotics: Second Edition, Revised and Expanded, *edited by William R. Strohl*

83. Mechanisms of Transdermal Drug Delivery, *edited by Russell O. Potts and Richard H. Guy*

84. Pharmaceutical Enzymes, *edited by Albert Lauwers and Simon Scharpé*

85. Development of Biopharmaceutical Parenteral Dosage Forms, *edited by John A. Bontempo*

86. Pharmaceutical Project Management, *edited by Tony Kennedy*

87. Drug Products for Clinical Trials: An International Guide to Formulation • Production • Quality Control, *edited by Donald C. Monkhouse and Christopher T. Rhodes*

88. Development and Formulation of Veterinary Dosage Forms: Second Edition, Revised and Expanded, *edited by Gregory E. Hardee and J. Desmond Baggot*

89. Receptor-Based Drug Design, *edited by Paul Leff*

90. Automation and Validation of Information in Pharmaceutical Processing, *edited by Joseph F. deSpautz*

91. Dermal Absorption and Toxicity Assessment, *edited by Michael S. Roberts and Kenneth A. Walters*

92. Pharmaceutical Experimental Design, *Gareth A. Lewis, Didier Mathieu, and Roger Phan-Tan-Luu*

93. Preparing for FDA Pre-Approval Inspections, *edited by Martin D. Hynes III*

94. Pharmaceutical Excipients: Characterization by IR, Raman, and NMR Spectroscopy, *David E. Bugay and W. Paul Findlay*

95. Polymorphism in Pharmaceutical Solids, *edited by Harry G. Brittain*

96. Freeze-Drying/Lyophilization of Pharmaceutical and Biological Products, *edited by Louis Rey and Joan C. May*

97. Percutaneous Absorption: Drugs–Cosmetics–Mechanisms–Methodology, Third Edition, Revised and Expanded, *edited by Robert L. Bronaugh and Howard I. Maibach*

98. Bioadhesive Drug Delivery Systems: Fundamentals, Novel Approaches, and Development, *edited by Edith Mathiowitz, Donald E. Chickering III, and Claus-Michael Lehr*

99. Protein Formulation and Delivery, *edited by Eugene J. McNally*

100. New Drug Approval Process: Third Edition, The Global Challenge, *edited by Richard A. Guarino*

101. Peptide and Protein Drug Analysis, *edited by Ronald E. Reid*

102. Transport Processes in Pharmaceutical Systems, *edited by Gordon L. Amidon, Ping I. Lee, and Elizabeth M. Topp*

103. Excipient Toxicity and Safety, *edited by Myra L. Weiner and Lois A. Kotkoskie*

104. The Clinical Audit in Pharmaceutical Development, *edited by Michael R. Hamrell*

105. Pharmaceutical Emulsions and Suspensions, *edited by Francoise Nielloud and Gilberte Marti-Mestres*

106. Oral Drug Absorption: Prediction and Assessment, *edited by Jennifer B. Dressman and Hans Lennernäs*

107. Drug Stability: Principles and Practices, Third Edition, Revised and Expanded, *edited by Jens T. Carstensen and C. T. Rhodes*

108. Containment in the Pharmaceutical Industry, *edited by James P. Wood*

109. Good Manufacturing Practices for Pharmaceuticals: A Plan for Total Quality Control from Manufacturer to Consumer, Fifth Edition, Revised and Expanded, *Sidney H. Willig*

110. Advanced Pharmaceutical Solids, *Jens T. Carstensen*

111. Endotoxins: Pyrogens, LAL Testing, and Depyrogenation, Second Edition, Revised and Expanded, *Kevin L. Williams*

112. Pharmaceutical Process Engineering, *Anthony J. Hickey and David Ganderton*

113. Pharmacogenomics, *edited by Werner Kalow, Urs A. Meyer, and Rachel F. Tyndale*

ADDITIONAL VOLUMES IN PREPARATION

Handbook of Pharmaceutical Analysis, *edited by Lena Ohannesian and Anthony J. Streeter*

Drug–Drug Interactions, *David Rodrigues*

Pharmaceutical Process Scale-Up, *Michael Levin*

Handbook of Drug Screening, *edited by Ramakrishna Seethala and Prabhavathi Fernandes*

Drug Targeting Technology: A Critical Analysis of Physical • Chemical • Biological Methods, *edited by Hans Schreier*

Pharmacogenomics

edited by

Werner Kalow
University of Toronto
Toronto, Ontario, Canada

Urs A. Meyer
University of Basel
Basel, Switzerland

Rachel F. Tyndale
University of Toronto
Toronto, Ontario, Canada

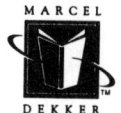

MARCEL DEKKER, INC.   NEW YORK · BASEL

FIRST INDIAN REPRINT 2008

ISBN: 0-8247-0544-0

Headquarters
Marcel Dekker, Inc.
270 Madison Avenue, New York, NY 10016
tel: 212-696-9000; Fax: 212-685-4540

Eastern Hemisphere Distribution
Marcel Dekker AG
Hutgasse 4, Postfach 812, CH-4001 Basel, Switzerland
tel: 41-61-261-8482; fax: 41-61-261-8896

World Wide Web
http://www.dekker.com

The publisher offers discounts on this book when ordered in bulk quantities. For more information, write to Special Sales/Professional Marketing at the headquarters address above.

Printed in India by Saurabh Printers Pvt. Ltd.

Preface

The term *pharmacogenomics* is a recent arrival in the literature, but it is a term that anyone interested in pharmacogenetics cannot overlook. The increasing prevalence of the term reflects the progressive transition from genetics to genomics that is taking place in pharmaceutical science. The most famous research in genomics is a worldwide program called the Human Genome Project,* a massive effort that is expected to change the science of human biology, including our understanding of human disease. For anyone concerned with drugs and pharmacology, the arrival of the term *pharmacogenomics* is a reflection of this broad change.

The genome of any organism is a complex structure built of almost innumerable molecules of deoxyribonucleic acid (DNA). Within any chromosome, the structure is a continuum made up of small sections called *genes*. It is interesting to note that some experts have recently questioned the scientific relevance of the subdivision of the genome structure into genes. Historically, this logical and useful subdivision came about through the realization that "one gene forms one protein" (but perhaps "peptide" is more accurate than "protein"). However, there is no question that the components of DNA that are not participating in the·

---

* S Collins et al. New goals for the U.S. Human Genome Project: 1998–2003. Science 282:682–689, 1998.

making of peptides at least play important roles by controlling gene expression, RNA splicing, chromatin domain formation, maintenance of chromosome structure, recombinations, and replications. The genome is more than the sum of the genes.

Current pharmacogenetics research deals mostly with inherited changes of protein structure (e.g., changes of drug-metabolizing enzymes) that affect the fate of and thereby the response to a particular drug. Future work in pharmacogenetics may also emphasize the often complex genetic control of the amounts of enzyme and receptor proteins. Although *pharmacogenetics* and *pharmacogenomics* are sometimes used interchangeably, the latter is understood to deal in addition with the identification of new drug targets. Although genetic diseases are generally rare, it is clear that other, more common diseases are usually associated with several or many genetic changes that cause disease in combination with environmental factors. The identification of such a genetic change means that, at least in some cases, drugs can be found that will reverse such a change or compensate for it.

Pharmacogenetics and pharmacogenomics are overlapping sciences, but in practice, pharmacogenomics introduces an additional element. For example, 20 genetic changes may contribute to cardiovascular disease, but only one or two of these changes may cause the disease in a given person. A given drug may alleviate the disease only in patients who are affected by these one or two changes. In addition, pharmacogenetics tells us that some drugs can be taken with safety only by persons without a particular genetic defect or alteration. Thus, there are two elements that point to the future usefulness of personalized medicine, provided that the genome of the patient can be scrutinized appropriately for the absence or presence of relevant mutations.

The effort of looking for relevant mutations has already led to many technical changes that allow examination of numerous genes in many people. A thorough discussion on pharmacogenomics should include a description of some of these new techniques to test genetic changes. Unfortunately, the knowledge of a genetic change may be useless until the affected protein or peptide is identified, and until the physiological or pathological significance of the protein or peptide is known. Therefore, this volume includes a look at the techniques that may provide that knowledge. The relevant techniques will give rise to masses of data that will be analyzed and organized with the help of a new science called bioinformatics. Thus, this book will provide the reader with a broad perspective on current topics as well as problems and solutions that may arise in pharmacogenomics in the future.

Werner Kalow

Contents

Preface   *iii*

Contributors   *ix*

1. Historical Aspects of Pharmacogenetics   1
   Werner Kalow

2. Pharmacogenomics, Biomarkers, and the Promise of
   Personalized Medicine   11
   B. Michael Silber

3. Current Status: Pharmacogenetics/Drug Metabolism   33
   Leif Bertilsson

4. Pharmacogenetics—Receptors   51
   Wendell W. Weber

5. Pharmacogenetics of Drug Transporters   81
   Richard B. Kim and Grant R. Wilkinson

6. Interethnic Differences in Drug Response   109
   Werner Kalow

7. Pharmacogenetics: Clinical Viewpoints   135
    Urs A. Meyer

8. Tools of the Trade: The Technologies and Challenges of
    Pharmacogenetics   151
    Glenn A. Miller

9. Molecular Diagnostics and Development of Biotechnology-
    Based Diagnostics   169
    Tracy L. Stockley and Peter N. Ray

10. Technologies for the Analysis of Single-Nucleotide
    Polymorphisms: An Overview   183
    Denis M. Grant and Michael S. Phillips

11. Multiplex Fluorescent Minisequencing Applied to the Typing
    of Genes Encoding Drug-Metabolizing Enzymes   191
    Gisela Sitbon and Ann-Christine Syvänen

12. Multiplex Genotyping by Specialized Mass Spectrometry   201
    Philip L. Ross, Laura Hall, Larry Haff, and Alex Garvin

13. Serial Analysis of Gene Expression: Transcriptional Insights
    into Functional Biology   223
    Stephen L. Madden, Clarence Wang, and Greg Landes

14. Proteomics   253
    Frank A. Witzmann

15. Bioinformatics: WWW Resources   291
    Siu Tang and Daiga Helmeste

16. Applied Bioinformatics   311
    David L. Hyndman and Masato Mitsuhashi

17. Mapping of Disease Loci   337
    Glenys Thomson

18. Positional Cloning and Disease Gene Identification   363
    *Mark S. Silverberg, Andrew P. Boright, and Katherine A.
    Siminovitch*

Contents

19. General Conclusions and Future Directions   389
    Werner Kalow and Arno G. Motulsky

Index   *397*

Contributors

Leif Bertilsson, Ph.D.   Department of Medical Laboratory Sciences and Technology, Division of Clinical Pharmacology at Karolinska Institutet, Huddinge University Hospital, Stockholm, Sweden

Andrew P. Boright, M.D., Ph.D.   Department of Genetics, University of Toronto, and Hospital for Sick Children, Toronto, Ontario, Canada

Alex Garvin, Ph.D.   Division of Pharmacology, Biocenter of the University of Basel, Basel, Switzerland

Denis M. Grant, Ph.D.   Orchid BioSciences Inc., Princeton, New Jersey

Larry Haff, Ph.D.   Applied Biosystems, Framingham, Massachusetts

Laura Hall   Applied Biosystems, Framingham, Massachusetts

Daiga Helmeste   Department of Psychiatry, University of California, Irvine, Irvine, California

David L. Hyndman   Hitachi Chemical Research Center, Irvine, California

ix

Werner Kalow, M.D.   Department of Pharmacology, University of Toronto, Toronto, Ontario, Canada

Richard B. Kim, M.D.   Department of Medicine and Pharmacology, School of Medicine, Vanderbilt University, Nashville, Tennessee

Greg Landes   Genzyme Corporation, Framingham, Massachusetts

Stephen L. Madden, Ph.D.   Genzyme Corporation, Framingham, Massachusetts

Urs A. Meyer, M.D.   Division of Pharmacology/Neurobiology, Biocenter of the University of Basel, Basel, Switzerland

Glenn A. Miller, Ph.D.   Genzyme Corporation, Framingham, Massachusetts

Masato Mitsuhashi, M.D., Ph.D.   Hitachi Chemical Research Center and Department of Pathology, University of California, Irvine, Irvine, California

Arno G. Motulsky   Department of Medicine and Genetics, University of Washington, Seattle, Washington

Michael S. Phillips, Ph.D.   Orchid BioSciences Inc., Princeton, New Jersey

Peter N. Ray, Ph.D.   Division of Molecular Diagnostics, Department of Pediatric Laboratory Medicine, Hospital for Sick Children, Toronto, Ontario, Canada

Philip L. Ross, Ph.D.   Applied Biosystems, Framingham, Massachusetts

B. Michael Silber, Ph.D.   Pharmacogenomics and Clinical Biochemical Measurements Department, Pfizer Global Research and Development, Groton, Connecticut

Mark S. Silverberg, M.D.   Department of Medicine, University of Toronto, and Samuel Lunenfeld Research Institute, Mount Sinai Hospital, Toronto, Ontario, Canada

Katherine A. Siminovitch, M.D.   Department of Medicine, University of Toronto, and Samuel Lunenfeld Research Institute, Mount Sinai Hospital, Toronto, Ontario, Canada

Gisela Sitbon, Ph.D.   PGL Professional Genetics Laboratory AB, Uppsala, Sweden

Tracy L. Stockley, Ph.D.   Division of Molecular Diagnostics, Department of Pediatric Laboratory Medicine, Hospital for Sick Children, Toronto, Ontario, Canada

Ann-Christine Syvänen, Ph.D.   Department of Medical Sciences, Molecular Medicine, Uppsala University, Uppsala, Sweden

Siu Tang   Department of Psychiatry, University of California, Irvine, Irvine, California

Glenys Thomson   Department of Integrative Biology, University of California, Berkeley, Berkeley, California

Clarence Wang   Genzyme Corporation, Framingham, Massachusetts

Wendell W. Weber, Ph.D., M.D.   Department of Pharmacology, University of Michigan, Ann Arbor, Michigan

Grant R. Wilkinson, Ph.D.   Department of Pharmacology, School of Medicine, Vanderbilt University, Nashville, Tennessee

Frank A. Witzmann, Ph.D.   Molecular Anatomy Laboratory, Indiana University–Purdue University, Columbus, Indiana

1

Historical Aspects of Pharmacogenetics

Werner Kalow
University of Toronto, Toronto, Ontario, Canada

1 INTRODUCTION

Pharmacogenetics deals with heredity and responses to drugs. It is a branch of science that attempts to explain variability of one or another drug responses, and to search for the genetic basis of such variations or differences. Early on, pharmacogenetics research examined differences between individual subjects, but as it developed, it also became concerned with genetic differences between populations. Although many pharmacogeneticists are primarily concerned with the human species, the science can, in principle, be applied to all subjects on earth, primitive or complex, that are capable of responding to a drug or to an environmental chemical.

Pharmacogenetics represents only one of many genetic responses to environmental impacts [1]. Human variation in pharmacogenetics is similar to human variation in response to foods [2]. For instance, modern salt intake causes members of populations who come from salt-poor areas to develop cardiovascular disease [3]. Populations adjusted to frequent periods of starvation tend to show a high incidence of type 2 diabetes [4]. There are different genetic mechanisms to fight infections. There is a gene conveying resistance to tuberculosis, acting before any immune response sets in [5]. AIDS resistance has been explained in Caucasians but not yet in Africans [6]. Thus, pharmacogenetics is not a unique affair, but let us still look at its development.

1

2 INITIAL PHASE OF PHARMACOGENETICS

2.1 My Unexpected Dive into Pharmacogenetics: A Personal Story

In Berlin in 1948, there were still incidences of malnutrition. Because of this, there were patients who suffered fatal poisoning from the generally safe, local anesthetic drug procaine. This became my impetus to study the esterase that hydrolyzed procaine [7]. When invited to Philadelphia, I continued these studies with the superior equipment there available to me. I found that the procaine-splitting esterase was butyrylcholinesterase, then called pseudo- or plasmacholinesterase, and I explored a method using UV spectrophotometry that elegantly and precisely indicated the esterase activity [8]. I then transferred to Toronto, where pseudocholinesterase had been discovered and where it was still being investigated. I proposed the use of my new UV method to replace the tedious gasometric method then in place. My proposal seemed acceptable to the responsible biochemist, provided I could demonstrate the efficiency of my method by comparing and testing plasma from patients with known high and low cholinesterase activity. Thus I came to test the esterase of patients known to show abnormal effects of succinylcholine, whose esterase had been designated by a government laboratory as having low activity. I was surprised to see that the cholinesterase activity was not low but that it displayed abnormal kinetics with grossly reduced affinity for its substrate, and thus appeared to be low. This could be explained only by an abnormal enzyme structure, and that could only be genetic; I could prove that point by family investigations [9]. I was excited by this observation of interplay between genetics and the abnormal effect of a drug. I tried to find out whether there were other established examples.

My literature search was successful. There was Waldenstrom's story on porphyria [10]. A major find was a report on hemolysis caused by the antimalarial drug primaquine in some American soldiers in the 1940s [11], later shown to be due to glucose-6-phosphate dehydrogenase (G6PD) deficiency. I became excited by a paper of Motulsky [12] entitled "Drug Reactions, Enzymes, and Biochemical Genetics," sponsored by the Council on Drugs of the American Medical Association. I found a report describing genetic differences of the metabolism of isoniazid [13], a then revolutionary antituberculosis drug. These and several other reports encouraged me to write a book on this new topic of pharmacogenetics [14], citing all examples I was able to find. Pharmacogenetics had become my scientific life blood.

2.2 Pharmacogenetics: A Growing Science

Many pertinent observations came in the following years. For instance, Vesell and Page [15] used twin studies to show genetic control of the metabolism of several drugs. Von Wartburg et al. [16] described a variant of alcohol dehydrogenase. However, a report from the laboratory of Dr. Robert Smith in London [17] became a milestone in pharmacogenetics. He described the deficient metabolism of debrisoquine, a deficiency he had personally experienced as a life-threatening drop of blood pressure after taking the drug [18]. Before that, Eichelbaum had reported in 1975 [19] in a thesis a metabolic deficiency of sparteine metabolism; both defects are now known to be due to deficiency of the P450 cytochrome CYP2D6. This deficiency affects the metabolism of more than 40 drugs; whether the deficiency is clinically important for any given drug depends on a number of drug-associated criteria and safety factors [20]. More than 70 different variants of CYP2D6 are known, many are completely without any trace of activity [21]. On the other hand, gene duplication or multiplication in some subjects causes extremely high CYP2D6 activity [22]. A recent Medline search quoted 1244 papers dealing with CYP2D6 variation. CYP2D6 is the most variable of human CYPs, but its variability is not unique: looking at 10 different CYPs, various observers found 144 alleles and 193 nucleotide changes among them [23].

It is not surprising that most initial discoveries in pharmacogenetics pertained to drug-metabolizing enzymes; measurements of drugs and drug metabolites required chemical analytical methods of more or less traditional nature. Investigation of receptor variation usually requires knowledge of the receptor's DNA sequence so that deviations can be discovered by testing the receptor genes in white blood cells [24]. Thus, most studies of the pharmacogenetics of receptors or, similarly, of ion channels and of transporters, have recent origins. Many of these topics will be covered in subsequent chapters.

It is only now that we can appreciate the magnitude of genetic variation. Let us look at a few numbers: The human genome contains about 3 billion base pairs, and single-base variations (called SNPs, for single nucleotide polymorphisms) are on the average as frequent as 1/1000 bases [25]. This means that many human proteins show genetic variation. There are known, e.g., more than 100 cancer-promoting oncogenes and about three dozen cancer-suppressing genes, and their functions may be controlled by genes determining DNA repair, cell division, metabolism, immune responses, embryonic development, and cell migration [26]. Thus, the number of opportunities and the magnitude of human genetic variation explain that there is what we call pharmacogenetics.

One should not forget that many environmental factors, including drugs, produce effects by altering gene expressions. This has been known for many years, when it was realized that certain drugs, besides foods and hormones, may induce formation of drug-metabolizing enzymes. Disregarding tradition, one might consider these drug-caused alterations of gene expression as an aspect of pharmacogenetics. This will not be further discussed here.

3   PHARMACOGENETICS AND POPULATIONS

Pharmacogenetics is still largely considered a story of person-to-person differences in drug metabolism and response. A broader view becomes effective when we look at simple organisms. To appreciate the fact that pharmacogenetic variation can be a protective commodity for a population, let us consider insect resistance to insecticides [1], or bacterial resistance to antibiotics [27]. Pharmacogenetic resistance of an individual insect to the killing effect of an insecticide causes this individual to survive an exposure, so that the offspring of that insect can multiply and in the long run create the resistant strain. Bacterial resistance to antibiotics represents the same mechanism. We cannot see this dramatic effect of pharmacogenetics in people because environmental hazards are usually not so directly killing, and the human generation time is too long. The initial emphasis upon differences between individuals is changing; we interprete them increasingly as diversities which characterize different human populations [28].

I knew early on of these and some other population differences [14], but let me tell the story how the importance of such differences was driven home to me. Toronto became more and more often the home of immigrants from China. In the early 1970s, there were a few Chinese in the class of 140 medical students at the University of Toronto. My colleagues and I were studying at the time the metabolism of the then frequently used drug amobarbital, a barbiturate, and we had found a family with impaired amobarbital metabolism [29]. We therefore asked the medical students to volunteer for an amobarbital study. After we had our laboratory results, I noticed that the data from seven subjects did not fit to the rest. I suspected an error of measurement and wanted to repeat the study of these subjects. I only knew the student numbers and asked a colleague for their names; after a while, he came back—visibly shaken—that all the student numbers came from students with Chinese names. Further investigations confirmed that one of the metabolic alterations of amobarbital was on the average distinctly faster in Chinese than in Caucasian students [29].

The deficiency of debrisoquine metabolism [17] was also tested in our laboratory, and we found a different metabolic ratio between Chinese and Caucasian students [30]. These observations, together with the old G6PD and NAT2 data and some additional comparisons, firmly planted in my mind the idea that differences in drug metabolism are not only a matter of individuals but also frequently occur between the human populations. I published a review article that probably was the first exclusively concerned with interethnic differences of drug metabolism [31]. Knowledge of such differences has become very important for the pharmaceutical industry.

4 MONOGENIC AND MULTIGENIC VARIATIONS OF DRUG RESPONSES

The occurrence of the response to a drug that differs between persons can have many different causes, for instance, variability of drug metabolism as indicated above. Other potential differences may lie in drug targets or receptors, or in the transporters of drugs that operate at sites of absorption, of the blood-brain barrier, or of cellular membranes in general.

Dealing with variation of specific genes is a relatively simple affair, and so far has characterised most aspects of pharmacogenetics. However, we cannot neglect the fact that most differences between people are due to differences between many genes, in addition to environmental influences. Pharmacology became a science only after the ever-present differences between subjects were recognized and the concept formalized by introduction of the term ED_{50} [32], indicating the dose sufficient to produce a given effect in 50% of a tested population. Whether somebody belongs to the 50% needing a lower or a higher dose may depend on many factors, including drug absorption, volume of drug distribution, drug transport, blood flow, target reaction, metabolic destruction, and elimination via kidney, bile, or gut. All may contribute to a difference between two people. Every one of these factors may depend on one or more gene products. Multigenic variation is important.

Let us consider a single reaction, the metabolic alteration of a drug. The metabolism may fail because of a genetic change in the enzyme structure, as discussed above. However, it may also fail because not enough enzyme was formed, perhaps due to a failure of transcription or translation. Was there the absence of an inducer or regulator, perhaps a hormone, not formed or too fast degraded? Perhaps a genetic abnormality of the promoting region prevented the normal response to the inducer. Perhaps the drug could not reach the enzyme. Thus, most genetic differences between people are complex and many genes contribute. Because of the complexity, the causes of such differences between individuals are usually ignored. The story changes if we have to deal with a multifactorial difference between populations.

As an example, let us consider a comparison between Swedish and Chinese populations and their capacity to metabolize codeine [33]. The drug undergoes three primary metabolic reactions: glucuronidation, N-demethylation to form norcodeine, and O-demethylation to form morphine. All these reactions differ between the two populations. The slow morphine formation in Chinese reflects the known ethnic variation of CYP2D6, but no single enzyme change is known to account for the metabolic differences in glucuronidation and in nor-codeine formation. Particularly the glucuronidation curves show a normal distribution in both populations, suggesting multifactorial variation. This raises the question how one should deal mathematically with multifactorial differences between population. As suggested in the chapter on interethnic differences in drug response, it is in such cases often better to compare the edges of two distribution curves rather than their means [34,35].

A problem with multifactorial variation is the question to what extent is it determined by heritable factors, and to what extent by environmental determinants; both are probably contributing to the variation. The answer may guide investigations of the problem: scientific inquiries may be directed to primarily look at genes or to search for environmental influences. Traditionally, twin studies were used to determine the heritability of any human variant. Since drug effects come and go, it is possible in pharmacology to avoid twins, to collect a group of people, and to give each subject a drug two or more times; this will allow a statistical comparison of inter- and intrasubject variation. The comparison can be used to calculate the genetic component contributing to any pharmacological variation [36–38].

5   ECOGENETICS AND PHARMACOGENOMICS

Observations of interindividual differences in metabolism of drugs, and therefore in different drug responses, led to the development of pharmacogenetics. However, it was not long before investigators without a particular interest in drugs noted similar differences in response to environmental toxicants. Thus, the term *ecogenetics* was coined by Brewer [39]. He asked whether geneticists with their exploding science were sufficiently concerned with humans ''facing an environmental crisis of such proportions that our very existence is threatened.'' The term was taken up and used when concerned with genetic differences in the tolerance of food items [2], such as lactose in milk products. Calabrese [40] was much concerned with occupational diseases, and wrote a book about ecogenetics. The World Health Organization arranged in 1989 a meeting on ecogenetics, which led to a subsequent book [41]. Thus, ecogenetics is firmly established as a term and a special branch of science. The principal concepts embodied by the terms *pharmacogenetics* and *ecogenetics* are indistinguishable.*

The word *pharmacogenomics* [42,43] reflects in the first place the change of the human technical ability to investigate and to pinpoint variations in DNA, a change that encouraged geneticists to study the genome [44,45] rather than merely single genes. This is an important change: It is now realized that only a

---

* There is an underlying linguistic problem: The word *pharmakon* in ancient Greek refers to both drugs and poisonous substances. Therefore, the term ''pharmacology'' means for many medical scientists a topic dealing with both therapeutic and toxic agents. For others, pharmacology invokes thoughts of drugs as therapeutic medicines, dispensed by pharmacists. Thus, some geneticists use the term ecogenetics, though the term seemed redundant to many pharmacologists.

few parts of the human genome are the standard protein-producing genes; functions of the total genome are being explored, with the trend to compare the genomes of different species [46]. From a medical point of view, it is mainly three aspects that will make pharmacogenetics and pharmacogenomics different subjects:

    1. The phenotyping methods which until recently governed most of pharmacogenetics will be more and more subservient to genotyping procedures. Phenotyping will remain important as a means to assess the medical significance of a genetic variation.

    2. Looking at the genome rather than at single genes improves the chances of finding variants that promote the occurrence of common diseases, that is, diseases like blood pressure elevation, asthma, or schizophrenia. This in turn will promote the discovery of new drug targets, the genes or proteins involved in disease production.

    3. Pharmacogenetics was historically most concerned with drug safety. Drug safety will remain a concern, but the main effect of pharmacogenomics promises to be an improvement of drug efficacy.

6 CONCLUSIONS

In summary, pharmacogenomics will in the long run lead to a better understanding of the interaction between drugs and gene products. The promise of pharmacogenomics is that the choice of drug to combat a disease will be determined more and more by which gene or genes contribute to the disease in a given subject; in other words, we can expect to see the development of individualized, gene-dependent drug therapy.

REFERENCES

1. W Kalow. Pharmacogenetics in biological perspective. Pharmacol Rev 49:369–379, 1997.
2. AG Motulsky. Pharmacogenetics and ecogenetics in 1991. Pharmacogenetics 1:2–3, 1991.
3. CE Grim, M Robinson. Blood pressure variation in blacks: genetic factors. Semin Nephrol 16:83–93, 1996.
4. JV Neel. The "thrifty genotype" in 1998. Nutr Rev 57:S2–S9, 1998.
5. E Skamene. The Bcg gene story. Immunobiology 191:451–460, 1994.
6. M Dean, LP Jacobson, G McFarlane, JB Margolick, FJ Jenkins, OM Howard, HF Dong, JJ Goedert, S Buchbinder, E Gomperts, D Vlahov, JJ Oppenheim, SJ O'Brien, M Carrington. Reduced risk of AIDS lymphoma in individuals heterozygous for the CCR5-delta32 mutation. Cancer Res 1:3561–3564, 1999.
7. H Herken, W Kalow. Photometometrische Bestimmung der Enzymatischen Novocain-Hydrolyse. Klin Wochenschr 29:90–91, 1951.

8. W Kalow. Hydrolysis of local anesthetics by human serum cholinesterase. J Pharmacol Exp Ther 104:122–134, 1952.
9. W Kalow. Familial incidence of low pseudocholinesterase level. Lancet 2:576–577, 1956.
10. J Waldenstrom. Studien uber Porphyrie. Acta Med Scand 82:1–254, 1937.
11. RJ Dern, E Beutler, AS Alving. The hemolytic effect of primaquine. J Lab Clin Med 44:171–176, 1954.
12. AG Motulsky. Drug reactions, enzymes, and biochemical genetics. JAMA 165:835–837, 1957.
13. R Bonicke, BP Lisboa. Uber die Erbeddingtheit der intraindividuellen Konstanz der Isoniazidausscheidung beim Menschen. Naturwissenschaften 44:314, 1957.
14. W Kalow. Pharmacogenetics. Heredity and the Response to Drugs. Philadelphia: W.B. Saunders, 1962.
15. ES Vesell, JG Page. Genetic control of dicumerol levels in man. J Clin Invest 47:2657–2663, 1968.
16. JP von Wartburg, PM Schurch. Atypical human liver alcohol dehydrogenase. Ann NY Acad Sci 151:936–946, 1968.
17. A Mahgoub, LG Dring, JR Idle, R Lancaster, RL Smith. Polymorphic hydroxylation of debrisoquine in man. Lancet 2:584–586, 1977.
18. RL Smith. Introduction: human genetic variations in oxidative drug metabolism. Xenobiotica 16:361–365, 1986.
19. M Eichelbaum. Ein neuentdeckter Defekt im Arzneimittel-stoffwechsel des Menshen: Die fehlende N-Oxidation des Spartein. Bonn: Medizinische Fakultat Rheinischen Friedrich-Wilhelms-Universitat, 1975.
20. UA Meyer, UM Zanger. Molecular mechanisms of genetic polymorphisms of drug metabolism. Annu Rev Pharmacol Toxicol 37:269–296, 1997.
21. D Marez, M Legrand, N Sabbagh, JM Lo Guidice, C Spire, JJ Lafitte, UA Meyer, F Broly. Polymorphism of the cytochrome P450 CYP2D6 gene in a European population: characterization of 48 mutations and 53 alleles, their frequencies and evolution. Pharmacogenetics 7:193–202, 1997.
22. ML Dahl, I Johansson, L Bertilsson, M Ingelman-Sundberg, F Sjoqvist. Ultrarapid hydroxylation of debrisoquine in a Swedish population. Analysis of the molecular genetic basis. J Pharmacol Exp Ther 274: 516–520, 1995.
23. Home Page. http://www.imm.ki.se/CYPalleles/. Internet 1999.
24. P Propping, MM Nothen. Genetic variation of CNS receptors—a new perspective for pharmacogenetics. Pharmacogenetics 5:318–325, 1995.
25. E Pennisi. Using the wildly popular genome markers called SNPs to track genes may be less straightforward than researchers expected. A closer look at SNPs suggests difficulties. Science 281:1787–1789, 1998.
26. K Garber. More SNPs on the way: genome research. Science 281:1788, 1998.
27. PM Bennett. The spread of drug resistance. In: S Baumberg, JPW Young, EMH Wellington JR Saunders, eds. Population Genetics of Bacteria. Cambridge: Cambridge University Press, 1995, pp 317–344.
28. W Kalow. Pharmacogenetics and evolution. Pharmacogenetics 10:1–3, 2000.
29. W Kalow, BK Tang, D Kadar, L Endrenyi, F-Y Chan. A method to study drug

metabolism in populations: racial differences in amobarbital metabolism. Clin Pharmacol Ther 26:766–776, 1979.

30. W Kalow, SV Otton, D Kadar, L Endrenyi, T Inaba. Ethnic difference in drug metabolism: debrisoquine 4-hydroxylation in Caucasians and Orientals. Can J Physiol Pharmacol 58:1142–1144, 1980.

31. W Kalow. Ethnic differences in drug metabolism. Clin Pharmacokinet 7:373–-400, 1982.

32. JW Trevan. The error of determination of toxicity. R Soc Lond Proc 1 Ser B 101: 483–514, 1927.

33. Q Yue, J Säwe. Interindividual and interethnic differences in codeine metabolism. In: W Kalow, ed. Pharmacogenetics of Drug Metabolism. New York: Pergamon Press, 1992, pp 721–727.

34. W Kalow. Pharmacoanthropology and the genetics of drug metabolism. In: W Kalow, ed. Pharmacogenetics of Drug Metabolism. New York: Pergamon Press, 1992, pp 865–877.

35. W Kalow, L Bertilsson. Interethnic factors affecting drug response. Adv Drug Res 25:1–59, 1994.

36. W Kalow, BK Tang, L Endrenyi. Hypothesis: comparisons of inter- and intra-individual variations can substitute for twin studies in drug research. Pharmacogenetics 8:283–289, 1998.

37. W Kalow, V Ozdemir, BK Tang, L Tothfalusi, L Endrenyi. The science of pharmacological variability: an essay. Clin Pharmacol Ther 66:445–447, 1999.

38. V Ozdemir, W Kalow, BK Tang, AD Paterson, SE Walker, L Endrenyi, ADM Kashuba. Evaluation of the genetic component of variability in CYP3A4 activity: a repeated drug administration (RDA) method. Pharmacogenetics 10:373–388, 2000.

39. GJ Brewer. Annotation: human ecology, an expanding role for the human geneticist. Am J Hum Genet 23:92–94, 1971.

40. EJ Calabrese. Ecogenetics: Genetic Variation in Susceptibility to Environmental Agents. New York: John Wiley & Sons, 1984.

41. P Grandjean, D Kello, G Rohrborn, S Tarkowski. Ecogenetics. Genetic Predisposition to the Toxic Effects of Chemicals. New York: World Health Organization/ Chapman & Hall, 1991.

42. DM Grant. Pharmacogenomics and the changing face of clinical pharmacology. Can J Clin Pharmacol 6:131–132, 1999.

43. WE Evans, MV Relling. Pharmacogenomics: translating functional genomics into rational therapeutics. Science 15:487–491, 1999.

44. FS Collins, A Patrinos, E Jordan, A Chakravarti, R Gesteland, L Walters. New goals for the U.S. human genome project: 1998–2003. Science 23:682–689, 1998.

45. SK Burley, SC Almo, JB Bonanno, M Capel, MR Chance, T Gaasterland, D Lin, A Sali, FW Studier, S Swaminathan. Structural genomics: beyond the human genome project. Nat Genet 23:151–157, 1999.

46. SJ O'Brien, M Menotti-Raymond, WJ Murphy, WG Nash, J Wienberg, R Stanyon, NG Copeland, NA Jenkins, JE Womack, JA Marshall Graves. The promise of comparative genomics in mammals. Science 15:458–481, 1999.

2

Pharmacogenomics, Biomarkers, and the Promise of Personalized Medicine

B. Michael Silber
Pfizer Global Research and Development, Groton, Connecticut

1 INTRODUCTION

In the postgenome era, identifying human DNA sequences, genomic structures, and human genetic variations, along with changes in gene and protein expression over time, in disease and health, will ultimately allow researchers and clinicians to more precisely define, stratify, and classify disease. In 2000, the human genome became fundamentally known and the information accessible, although refinements are still outstanding. It is now likely that sequencing of the human genome will be complete by 2001 by the publicly funded Human Genome Project (HGP), the private sector, or both. Access to these data should ultimately lead to the identification of all genes, therapeutic targets, and proteins (i.e., receptors, enzymes, ion channels, transporters, nuclear receptors, hormones, factors) that make up or contribute to a specific disease process. This will lead to "drugable" and "nondrugable" targets put into high-throughput screens, allowing the selection of new chemical entities for drug development. These candidates will then be evaluated in Phase I–III clinical trials to identify new medicines.

Drugable targets are those that can be successfully approached with conventional small-molecule, protein, or antibody therapeutic interventions. Non drugable targets will likely require unconventional approaches, including anti-sense or gene therapy. While 5000 to 10,000 drugable targets have been proposed [1], this is speculative. Meanwhile, the pharmaceutical and biotechnology industries currently focus on a combined total of less than 500 targets, which is about 10% of the total number of (speculative) targets [2]. For each complex, common, and chronic disease, the pharmaceutical and biotechnology industries currently have one or more approved drugs. There are likely to be many more targets related to the prevention, treatment, or cure of such diseases that have not yet been identified. This will ultimately lead to a multitude of novel drugs for each of these targets.

Until very recently, genetic research in the pharmaceutical and biotechnology industries has largely focused on the use of genomics and genetics to discover novel targets and genes related to disease susceptibility. Because most common, complex, and chronic disease is polygenic and influenced by environmental factors, it has been difficult to identify all of the genes that contribute to these diseases. This will change dramatically with the unraveling of the complete human genome.

It is widely believed that the polygenic nature of disease, coupled with environmental influences, is the fundamental reason we often see large differences in the effectiveness of medicines from one individual to the next. Similar reasoning probably explains why disparate profiles in adverse experiences from one individual to the next may be observed, especially rare serious adverse experiences (SAEs) that occur at very low frequencies. The improved basis for disease classification will ultimately facilitate a substantially improved ability to characterize an individual at the molecular disease level. This enhanced capability will ultimately spawn the development of diverse drugs to address the many causes of what had traditionally been thought of as a single disease. Ultimately, this molecular characterization together with improved diagnostic methods will lead to therapies targeting the individual patient, or personalized medicine. Fundamental to this thesis is the assumption that at least some of the interpatient variation in the response to drugs is genetic.

The perfect medicine is one that effectively treats, or ideally prevents, disease and is free of unwanted side effects. Newer drugs have unquestionably led to important breakthroughs in medicine and therapeutics in a variety of diseases, and overall have had a profound effect on healthcare (i.e., selective serotonin reuptake inhibitor [SSRI] anti-depressants, histamine-2 [H_2] blocker antiulcer medicines). However, even the most effective and successful drugs provide optimal therapy only to a subset of those treated. Some individuals with a particular disease may receive little to no benefit from a drug, while others may experience confirmed drug-related SAEs, consistent with the labeling. If the drug-related SAE is life-threatening, the drug may be withdrawn from that particular patient, but may also be withdrawn from wider use in the population, thus preventing a majority of individuals access to a valuable therapeutic option.

A great deal of attention is being directed to developing a better understanding of heterogeneity in disease, in patients and in drug response profiles. Researchers are advocating the identification and use of various biomarkers to characterize disease and patient heterogeneity, as well as heterogeneity of drug response. Biomarkers include laboratory-based markers such as genetic variations, those based on changes in gene and protein expression in relevant tissues or biofluids, or other biochemical measures in disease, to name a few. Non-laboratory-based biomarkers might include one or more imaging-based approaches (i.e., magnetic resonance imaging [MRI], positron emission tomography [PET], etc.), as well as assessments based on behavior and function. Newer biomarkers may prove superior to conventional ones in certain disease [3]. However, researchers can be misled by biomarkers, especially if they are being used as a surrogate to predict the benefit of a particular therapy [4], since we often don't understand relationships between the biomarker, disease causes(s) and interventions.

Over the past few years, single nucleotide polymorphisms (SNPs) have been identified as the best marker of genetic variation. SNPs have been identified because they are widely distributed throughout the genome, they involve mostly substitutions, they have low rates of mutation, and their measurement is amenable using high-throughput genotyping methods. Under certain circumstances, SNPs may be less informative than other markers of genetic variation (i.e., microsatellite markers). Nevertheless, they have been widely embraced as the most important markers of genetic variation. For example, SNPs in drug metabolizing enzymes have long been informative and useful in guiding therapeutic decisions regarding dose selections. The ideal for providers and payers of healthcare, as well as patients that receive medicines, is to find a way to give the right medicine to the right individual at the right dose and at the right time: personalized medicine. Personalized medicine is a long-term vision, a formidable challenge, and will require varied approaches to achieve success. Discoveries from emerging information and knowledge from genomic, genetic, and proteomic sciences will contribute significantly to achieving personalized medicine. This may apply both to medicines already approved, as well as to drug candidates under evaluation in clinical trials during the drug development process.

Pharmacogenomics seeks to identify genomic, genetic, and proteomic data and to develop associations between these data and drug response patterns. This is intended to explain interpatient variability in drug response, and to predict likely response in individuals receiving a particular medicine. Pharmacogenomics has the potential to influence the way approved medicines are used, as well as impact how clinical trials are designed and interpreted during the drug development process. Relevant information may be derived during the clinical trial recruitment phase, following the treatment phase, or both. In addition, because pharmacogenomics may also uncover patterns associated with a lack of any response to a particular medicine, it may be possible to uncover novel discovery target opportunities. Today, pharmacogenomic studies explore correlations between patient outcomes with genetic variations in genes involved in a drug's mechanism of action (MOA), biochemical pathway, or metabolic pathway. This involves a candidate gene-specific approach, which is largely hypothesis dependent. Newer approaches have been proposed using genetic variation data in a hypothesis-independent approach.

Important genetic variations are in DNA (SNPs) in regions of genomic or nongenomic structure at the germ line level, the somatic level (i.e., cancer), or both. Genotypes or haplotypes within specific candidate genes may be informative. SNPs may also be found outside gene regions. Genomewide SNP maps, including SNPs inside and outside of gene regions, may also prove to be valuable in delineating drug response patterns especially when the map includes >500,000 SNPs. This will provide an opportunity to explore the utility of linkage disequilibrium (LD) at distances of 5–10 kb or less [5,6].

Changes in the expressed human genome (i.e., mRNA) in relevant tissues may be especially important in diseases where access to that tissue could bear on disease diagnosis, treatment, or both. The information could include changes in the expressed human proteome in relevant biological fluids (i.e., blood, serum, plasma, urine, cerebrospinal, synovial) or tissues in relation to disease diagnosis, treatment, or both. These data may also identify new targets or confirm the relevance of previously identified targets.

The key to translating information into useful knowledge is the development of comprehensive strategies and databases linking laboratory-derived data with clinically derived data collected from well-characterized patients, providing an opportunity for exhaustive data mining, including appropriate statistical evaluations. This approach may be useful for drugs already approved, during the drug development process, or both. While desirable in many circumstances, some of these approaches may be impractical or impossible to achieve today because of existing or emerging obstacles and barriers to developing personalized medicine. These include issues of confidentiality, collection of DNA (or relevant biofluids or tissues) or tissues from patients enrolled in clinical trials, and collection of accurate clinical information from patients treated after drug approval in the postmarketing phase.

In this regard, it is important to recognize that pharmacogenomics is not about disease diagnosis or disease genetics; it targets the development of medicine response profiles. The importance of this distinction has recently been emphasized [7,8].

2 DRIVERS FOR PERSONALIZED MEDICINE

2.1 Completion of the Sequencing of the Human Genome

The principal driver for personalized medicine will be the emergence of information and knowledge delineating the causes of disease and patient heterogeneity, and heterogeneity in drug response. There will always be a goal to improve the benefit to risk ratio associated with the use of a particular medicine in a particular patient and to discover newer, more specific, and safer medicines.

The burgeoning scientific evidence uncovering the heterogeneity of both diseases and patients will undoubtedly lead to the emergence of newly discovered disease-related targets and more sensitive and specific methods of diagnosis. It has been estimated that as many as 10 different genes on average may contribute to a common, complex, chronic disease [1,2]. This should ultimately lead to multiple novel and improved therapeutic approaches and earlier interventions. Consequently, health care providers will have a variety of drug options to treat each patient with a heterogeneous disease. When diagnostics bundled to drugs become available, they will provide guidance for decisions about the drug option that is best suited to an individual patient and the health care provider will then prescribe appropriately. This selection will take into account issues of drug efficacy, safety, or both. Although no one knows when this will become feasible, it is undoubtedly many years into the future for many, if not most, diseases.

2.2 Molecular Characterization of Disease

Relevant genomic, genetic, and proteomic data linked to clinical information in well-characterized individuals will be collected and exhaustively mined using bioinformatic and statistical tools as more information emerges about disease and patient heterogeneity. This will be made possible using high-throughput genotyping, and gene and protein expression methods, to name a few. This is already being done in various diseases, especially in cancer; it defines somatic differences in gene expression, and linking these differences to interpatient variability in drug response, as well as to select suitable therapeutic interventions.

This could lead to many targets and eventually medicines that will have the greatest benefit for the patient, as a function of timing of the intervention. Disease classification will further stratify at-risk patient populations, leading to earlier diagnosis or prevention of disease, more targeted therapies, and markers to suggest decisions regarding drug therapy. It may soon be possible in some diseases to identify the genes and targets that contribute substantially to the development or penetrance of a particular disease.

It will take many years to define all of the genes and targets contributing to the penetrance of a disease. However, it is possible even now using SNP maps to compare differences in genotypes in responders and nonresponders to drugs. This may soon have an effect on how clinical trials are designed and how drug development is carried out in certain diseases. Similarly, with a growing demand for safer drugs, especially in the treatment of chronic disease, there will be a growing demand to use drugs in those individuals most likely to derive benefit and not to use drugs in those patients who would merely incur side effects. Taken together, this will lead to the need for a variety of markers that will identify the molecular basis for disease in a given individual, along with correlates of safety.

2.3   Search for Biomarkers of Drug Response

As previously discussed, significant heterogeneity is frequently observed in the way individuals respond to a drug in terms of efficacy and SAEs [9]. The cause for this heterogeneity includes the molecular basis of the disease, the influence of environment, the status and severity of the disease at a particular time, the influence of drug-drug interactions, the individual's overall health, including function of vital organs, and disease comorbidities.

The first systematic account of pharmacogenetics was given in 1962 [10]. Since then, genetic variations within drug metabolizing enzymes, as well as in drug target genes (i.e., enzymes, ion channels, transporters, hormones, and receptors), have been described and this process will likely continue. One strategy for personalized medicine may be to achieve improved efficacy, safety, or both for an approved drug, since even the best medicines do not lead to robust efficacy or safety in 100% of treated patients.

Table 1 provides some examples where approved therapies have not been effective in all patients. For example, β_2-adrenoreceptor genotype had a profound effect on the percent of asthmatic patients that had a favorable improvement in FEV_1 following treatment with a β_2-adrenoreceptor agonist [32]. Similarly, there was a clear relationship between genotype in the ALOX5 promoter and failure to respond to a 5-lipoxygenase inhibitor [33]. Patients with rheumatoid arthritis and positive for certain HLA subtypes had substantially better response rates following methotrexate than patients lacking these markers [34,35]. A recent example of a clinically significant variation in a drug-metabolizing enzyme gene was published that showed a clear relationship between genotype and cure rates [22], where *CYP2C19* genotype had a dramatic effect on cure rate following a proton pump inhibitor.

In addition to examples of where genetic variation has led to heterogeneity in drug efficacy, SAEs have been responsible for the discontinuation of drug candidates during drug development, as well as removal of approved drugs post-launch. In most of these cases, genetic factors may have played a predominant role in determining susceptibility to SAEs. For example, as shown in Table 2, two of the most common reasons for the removal of drugs postapproval are excessive prolongation of the QTc interval as measured by electrocardiogram, and hepatotoxicity. In the case of excessive QTc prolongation, the effect may be dichotomous, with some cases leading to life-threatening torsades de pointes (TdP). Familial non-drug-induced TdP is a rare Mendelian disease; drug-induced TdP has also been reported recently [36]. Specific genetic variations have been described relating to drug-induced TdP. Drug-induced excessive QTc prolongation may be

TABLE 1 Examples of Poor or Nonresponders (Efficacy) Following Drug Therapy

Disease	Drug class	Poor/non-responders (%)	References
Asthma	Beta-2 adrenergic agonist, 5-LO, LTD4	40–75	11,12
Cancer (breast, lung, brain)	Various	70–100	13–15
Depression	SSRIs, tricyclics, MAOs	20–40	16–19
Diabetes	Sulfonylureas, biguanides, glitazones	50–75	20–21
Duodenal ulcer	H_2 antagonists, proton pump inhibitors	20–70	22
Hyperlipidemia	HMGCoA reductase, resins, niacin	30–75	23,24
Hypertension	Thiazide diuretics, beta-blockers, ACE inhibitors, all antagonists	10–70	25,26
Migraine	Triptans, NSAIDs, ergots	30–60	27
Osteo/rheumatoid arthritis	NSAID, COX-2, antimetabolites	20–50	28,29
Schizophrenia	Tricyclic dibenzodiazepines, benzisoxazoles, butyrophenones	25–75	16,30,31

a continuous SAE, dose, or concentration related [37]. For the other major cause of drug withdrawal, drug-induced hepatotoxicity, the incidence is exceedingly low and believed to have a genetic basis, but no definitive evidence for this exists. Therefore, efficacy, SAEs, or both could drive personalized medicine.

3 STRATEGIES

3.1 Focus on Approved Drugs

One approach to personalized medicine is to comprehensively collect drug response profiles in patients following drug approval and widespread use in disease populations. This can be done in conjunction with the development and use of

TABLE 2　Drugs Withdrawn Following
Approval Because of QTc or Hepatotoxicity

Drug	Cause of withdrawal
Grepafloxacin	QTc
Cisapride	QTc
Terfenadine	QTc
Astemizole	QTc
Mibefradil	QTc
Encainide	Arrhythmias
Temafloxacin	Renal toxicity/hepatotoxicity
Zomepirac	Hepatotoxicity
Bromfenac	Hepatotoxicity
Benoxaprofen	Hepatotoxicity
Ticrynafen	Hepatotoxicity

diagnostic assays, as currently used in the treatment of acute myeloid leukemia (AML) and acute lymphoblastic leukemia (ALL) [38–42]. In cancer, a comprehensive approach can use diagnostics based on tumor tissue and focus on genetic analysis, gene and protein expression analyses, or both.

In the future, it may be possible to use SNP maps to look for patterns that distinguish those patients that develop the SAEs from those that do not. If this strategy can identify patients that are, and those that are not, at risk from developing these SAEs, a valuable drug may serve as a therapeutic option for the majority of patients who stand to benefit from it. Another approach after drug approval is the collection of DNA samples from patients enrolled in postmarketing trials. Genetic association studies could be used, if warranted, to better understand interpatient variability in efficacy, SAEs, or both. This could be especially useful in addressing SAEs that occur with a very low incidence that would not be detected in clinical trials during drug development, especially for drugs that are threatened by removal postapproval because the SAEs are life-threatening. This would provide a mechanism to access hundreds of thousands, or millions, of DNA samples for possible genetic analysis, should it be required retrospectively.

3.2　Applications During Drug Development Prior to Drug Approval

Another approach would incorporate pharmacogenomics into the drug development process early in development [7,8]. In this approach, SNP-LD profiles would be determined in Phase II trials. These results would be used to determine whether SNP profiles could be identified for those patients who show efficacy for a particular drug from those who don't, those who show SAEs from those who don't, or both. These results can then be used to design Phase III trials, including recruitment of patients for pivotal clinical trials [43]. In principle, Phase III would enroll a high percentage of patients that would respond favorably and not expose nonresponders to potential SAEs. The benefit-to-risk ratio in this type of study would, theoretically, be increased over that in traditional trials.

The use of SNP-LD profiles could lead to drug approval limited to patients with specific SNP-LD profiles, which has inherent disadvantages. On the other hand, it may provide a mechanism of identifying a patient population where efficacy can be clearly demonstrated and allow for early registration. Such an approach may be possible near term with the development of cost-effective high-throughput technologies, after construction of SNP-LD maps. These maps may be available in ~1 year because of an initiative sponsored by the SNP Consortium (TSC). This approach is also applicable postmarketing to development of a medicine response profile in relation to SAEs [8]. Further, this approach may also lead to the identification of SNP patterns that may ultimately uncover new target opportunities. While such an approach may prove useful, it is unproven at this time and it faces many hurdles and obstacles to implementation. Genetic association and linkage analysis studies are being used by pharmacogenomic researchers as a means of identifying important relationships between haplotypes linked to important phenotypes both to understand disease and patient heterogeneity, and to understand heterogeneity in drug response.

3.3 Early Use of Biomarkers

As previously discussed, one strategy receiving greater attention now to address issues surrounding patient heterogeneity in disease and patients, and in relation to heterogeneity in response to medicines, is the use of biomarkers with ideal features identified in Table 3. Biomarkers will facilitate the concept of prescribing the right drug for the right patient at the right time.

Clearly, a drug will ultimately be selected based on whether it is being used preventively, to modify the course of the disease, or for symptomatic treatment. While the use of genetic markers has already been discussed, pharmacogenomic-based markers include other types of biomarkers. A biomarker could provide evidence that a drug is acting on the intended mechanism of action (MOA), or evidence that a drug is eliciting a desired pharmacodynamic (PD) response. The MOA and PD biomarkers may be similar or different, depending on the disease and/or the intervention. In addition to the need for biomarkers of drug efficacy, there is a similar need for biomarkers associated with drug safety. Recently, in the United States, the Food and Drug Administration sponsored sympo-

TABLE 3 Ideal Biomarkers in Relation to the
Process of Disease, from DNA ⇒ RNA ⇒
Protein ⇒ Posttranslationally Modified
Protein ⇒ Clinical Phenotype

Predict disease risk
Predict disease prevention
Predict disease severity
Predict disease progression
Relate to accepted outcome measures
Confirm drug activity in short-term trials
Provide patient-specific disease monitoring
Provide patient-specific drug monitoring
Facilitate review/approval of drugs
Identify new disease-relevant targets
Confirm relevance of known targets

sia in two specific areas relating to biomarkers, drug-induced QTc changes, and drug-induced hepatotoxicity, leading to further initiatives to address these important issues.

Providing relevant and appropriately valid biomarkers could conceivably contribute to a better understanding of interpatient variability. Such a better understanding could reduce unnecessary investments for a given drug candidate entering or proposed for development, while providing improved rationale for accelerated investments for others. We need to consider which research tools are needed to understand and interpret the different biological processes at the relevant molecular, cellular, tissue, and organ levels. These tools should uncover critical information and enable the development of clinically relevant biomarkers of different types—namely, diagnostic, progression, and severity (Table 4).

Biomarkers that provide information related to the prediction of disease risk or susceptibility would be important for new therapeutic approaches targeting disease prevention. These pathophysiologically relevant tools could uncover new disease-relevant targets or markers that could better define the disease process. Alternatively, for new therapeutic approaches targeting disease progression, the goal is to alter the course of disease, biomarkers that monitor various clinically relevant endpoints. Finally, for new approaches targeting symptomatic treatment, biomarkers that demonstrate disease stabilization or regression would be important. Research tools and technologies can be used to identify biomarkers that meet these individual needs. The biomarkers identified either will be unique or will show some overlap.

DNA and RNA expression-based approaches require cells in order to isolate relevant material. Protein-based approaches (i.e., proteomics) seek to define

Table 4 Types of Disease Biomarkers

Diagnostic
specific to disease, appearing *prior to* clinical diagnosis
identify and select subjects for earlier treatment
identify potential targets for Discovery
high specificity and sensitivity
Progression
predict future progression of disease
endpoint for rapid decisions in early development
selection of subjects in trials with traditional endpoints
high specificity
Severity
pattern of markers that are disease-specific
high specificity and sensitivity

and understand the significance of pattern differences in protein expression in cells, tissues, or fluids of the body. In contrast to DNA- and RNA-based approaches, proteomics does not require cells to be informative, since biofluids such as blood, plasma, serum, cerebrospinal fluid, urine, and synovial fluid can be used to delineate pattern expression differences. Since proteins mediate the complex processes involved in health and disease, changes in protein expression levels or structural modifications (e.g., in the amino acid sequence or by post-translational modifications) may be the most important biologically and hence the most useful for detecting and in monitoring of changes in patients involved in clinical trials. Plasma-based markers believed to be linked to various diseases are also informative.

4 CHALLENGES, BARRIERS, AND OBSTACLES

4.1 Technological

4.1.1 Finding the Right Markers

The challenges, barriers, and obstacles can be categorized into those that are technological and those that are nontechnological. On the technological side, researchers will need to have access to the human genome sequence, including knowledge of genetic variations and their frequencies in different populations. This will include information regarding SNPs in candidate genes, as well as access to a very dense set of SNPs across the human genome. Recently, investigators reported on the characterization and patterns of SNPs in approximately 180 genes believed to be important in a variety of human diseases [44,45]. This type of data would be needed for a much larger number of genes in different populations to identify SNPs with high and low frequencies. TSC will be making ~800,000 SNPs, with ~90% of these mapped, via a publicly accessible website [46] by the end of 2000, in part because of a recent collaboration with the HGP. However, the allelic frequencies of only a fraction of these (~60,000) will be determined by TSC in three major populations. Therefore, the allelic frequency of a larger fraction of mapped SNPs will be needed in different ethnic, racial, and diseased populations.

The bigger challenge today is the unavailability of scoring methods to genotype thousands of individuals with tens of thousands of SNPs. It is not feasible to genotype 1000 individuals in a single study, since there would be a need to perform ~1 million genotypes per day for months. Specifically, the time and resources required to perform such an analysis using today's technologies would make such an analysis prohibitively expensive. Only when robust analytical tools, platforms, and technologies, capable of performing very high-throughput genotyping, at very low cost, are available, will it become practical to consider large-scale genotyping in support of clinical trials. Today, technologies limit researchers to do targeted candidate-specific genotyping for testing very specific hypotheses involving candidate genes. However, it is anticipated that high-throughput and low-cost platforms for large-scale genotyping will be available in as little as 1–2 years. TSC is currently performing an analysis to define the specifications for high-throughput genotyping platforms.

It is also not feasible to perform gene or protein expression analysis routinely in support of clinical trials. While some cancer investigators are already using gene expression analysis to accurately determine the type of cancer and to select the optimal treatment, these studies are complex, not routine, and costly. Therefore, these approaches are used very carefully under controlled experimental conditions. Similarly, performing protein expression analysis on tissue or biofluid samples is extremely complex, requires highly skilled researchers, is not routinely available, requires highly complex analysis, and is costly. A major hurdle would be removed if these tools were accessible to a wider number of investigators, were more user-friendly, and were available at a much lower cost. Competition and expanded use should lower the costs of many of these tools.

4.1.2   Need for Diagnostic Assays

In addition to becoming more available and more affordable for researchers to use once molecular correlates have been identified and validated, associated with, or predictive of drug response outcomes, hospital-based or point-of-care diagnostic assays can potentially be made available for bundling with a drug. While diagnostic assays based on genetic variations, gene expression, or protein expression are currently available for a small number of selected molecular targets, personalized medicine will require new platforms and technologies to be developed, implemented, and validated for these advances to be applied broadly. One of the biggest challenges will be to have these diagnostic tests available in time to be used when the drug is ready to be launched, where so desired.

4.2 Nontechnological

4.2.1 Collecting DNA, RNA, Tissues, and Biofluids

The second major area representing challenges, barriers, and obstacles to achieving personalized medicine involves non-technology-related issues. Collection of DNA, RNA, tissues, and certain biofluids in clinical trials can be difficult, as it requires a well-organized and systematic approach and involves a variety of issues. While academic and government investigators have collected DNA and other tissues for a variety of purposes for many years, a recent focus on how these samples were collected has raised doubts about the adequacy of the informed consent process used. The President's National Bioethics Advisory Council (NBAC) has recently stipulated guidelines for the use of research samples from human subjects [47].

The pharmaceutical and biotechnology industries are routinely collecting DNA during clinical trials before drug approval and in some cases postapproval for a variety of purposes. Depending upon the purpose of the study, the samples may undergo anonymization or may be analyzed nonanonymously. An example of the latter may be the analysis of *CYP450* genotypes in order to understand how metabolizer status, poor or extensive, affects the drug metabolism or pharmacokinetic profile of the drug. To accomplish this, suitable safeguards were put in place to ensure confidentiality, privacy, and security for both the samples and the databases. While this has resulted in general acceptance by institutional review boards (IRBs) in most countries reviewing protocols calling for the collection of DNA, RNA, and other tissues or biofluids, difficulties remain in gaining approval with certain IRBs. This may be due to an incomplete understanding by the given IRB of the safeguards to be used, including matters related to confidentiality, privacy, and security. Nevertheless, this represents a significant hurdle in some parts of the world. If we are to establish an understanding of drug response profiles in various populations, dependent on racial, ethnic, ancestral, or geographic differences, it is necessary to be able to collect DNA or other tissues or biofluids in each of these populations, while ensuring that these individuals are protected against discrimination.

4.2.2 Pharmacogenomics Versus Disease Genetics

The importance of distinguishing between pharmacogenomics, which targets the development of medicine response profiles, and disease genetics, which targets the identification and development of disease prognostics and diagnostics, has recently been emphasized [7,8]. This is crucial because it illustrates the importance of distinguishing between "genetic testing" in the traditional sense and the types of research that make up pharmacogenomics. There is a heightened sense of concern and risk perceived by the public and by ethicists in relation to genetic testing. Since pharmacogenomics focuses on medicine response profiles, it should not present the same risks as those raised for genetic testing. If research is to be successful in identifying the causes of heterogeneity in drug response, we must be able to collect relevant biological samples to identify relevant biomarkers, including those that are genetically based. It is critical that we succeed in convincing investigators, IRBs, and patients that having access to these materials is warranted and fundamental to the goal of personalized medicine. To ensure continued access, researchers must ensure that these samples as well as any data derived from or based upon the samples are maintained in a confidential and secure manner, providing safeguards to prevent discrimination.

5 FUTURE TRENDS TOWARD PERSONALIZED MEDICINE

5.1 Emerging Science: Target Validation and Biomarkers

Investments continue in the public and private (pharmaceutical, biotechnology, and genomic industries) sectors to use genomic, genetic, and proteomic strategies in the discovery of clinically relevant targets, to understand disease and patient heterogeneity, to discover and develop novel drug candidates, to understand the causes of drug attrition, and to develop tools, diagnostics, and/or biomarkers. These tools and diagnostics will be useful for a variety of purposes, including a means of classifying patients according to disease heterogeneity and their response to medications.

Better diagnosis of disease, especially the molecular genetic basis of disease, will lead to precise diagnosis and classification of disease, or at least an assessment of an individual's relative risk of disease development. This will be made possible by the development of diagnostic tools and tests that will look at an individual more precisely over time, focusing on gene, genetic, protein, and biochemical differences, changes, or both. Likewise, similar clinical phenotypes will have different underlying mechanisms and these tools will provide an opportunity to stratify disease classifications that otherwise appear to be identical in the clinic. Moreover, much more knowledge is needed regarding environmental contributions to disease, especially complex, chronic, common disease.

Completion of the sequencing of the human genome is only the first step in a long road toward understanding the molecular genetic basis of disease. The next major challenge is the identification of all genes and the full genomic structure for each, along with all genetic variations, across all population groups globally. A parallel road will be the identification of the sequence and structure of the products of genes and proteins, together with all posttranslational modifications (PTMs) of these proteins, and changes in certain PTMs in various diseases. Similar unanticipated rates of progress in the identification of genes, genomic structures, proteins, protein structures, and genetic variations, and in the understanding of changes in gene and protein expression patterns in disease versus health may also be stimulated by greater access to enabling information, new technologies, and competition. Ultimately, an important achievement from this collaboration among the pharmaceutical industry, academia, and a charitable trust may be the ability for disparate groups to engage important research and prevail.

These trends of cooperativity will enable more targets to be identified and more disease stratification. Some speculate that this will lead to a boom in the development of novel drugs over the next 10–20 years, which should facilitate personalized medicine [48]. The central question is the specifics of when this will happen for each important disease. A leader in the HGP has provided a glimpse of how an individual may be treated in 2010 [49], as well as speculated where we will be over the next 40 years (Table 5) (F.S. Collins, personal communication, 2000).

5.2 Toward Personalized Medicine

One example of where this principle is already being employed is in the treatment of certain cancers. As previously discussed, researchers have shown that various genes can be genotyped to guide the selection and dosing of chemotherapy [38–42]. It is well established that genetic polymorphisms in drug metabolizing enzymes can have a profound effect on efficacy and toxicity of medications used to treat ALL and that individualizing drug dosages can improve clinical outcome. Genotype of leukemic lymphoblasts is an important prognostic variable that can be used to guide the intensity of treatment. While other genetic polymorphisms exist, other determinants of host susceptibility to pathogens, to polymorphisms in other diseases, and to other receptors may be important determinants of an individual's susceptibility to SAEs. Ultimately, putting all of these molecular diagnostics on an "ALL chip" or its equivalent would provide the basis for rapidly, and objectively, selecting therapy for each patient [42].

5.3 Pharmacogenomics in Drug Development

Alzheimer's disease provides a useful example of what future trends may bring, especially in the drug development process [7,8]. The diagnosis of Alzheimer's disease is subjective, based on clinical criteria established by groups of clinicians,

TABLE 5   Selected Medical and Societal Consequences of the Human
Genome Project

Decade	Key milestones in medicine, therapeutics, and society
2010	Predictive genetic tests available for 25 conditions Interventions to reduce risk available for most of these 25 conditions Small molecule drugs prevail; some examples of biologicals, including antisense/gene therapies Diagnostic/therapeutic pharmacogenomic approach is used for a few drugs Primary care providers begin to practice genetic medicine Effective legislation solutions to genetic discrimination and privacy in place in U.S.
2020	Pharmacogenomic-based designer drugs for diabetes, hypertension and other common, chronic, complex disease coming to the market Diagnostic/therapeutic pharmacogenomic approach is standard practice for many drugs Mental illness diagnosis transformed, new therapies arriving, societal views shifting Homologous recombination technology suggests germline gene therapy could be safe
2030	Genes involved in human aging process fully catalogued Clinical trials underway to extend maximum human life span Full computer model of human cell replaces many laboratory experiments Complete genomic sequencing of an individual is routine, costs less than $1,000 Major antitechnology movements active in U.S. and elsewhere
2040	Comprehensive genomics-based healthcare is the norm Disease predisposition determined (? at birth) Individualized preventive medicine available and largely effective Illnesses are detected early by molecular surveillance Gene therapy and gene-based drug therapies available for most diseases Average life span reaches 90 years, stressing prior socioeconomic norms Worldwide inequities remain, contributing to international tensions Serious debate is underway about humans possibly taking charge of their own evolution

Source: F.S. Collins, personal communication.

while confirmation awaits brain biopsy, postmortem. Alzheimer's disease has variable pathology, with gene mutations in at least several genes, including amyloid precursor protein, presenilin 1, and presenilin 2. If an effective treatment were developed for a common form of Alzheimer's disease, it might not work for all patients. Conversely, a treatment developed for a specific gene mutation may have no effect in common Alzheimer's disease phenotypes. While the clinical description of the phenotype will be identical, what will have changed is the ability to define disease and patient heterogeneity, or to define heterogeneity in drug response. The tools for defining patient heterogeneity will hopefully become available over the next decade.

If a new drug candidate for the treatment for Parkinson's, Alzheimer's, osteoarthritis, diabetes, osteoporosis, depression, schizophrenia, or other chronic disease goes into early clinical development, Phase Ia, it may be possible to confirm that the drug is successfully affecting the MOA. However, it may be necessary to wait until Phase Ib or Phase IIa to determine whether the drug is achieving any PD effect that is directly or indirectly linked to drug efficacy. This would be enhanced by the availability of one or more biomarkers linked to disease progression—a goal currently under investigation by many. If the drug candidate showed clear signs of efficacy in a small percentage of those treated in Phase II, a Phase III study with this drug would in effect be studying only the safety profile of the drug in the large percentage of those receiving treatment. One future approach might be to use the biomarkers for the purpose of recruitment of those patients that would be predicted to respond. An approach using an SNP-LD profile has recently been proposed [7,8], and the statistical rationale for such a design has also been described [43].

Better treatment options will ultimately lead to personalized medicine, but must include the role of environmental influences on disease pathogenesis, susceptibility, resistance mechanisms, and the interplay between genes and the environment. This emerging science will drive the identification of therapeutics, which will in turn drive the practice of medicine.

Unanticipated rapid rates of progress have occurred and continue to occur in understanding the molecular pathogenesis of disease. One of the best examples of this principle is the completion of the sequencing of the human genome, involving the publicly funded HGP, as well as the private industry-funded initiatives. While original projections were made for completion by 2005, it now appears that this gargantuan task will be completed by the end of 2001—approximately 4 years ahead of the schedule originally set out by the HGP. A recent excellent review provided insight into how medicine will change because of pharmacogenetics/pharmacogenomics and how knowledge derived from these sciences will impact how new medicines are discovered and developed [8].

6 CONCLUSIONS

True personalized medicine is limited today, largely due to a lack of sufficient basic knowledge regarding disease and patient heterogeneity, and limited diagnostic tools to identify such heterogeneity. For most diseases, we are a long way from achieving personalized medicine. In addition, the issues that recent advances in the postgenome era have brought to the forefront of therapeutics that impact on the attainment of personalized medicine are burdensome and complex.

The disparate goals of pharmacogenomics from disease genetics or gene therapy must become clearer and more transparent to ensure access to patients and relevant biological tissues to perform and validate the research. To ensure that personalized medicine can ultimately be an achievable goal, an even better approach would be for researchers, clinicians, and ethicists in academia, industry, and regulatory authorities to work together to address ethical, legal, social, and regulatory concerns. This would be intended to address the potential for individual harm that accompanies these advances, while not placing undue barriers, obstacles, or burdens on the research process. While personalized medicine will be a one-off process for the immediate future, there will ultimately be advantages to the harmonization of approaches used by the pharmaceutical and biotechnology industries.

Given all of the uncertainties in this rapidly changing world, it is challenging to predict exactly when personalized medicine will be commonplace in medicine and therapeutics. What is certain, though, is how difficult this challenge will be. It will likely be achieved one victory at a time and will include diagnostic information from one or more biomarkers, based on genetic variations in drug metabolizing enzymes, drug targets, drug transporters, biochemical pathways, gene or protein expression changes in relevant tissues or biofluids, biochemical data, functional scores or scales, imaging data, or some combination of such information. A systems biology approach will probably be key to developing an understanding of the complex biological processes involved in disease and in ultimately developing more personalized medicines.

In the meantime, pharmacogenomic or biomarker data can potentially contribute to confirming a drug's MOA, provide unambiguous evidence of PD activity, or provide clinically relevant disease severity or progression information. Such information will be valuable during the drug discovery and development process, since it could increase the confidence in rationale for a given target, provide earlier proof of concept, or both, thereby contributing to the development of personalized medicines.

REFERENCES

1. J Drews. In: J Drews, S. Ryser, eds. Human Disease from Genetic Causes to Biochemical Effects. Berlin: Blackwell, 1997, pp 5–9.

2. J Drews. Drug discovery: a historical perspective. Science 287:1960–1964, 2000.

3. PM Ridker, CH Hennekens, JE Buring, N Rifai. C-reactive protein and other markers of inflammation in the prediction of cardiovascular disease in women. N Engl J Med 342:836–843, 2000.

4. TR Fleming, DL DeMets. Surrogate end points in clinical trials: are we being misled? Ann Intern Med 125:605–613, 1996.

5. L Kruglyak. Prospects for whole-genome linkage disequilibrium mapping of common disease genes. Nat Genet 22:139–144, 1999.

6. J Ott. Predicting the range of linkage disequilibrium. Proc Natl Acad Sci USA 97: 2–3, 2000.

7. AD Roses. Pharmacogenetics and future drug development and delivery. Lancet 355:1358–1361, 2000.

8. AD Roses. Pharmacogenetics and the practice of medicine. Nature 405:857–865, 2000.

9. J Lazarou, BH Pomeranz, PN Corey. Incidence of adverse drug reactions in hospitalized patients: a meta-analysis of prospective studies. JAMA 279:1200–1205, 1998.

10. W Kalow. Pharmacogenetics—Heredity and the Response to Drugs. Philadelphia: W.B. Saunders, 1962.

11. AM Karnik. Update in pulmonary diseases. Ann Intern Med 131:596–604, 1999.

12. LJ Smith. Newer asthma therapies. Ann Intern Med 130:531–532, 1999.

13. JC Ruckdeschel. Update in oncology. Ann Intern Med 131:760–767, 1999.

14. KH Antman, DF Heitjan, GN Hortobagyi. High-dose chemotherapy for breast cancer. JAMA 282:1701–1703, 1999.

15. PC Hoffman. Lung cancer. Lancet 355:479–485, 2000.

16. RK Schneider, JL Levenson. Update in psychiatry. Ann Intern Med 131:514–521, 1999.

17. SJ Fredman, M Fava, AS Kienke, CN White, AA Nierenberg, JF Rosenbaum. Partial response, nonresponse, and relapse with selective serotonin reuptake inhibitors in major depression: a survey of current ''next steps'' practices. J Clin Psychiatry 61: 403–408, 2000.

18. MB Keller, JP McCullough, DN Klein, B Arnow, DL Dunner, AJ Gelenberg, JC Markowitz, CB Nemeroff, JM Russell, ME Thase, MH Trivedi, J Zajecka. A comparison of nefazodone, the cognitive behavioral-analysis system of psychotherapy, and their combination for the treatment of chronic depression. N Engl J Med 342: 1462–1470, 2000.

19. J Scott. Treatment of chronic depression. N Engl J Med 342:1518–1520, 2000.

20. RA DeFronzo. Pharmacologic therapy for type 2 diabetes mellitus. Ann Intern Med 131:281–303, 1999.

21. MI Harris. Health care and health status and outcomes for patients with type 2 diabetes. Diabetes Care 23:754–758, 2000.

22. T Furata, K Ohashi, T Kamata, M Takashima, K Kosuge, T Kawasaki, H Hanai, T Kubota, T Ishizaki, E Kaneko. Effect of genetic differences in omeprazole metabolism on cure rates for helicobacter pylori infection and peptic ulcer. Ann Intern Med 129:1027, 1998.

23. RS Rosenson, CC Tangney. Anti-atherothrombotic properties of statins: implications for cardiovascular event reduction. JAMA 279:1643–1650, 1998.

24. P Jones, S Kafonek, I Laurora, D Hunninghake. Comparative dose efficacy study of atorvastatin versus simvastatin, pravastatin, lovastatin, and fluvastatin in patients with hypercholesterolemia (the CURVES study). Am J Cardiol 81:582–586, 1998.

25. RE Schmieder, MP Schlaich, AU Klingbeil, P Martus. Update on reversal of left ventricular hypertrophy in essential hypertension (a meta-analysis of all randomized double-blind studies until December 1996). Nephrol Dial Transplant 13:564–569, 1998.

26. TG Pickering. Advances in the treatment of hypertension. JAMA 281:114–116, 1999.

27. MD Ferrari. Migraine. Lancet 351:1043–1051, 1998.

28. R Wernick, SM Campbell. Update in rheumatology. Ann Intern Med 132:125–133, 2000.

29. M Feldman, AT McMahon. Do cyclooxygenase-2 inhibitors provide benefits similar to those of traditional nonsteroidal anti-inflammatory drugs, with less gastrointestinal toxicity? Ann Intern Med 132:134–143, 2000.

30. WT Carpenter, RW Buchanan. Medical progress: schizophrenia. N Engl J Med 330: 681–688, 1994.

31. RW Kerwin, D Taylor. New antipsychotics, a review of their current status and clinical potential. CNS Drugs 6:71–82, 1996.

32. FD Martinez, PE Graves, M Baldini, S Solomon, R Erickson. Association between genetic polymorphisms of the beta sub-2 adrenoceptor and response to albuterol in children with and without a history of wheezing. J Clin Invest 100:3184–3188, 1997.

33. CN Yandava, L Dubeacute, N Szczerback, R Hippensteel, A Pillari, E Israel, N Schork, E Silverman, DA Katz, J Drajesk, JM Drazen. Pharmacogenetic association between ALOX5 promoter genotype and the response to anti-asthma treatment. Nat Genet 22:168–170, 1999.

34. CM Weyand, G McCarthy, JJ Goronzy. Correlation between disease phenotype and genetic heterogeneity in rheumatoid arthritis. J Clin Invest 95:2120–2126, 1995.

35. JR O'Dell, BS Nepom, C Haire, VH Gersuk, L Gaur, GF Moore, W Drymalski, W Palmer, PJ Eckhoff, LW Klassen, S Wees, G Thiele, GT Nepom. HLA-DRB1 typing in rheumatoid arthritis: predicting response to specific treatments. Ann Rheum Dis 57:209–213, 1998.

36. GW Abbott, F Sesti, I Splawski, ME Buck, MH Lehmann, KW Timothy, MT Kenting, N Goldstein. MiRP1 forms Ikr potassium channels with HERG and is associated with cardiac arrhythmia. Cell 97:175–187, 1999.

37. B Drolet, M Khalifa, P Daleau, BA Hamelin, J Turgeon. Block of the component of the delayed rectifier potassium current by the prokinetic agent cisapride underlies drug related lengthening of the QT interval. Circulation 97:204–210, 1998.

38. EY Krynetski, WE Evans. Pharmacogenetics of cancer therapy: getting personal. Am J Hum Genet 63:11–16, 1998.

39. WE Evans, MV Relling, JH Rodman, WR Crom, JM Boyett, CH Pui. Conventional compared with individualized chemotherapy for childhood acute lymphoblastic leukemia. N Engl J Med 338:499–505, 1998.

40. CH Pui, WE Evans. Drug therapy: acute lymphoblastic leukemia. N Engl J Med 339:605–615, 1998.

41. TR Golub, DK Slonim, P Tamayo, C Huard, M Gaasenbeek, JP Mesirov, H Coller,

ML Loh, JR Downing, MA Caligiuri, CD Bloomfield, ES Lander. Molecular classification of cancer: class discovery and class prediction by gene expression monitoring. Science 286:531–537, 1999.

42. WE Evans, MV Relling. Pharmacogenomics: translating functional genomics into rational therapeutics. Science 286:487–491, 1999.

43. BA Fijal, JM Hall, JS Witte. Clinical trials in the genomic era: effects of protective genotypes on sample size and duration of trial. Contr Clin Trials 21:7–20, 2000.

44. M Cargill, A Altshuler, J Ireland, P Sklar, K Ardlie, N Patil, CR Lane, EP Lim, N Kalyanaraman, L Ziaugra, L Friedland, A Rolfe, J Warrington, R Lipshutz, GQ Daley, E Lander. Characterization of single-nucleotide polymorphisms in coding regions of human genes. Nat Genet 22:231–238, 1999.

45. MK Halushka, JB Fan, K Bentley, L Hsie, N Shen, A Weder, R Cooper, R Lipshutz, A Chakravarti. Patterns of single-nucleotide polymorphisms in candidate genes for blood-pressure homeostatis. Nat Genet 22:239–247, 1999.

46. SNP Consortium (TSC) website. http://snp.cshl.org/.

47. U.S. National Bioethics Advisory Commission. Research involving human biological materials. http://bioethics.gov, 1999.

48. W Sadee. Genomics and drugs: finding the optimal drug for the right patient. Pharm Res 15:959–963, 1998.

49. FS Collins. Medical and societal consequences of the human genome project. N Engl J Med 341:28–37, 1999.

3

Current Status: Pharmacogenetics/Drug Metabolism

Leif Bertilsson
Huddinge University Hospital, Stockholm, Sweden

1 INTRODUCTION

The interindividual variation in the effect of drug treatment is pronounced. A major part of this is due to variation in drug metabolism, but also due to variation in drug targets such as receptors and transporters, which is evident from other chapters in this volume. The rate of drug metabolism is regulated by environmental factors such as food intake and smoking habits, but genetic factors are of utmost importance.

The pharmacogenetics of drug metabolism was established in the 1950s by the demonstration of the polymorphisms of plasma cholinesterase and N-acetyltransferase. The area of pharmacogenetics of drug metabolism has expanded tremendously and is now recognized in drug development and by drug regulatory authorities. This area of research has been reviewed extensively for example in the volume edited by Kalow and published in 1992 [1]. Dr. Kalow and I have recently reviewed the interethnic differences in drug disposition and effects [2]. There are also many other reviews to consult in this area [3–7]. Table 1 gives same examples of firmly established polymorphic drug-metabolizing enzymes and substrates. To cover the details of the individual polymorphic enzymes cata-

TABLE 1   Some Examples of Firmly Established Polymorphic Drug-Metabolizing Enzymes and Substrate Drugs

Polymorphic enzymes	Drug substrates
N-acetyltransferase 2 (NAT2)	Isoniazid, procainamide
Cytochrome P450 CYP2C9	S-Warfarin, losartan, phenytoin, tolbutamide, NSAIDs
Cytochrome P450 CYP2C19	Diazepam, omeprazole, proguanil
Cytochrome P450 CYP2D6	Most antidepressants and neuroleptics, antiarrhythmics
Thiopurine methyltransferase (TPMT)	6-Mercaptopurine, azathioprine

For individual references the reader is referred to recent books and reviews [1–7].

lyzing drug metabolism, references [2] and [3] are recommended. In the present review I will focus on two polymorphisms, which I consider both illustrative and clinically important—the cytochrome P450 CYP2D6, and the thiopurine methyltransferase (TPMT).

Until recently polymorphisms in drug metabolism were discovered by phenotypic analysis detecting a bi- or trimodality of an index of enzymatic activity. This was the case for slow and rapid acetylators of isoniazid and extensive and poor metabolizers (EM and PM, respectively) of debrisoquine/sparteine. This area of research is a good example of what is now popularly called *functional genomics*. With the molecular genetics techniques available today, single-nucleotide polymorphisms (SNPs) are easily detected, and later on their biochemical and clinical consequences may or may not be demonstrated. As examples of this, mutated alleles of both *CYP1A2* [8,9] and *CYP3A4* [10] have been demonstrated, but their functional importance needs to be validated. A recent study [11] strongly suggests a genetic component in the variability of the activity of the important enzyme CYP3A4 and therefore further genetic investigations are warranted.

2   THE CYP2D6 POLYMORPHISM

2.1   The Discovery and Incidence of the PM Phenotype

Mahgoub et al. [12] and Tucker et al. [13] described in 1977 that the hydroxylation of the antihypertensive drug debrisoquine is polymorphic in nature. Independently Eichelbaum et al. [14] showed that the oxidation of sparteine also is polymorphic. The metabolic ratios (MR; parent drug/metabolite) of the two

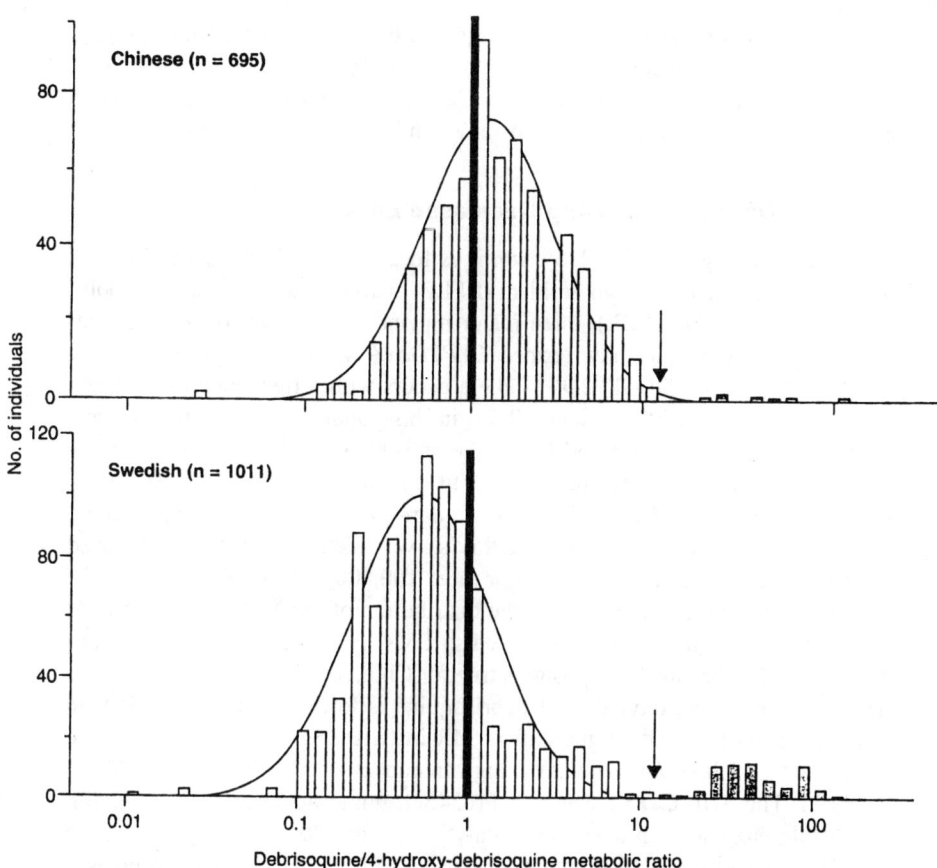

FIGURE 1 Distribution of the urinary debrisoquine/4-hydroxydebrisoquine metabolic ratio (MR) in 695 Chinese and 1011 Swedish healthy subjects. The arrows indicate MR = 12.6, the antimode between EM and PM established in Caucasians. A line is drawn at MR = 1. Most Chinese EM have MR > 1, while most Swedish EM have MR < 1. (From Ref. 18.)

drugs were closely correlated [15], showing that the same enzyme, now termed CYP2D6, is responsible for the two metabolic reactions.

The incidence of PMs of debrisoquine/sparteine has been investigated in many populations, most of them with a fairly small numbers of subjects [16,17]. Among 1011 Swedish Caucasians we found 69 (6.8%) PMs of debrisoquine (Fig. 1) [18]. This incidence is very similar to other European [16,17] and American

[19] Caucasian populations. In collaboration with Lou and associates in Beijing, we showed that the incidence of PM among 695 Chinese was only 1.0% using the antimode MR = 12.6 established in Caucasian populations (Fig. 1) [18]. A similar low incidence of PM has been shown in Japanese [19] and Koreans [20].

2.2   CYP2D6 Alleles Causing Decreased Enzyme Activity

The gene encoding the CYP2D6 enzyme is localized on chromosome 22 [21]. Using restriction length polymorphism (RFLP) analysis and allele-specific polymerase chain reaction (PCR), three major mutant alleles were found in Caucasians [22–25]. These are now termed *CYP2D6*3, 4,* and *5* [26] (Table 2). In Swedish Caucasians the *CYP2D6*4* allele occurs with a frequency of 22% and accounts for >75% of the mutant alleles in this population [27]. The *4 allele is almost absent in Chinese and this is the reason for the low incidence of 1% PM in this population compared to 7% in Caucasians [18]. The occurrence of the gene deletion *(CYP2D6*5)* is very similar—4–6% (Table 2)—in Sweden, China, and Zimbabwe. This shows that this is a very old mutation, which occurred before the separation of the three major races 100,000 to 150,000 years ago [2].

It is apparent in Figure 1 that the distribution of the MR of Chinese EMs is shifted to the right compared to Swedish EMs (*P* < .01) [18]. Most Swedes have MR < 1, whereas the opposite is true for Chinese subjects. This shows that the mean rate of hydroxylation of debrisoquine is lower in Chinese EMs than Caucasian EMs [18]. This right shift in MR in Orientals is due to the presence of a mutant *CYP2D6*10* allele at the high frequency of 51% in Chinese [28,29] (Table 2). The SNP C188T causes a Pro34Ser amino acid substitution, giving an unstable enzyme with decreased catalytic activity [29]. As shown in Figure 2, the presence of this C188T mutation causes the right shift among the investigated 152 Koreans [30]. The high frequency of this *CYP2D6*10* allele is similar in Chinese, Japanese, and Koreans.

Masirembwa et al. [31] found a right shift of MR in black Zimbabweans similar to that found in Orientals. A mutated allele was subsequently identified and named *CYP2D6*17*, which encodes an enzyme with decreased activity. Among black Africans the frequency of this allele was found to be 34% in Zimbabweans [31] (Table 2), 17% in Tanzanians [32], 28% in Ghanaians [33] and 9% in Ethiopians [34]. This study and many others demonstrate the genetic heterogeneity of populations in Africa.

There are thus population-specific *CYP2D6* alleles with the *4 in Caucasians with a C1934A mutation giving a splicing defect and thus no enzyme is encoded. The *CYP2D6*10* and *17* in Orientals and Africans, respectively, encode two different enzymes with decreased activity. In Caucasians and Orientals a close geno- and phenotype relationship has been demonstrated in several studies [27,29,30]. However, in studies in Ethiopia [34], Ghana [33], and Tanzania [32]

TABLE 2 Frequency of Normal CYP2D6*1 or *2 Alleles and Some Alleles Causing No or Deficient CYP2D6 Activity in Three Different Populations

CYP2D6 alleles	Functional mutation	Consequence	Allele frequency (%)		
			Swedish	Chinese	Zimbabwean
*1 or *2 (wt)			69	43	54
*3 (A)	A2637 del	Frame shift	2	0	0
*4 (B)	G1934A	Splicing defect	22	0–1	2
*5 (D)	Gene deletion	No enzyme	4	6	4
*10 (Ch)	C188T	Unstable enzyme	n.d.	51	6
*17 (Z)	C1111T	Reduced affinity	n.d.	n.d.	34

n.d. = not determined. Data are from original publications [27–29,31] and reviews [3–5].

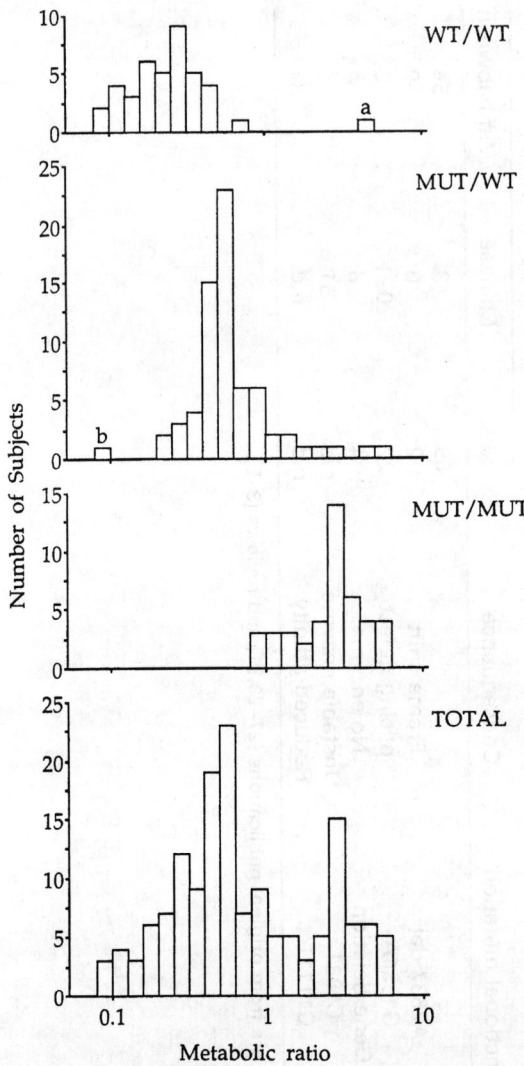

FIGURE 2 Distribution of the debrisoquine MR in three genotype groups related to the *CYP2D6*10* allele in 152 Korean subjects. wt = *CYP2D6*1* (or *2*) and mut = *CYP2D6*10*. (From Ref. 30.)

a lower CYP2D6 activity in relation to genotype has been demonstrated indicating that environmental factors in Africa; e.g. infections and food intake are of importance in addition to genetic factors.

2.3 Gene Duplication, Multiduplication, and Amplification

The problems in treating PMs of debrisoquine with various drugs have been extensively discussed over the years since the discovery of the CYP2D6 polymorphism [17]. Much less attention has been given to patients at the other extreme of the distribution of MR, i.e., ultrarapid hydroxylators. Fifteen years ago we described a women with depression having an MR of debrisoquine of 0.07, who had to be treated with 500 mg nortriptyline daily [35]. This is three to five times higher than the recommended dose. Due to the fruitful collaboration with Ingelman-Sundberg's group, we could identify the molecular genetic basis for the ultrarapid metabolism in this patient and in another patient, who had to be treated with megadoses of clomipramine [36]. These two patients had an *XbaI* 42-kb fragment containing two different functionally active *CYP2D6* genes in the *CYP2D* locus, causing more enzyme to be expressed. The same year, 1993, a father and his daughter and son with 12 extra copies of the *CYP2D6* gene were described [37]. This was the first demonstration of an inherited amplification of an active gene encoding a drug-metabolizing enzyme. These subjects were ultrarapid hydroxylators of debrisoquine with MR 0.01–0.02. The 12.1-kb fragment obtained by *EcoRI* RFLP analysis corresponds to the presence of a duplicated or multiduplicated *CYP2D6*2* gene [37]. There are now also a few examples of duplicated *CYP2D6*1* and *4* genes [38].

In Swedish Caucasians the frequency of subjects having duplicated/multiduplicated genes is about 1–2% [39]. Going south in Europe the frequency increases, being 3.6% in Germany [40], 7–10% in Spain [38,41], and 10% on Sicily in Italy [42]. The frequency is as high as 29% in black Ethiopians [34] and 20% in Saudi Arabians [43]. There is thus a European-African north-south gradient in the incidence of *CYP2D6* gene duplication. The high incidence among Ethiopians and Saudi Arabians indicates that the high incidence in Spain and Italy may have an ancestry in the Arabian conquest in the Mediterranean area [38]. The high frequency of duplicated genes among Ethiopians might be the result of a dietary pressure favoring the preservation of duplicated *CYP2D6* genes because of the ability of the enzyme to metabolize plant toxins including alkaloids [5,43]. Caucasian subjects with a *CYP2D6* gene duplication have been shown to be ultrarapid metabolizers of debrisoquine with MR usually between 0.01 and 0.15 [37–39]. In the study of Aklillu et al. [34], black Ethiopians with multiple *CYP2D6* genes had higher MR, usually between 0.1 and 1. These subjects do thus not have the ultrarapid metabolism of debrisoquine demonstrated for Caucasians with multiple genes. This might be due to environmental factors in Africa causing a decreased activity as discussed for Ghanaians [33] and Tanzanians above [32]. Support for this hypothesis has recently been obtained by Aklillu et al. (unpublished) showing that black Ethiopians living in Sweden have a more rapid metabolism of debrisoquine than black Ethiopians living in Ethiopia with the same genotype.

2.4 Metabolism of CYP2D6 Drug Substrates in Relation to Genotypes

Since the discovery of the CYP2D6 polymorphism almost 100 drugs have been shown to be substrates of this enzyme. Some of these drugs are shown in Table 3. CYP2D6 substrates are all lipophilic bases. To study whether a drug is metabolized by CYP2D6 or not, both in vitro and in vivo techniques may be employed. To establish the quantitative importance of this enzyme for the total metabolism of the drug, in vivo studies need to be performed. I will here give two examples with the tricyclic antidepressant nortriptyline and the neuroleptic haloperidol.

Nortriptyline was one of the first clinically important drugs to be shown to be metabolized by CYP2D6 [44,45]. These early studies (before the era of genotyping) were performed in phenotyped panels of healthy subjects, and the results have been confirmed in vivo in patients as well as in vitro using human liver microsomes and expressed enzymes. In a recent study by Dalén et al. [46], nortriptyline was given as a single oral dose to 21 healthy Swedish Caucasian subjects with different genotypes. As seen in Figure 3 there was a decrease in the plasma concentration of nortriptyline from subjects with 0 functional genes (5

TABLE 3 Some Drugs Whose Metabolism Is Catalyzed by the CYP2D6 Enzyme, i.e., the Debrisoquine/Sparteine Hydroxylase

β-Adrenoceptor blockers	Antidepressants	Neuroleptics
Metoprolol	Amitriptyline	Haloperidol
Propranolol	Clomipramine	Perphenazine
Timolol	Desipramine	Risperidone
	Fluoxetine	Thioridazine
Antiarrhythmic drugs	Fluvoxamine	Zuclopenthixol
Encainide	Imipramine	
Flecainide	Mianserin	Miscellaneous
Perhexiline	Nortriptyline	Codeine
Propafenone	Paroxetine	Debrisoquine
Sparteine		Dextromethophan
		Phenformin
		Tramadol

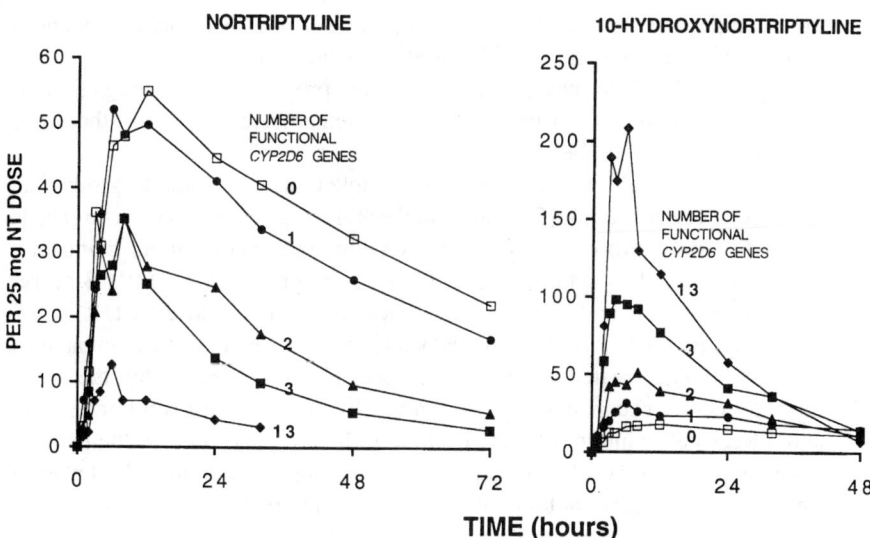

FIGURE 3 Mean plasma concentrations of nortriptyline (left) and 10-hydroxy-nortriptyline (right) in different genotype groups after a single oral dose of nortriptyline. The numerals close to the curves represent the number of functional *CYP2D6* genes in each genotype group. In groups with 0–3 functional genes, there were five subjects in each group. There was only one subject with 13 functional genes. (From Ref. 46.)

PM with the *CYP2D6*4/*4* genotype) to those with 1, 2, and 3 (gene duplication) functional genes (5 in each group). The plasma concentrations of the parent drug were extremely low in one subject with 13 *CYP2D6* genes. This is the son in the family mentioned above (genotype *CYP2D6*2 × 13/*4*). The plasma concentrations of the formed metabolite 10-hydroxynortriptyline show the opposite pattern—highest concentrations in the subject with 13 genes and lowest in the PMs (Fig. 3, right). This study clearly shows the impact of the detrimental *CYP2D6*4* allele as well as the duplication/amplification of the *CYP2D6*2* gene on the metabolism of nortriptyline [46]. A relationship between *CYP2D6* genotype and steady-state plasma concentration of nortriptyline and its hydroxy metabolite has been shown in Swedish depressed patients treated with the drug [47].

Using the same protocol as in the study of Dalén et al. in Caucasians [46], we investigated the influence of the Asian-specific *CYP2D6*10* allele on the disposition of nortriptyline in Chinese subjects living in Sweden [48]. Recently Morita et al. [49] related the *CYP2D6*10* allele to steady-state plasma levels of nortriptyline and its metabolites in Japanese depressed patients. From these two studies it may be concluded that the Asian *CYP2D6*10* allele encodes an enzyme with decreased activity to metabolize nortriptyline. This effect is less pronounced than the Caucasian-specific *CYP2D6*4* allele, which encodes no enzyme at all. Genotyping of *CYP2D6* may be a tool to predict proper dosing of drugs such as nortriptyline in individual patients. It must be remembered, however, that there are population-specific alleles.

Haloperidol will serve as a second example of an important drug substrate of CYP2D6. Llerena et al. [50] gave single oral doses of haloperidol to panels of six EMs and six PMs of debrisoquine. PMs eliminated haloperidol significantly slower than EMs, the mean plasma half-life being longer (29.4 and 16.3 hr, respectively; $P < .01$) and the mean clearance lower (1.16 and 2.49 $L \cdot h^{-1} \cdot kg^{-1}$, respectively; $P < .05$) [50]. In a clinical study involving eight Caucasian patients with schizophrenia treated with depot haloperidol (as the decanoate), the dopamine D2 receptor occupancy was determined by positron emission tomography 1 and 4 weeks after intramuscular injection of the drug [51]. One of the patients was genotypically a PM of debrisoquine. Of the group, he had the highest plasma concentration of haloperidol and also the highest D2 receptor occupancy.

Two studies from Hirosaki in Japan [52,53] have shown a relationship between increased haloperidol plasma concentrations and the presence of *CYP2D6*10* (and*5*) alleles in Japanese patients treated with oral doses of haloperidol. The dose used was 12 mg daily. In a recent study in Korea (Roh et al., in preparation) a relationship between haloperidol concentration and *CYP2D6* genotype was established in patients receiving <20 mg daily, but not in patients receiving higher doses. We believe that the high-affinity low-capacity CYP2D6 is the predominant enzyme at low concentrations/doses of haloperidol, while the low-affinity high-capacity CYP3A4 becomes more important at higher doses. We could thus conclude that at least at low doses haloperidol is metabolized by CYP2D6. The metabolic pathway of haloperidol catalysed by CYP2D6 is not known. Also, other neuroleptics, such as perphenazine, risperidone, thioridazine, and zuclopenthixol, are metabolized by CYP2D6 (Table 3) [4].

3 THE TPMT POLYMORPHISM

In contrast to drug metabolism catalyzed by CYP enzymes, I have no experience of TPMT. However, gastroenterologists at our university hospital use azathioprine quite extensively as an immunosuppressant for, e.g., Crohn's disease, and have consulted me on this. I have thus been impressed by the work on TPMT by several research groups.

TPMT is a cytosolic enzyme which methylates thiols using S-adenosine methionine as a methyldonor [54]. The TPMT activity in red blood cells is polymorphic, and a trimodal distribution has been demonstrated in Caucasians [55]. About one subject in 300 is homozygous for a defect *TPMT* allele with very

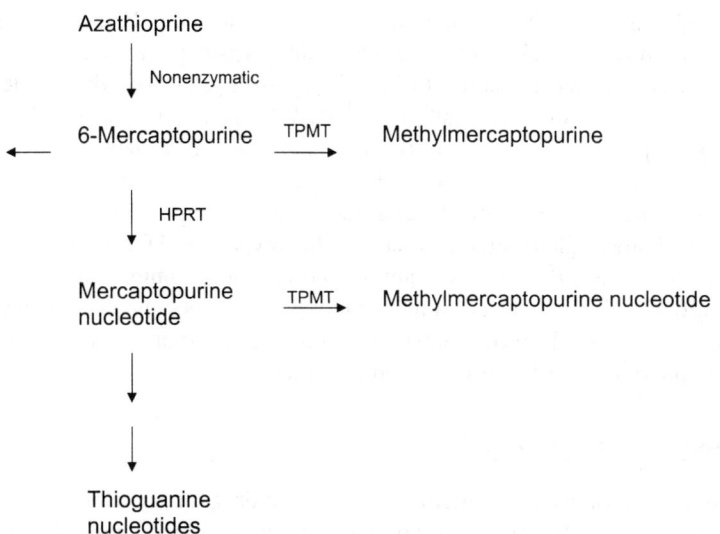

FIGURE 4 Metabolism of azathioprine and 6-mercaptopurine. TPMT = thiopurine methyltransferase; HPRT = hypoxantine–guanine phosphoribosyltransferase.

low enzyme activity [55]. Eleven percent are heterozygotes with an intermediate activity.

Azathioprine is an imidazole derivative of and metabolized nonenzymatically to 6-mercaptopurine (Fig. 4). 6-Mercaptopurine is metabolized by several pathways, one of which is catalyzed by TPMT. Another pathway leads to the active metabolite thioguanine nucleotides, which at high concentrations may cause toxicity (low TPMT) and at low concentrations (high TPMT) may give a high risk of therapeutic failure (Fig. 4). Several studies have shown a relationship between therapeutic effects and TPMT activity or thioguanine nucleotides concentration in red blood cells. The use of these two measures to optimize the dosage of such drugs has been reviewed by Lennard [56]. Lennard et al. [57] showed that three adult dermatology patients, who had low TPMT activity and also high 6-thioguanine nucleotide concentration in red blood cells, developed azathioprine-induced myelosuppression. Also in children treated with thiopurines for leukemia, these measures in red blood cells may be used to identify patients receiving suboptimal chemotherapy [56,57]. Evans and Relling [6] further discuss the use of pheno- and genotyping for TPMT to optimize the dosing of thiopurine drugs.

The *TPMT* gene is located on chromosome 6 and includes 10 exons [58]. *TPMT*3A*, the most common mutated allele, contains two point mutations in exons 7 (G460A; Ala154Thr) and 10 (A719G; Tyr240Lys). Two other alleles contain a single mutation, the first SNP (*TPMT*3B*) and the second SNP (*TPMT*3C*) [58]. Aarbakke et al. [59] have reviewed the variant alleles of the *TPMT* gene and the relationship to TPMT deficiency. In Caucasians the *TPMT*3A* accounts for ~85% of mutated alleles, and in such populations the analysis of the known alleles may predict the phenotype (TPMT activity). In a Korean population the *TPMT*3A* was absent and the most common allele was *TPMT*3C* [56,60]. Continued studies in different populations seem necessary to generally use genotyping instead of phenotyping for TPMT to predict the proper dosage of thiopurines to be used in individual patients.

4   FUTURE PERSPECTIVES

The pronounced interindividual variation in the rate of drug metabolism has been known for many years. It was initially only of academic interest, but today the pharmaceutical industry has to document the metabolism of a new drug in development before registration. This is a requirement of the U.S. Food and Drug Administration and similar authorities. The knowledge of how a drug is metabolized and which enzymes are involved may help to predict drug-drug interactions and how fast an individual patient may metabolize a specific drug.

With the high-throughput screening techniques available today, pharmaceutical industries may screen for drug candidates which are metabolized by and/ or inhibitors of, e.g., CYP2D6. Such drugs are in the hands of many companies not further developed. If this had been the case in the past, we would not have many of the important drugs available today (see Table 3). I see a danger in deleting potential drugs from development, if CYP2D6 is involved in their metabolism. The novel antimuscarinic drug tolterodine may serve as an example of a drug metabolized by CYP2D6, but not discontinued for development. It is now used as a valuable drug for the treatment of urinary incontinence. In early Phase I studies, it was discovered that tolterodine is hydroxylated by CYP2D6, but the surrogate antimuscarinic effect on salivation was the same in EM and PM [61]. The reason is that 5-hydroxytolterodine is an active metabolite and responsible for some of the effect in EM. After some well-planned studies [62] this drug was soon approved in both Europe and in the United States.

Phenotype analysis with, e.g., debrisoquine or sparteine may be performed to predict a proper dosage schedule before starting treatment with a CYP2D6 substrate drug. Phenotyping should be avoided during treatment as many drugs, especially psychotropic drugs such as imipramine and levomepromazine, may inhibit the test drug [63]. Genotyping may of course be performed independent of ongoing drug treatment. In many cases a nice geno-phenotype relationship has been established, but as pointed out above, interethnic differences must be considered. With the development of new, less expensive genotyping methods, the use of such techniques will increase in the future. The measurement of the active species of a drug in plasma (i.e., therapeutic drug monitoring) is maybe the best tool to optimize prescription in the individual patient. I consider TPMT the best-documented polymorphic drug-metabolizing enzyme, which requires personalized medication. In this case the best is to determine TPMT activity in red blood cells, but active thioguanine nucleotides may be measured as an alternative. Genotyping might here be a valuable tool in the future (see references above).

The need for personalized medication has been discussed in many recent articles. One often quoted is by Lazarou et al. [64], who performed a meta-analysis of the incidence of adverse drug reactions (ADRs). They found the extremely high incidence of serious ADRs of 6.7% and of fatal ADRs of 0.32% among hospitalized patients in the United States. This means that about 100,000 U.S. citizens die every year from drug side effects and about 2 million get seriously ill because of drug intake. At least some of these patients might have had low activity of polymorphic drug-metabolizing enzymes such as CYP2D6 or TPMT, but this can only be speculated upon. Partial support for such a speculation comes from a pilot study by deLeon et al. [65]. They determined the *CYP2D6* genotype in 100 consecutive patients in a psychiatric hospital in Kentucky and found that 14% were PM, which is twice that of the U.S. population (7%). The patients with CYP2D6 deficiency also appeared more likely to experience side effects in response to CYP2D6 medications [65].

ACKNOWLEDGMENTS

The studies performed in the author's laboratory were supported by the Swedish Medical Research Council (3902) and Karolinska Institutet.

REFERENCES

1. W Kalow. Pharmacogenetics of Drug Metabolism. New York: Pergamon Press, 1992.
2. L Bertilsson, W Kalow. Interethnic differences is drug disposition and effects. In: GM Pacifici, O Pelkonen, eds. Interindividual Variability in Drug Metabolism in Humans. London: Taylor & Francis, 2000. In press.
3. GM Pacifici, GN Fracchia. Advances in Drug Metabolism in Man. Brussels: European Commission, 1995.
4. L Bertilsson, M-L Dahl. Polymorphic drug oxidation: relevance to the treatment of psychiatric disorders. CNS Drugs 5:200–223, 1996.
5. M Ingelman-Sundberg, M Oscarsson, RA McLellan. Polymorphic human cytochrome P450 enzymes: an opportunity for individualized drug treatment. Trends Pharmacol Sci 20:324–349, 1999.

6. WE Evans, MV Relling. Pharmacogenomics: translating functional genomics into rational therapeutics. Science 286:487–491, 1999.

7. CR Wolf, G Smith, RL Smith. Clinical review. Pharmacogenetics. BMJ 320:987–990, 2000.

8. SL McLeod, Y-M Tang, T Yokoi, T Kamataki, S Doublin, B Lawson, J Massengill, FF Kadlubar, NP Lang. The role of recently discovered genetic polymorphism in the regulation of the human CYP1A2 gene. Proc Am Assoc Canc Res 396, 1998.

9. C Sachse, J Brockmöller, S Bauer, I Roots. Functional significance of C-A polymorphism in intron 1 of the cytochrome P450 CYP1A2 gene tested with caffeine. Br J Clin Pharmacol 47:445–449, 1999.

10. F Sata, A Sapone, G Elizondo, P Stocker, VP Miller, W Zheng, H Raunio, CL Crespi, FJ Gonzalez. CYP3A4 allelic variants with amino acid substitution in exons 7 and 12: evidence for an allelic variant with altered catalytic activity. Clin Pharmacol Ther 67:48–56, 2000.

11. V Özdemir, W Kalow, B-K Tang, AD Paterson, SE Walker, L Endrenyi, APM Kashuba. Evaluation of the genetic component of variability in CYP3A4 activity: a repeated drug administration method. Pharmacogenetics 10:373–388, 2000.

12. A Mahgoub, JR Idle, DG Dring, R Lancaster, RL Smith. Polymorphic hydroxylation of debrisoquine in man. Lancet 2:584–586, 1977.

13. GT Tucker, JH Silas, AO Iyun, MS Lennard, AJ Smith. Polymorphic hydroxylation of debrisoquine in man. Lancet 2:718, 1977.

14. M Eichelbaum, N Spannbrucker, B Steinke, HJ Dengler. Defective N-oxidation of sparteine in man: a new pharmacogenetic defect. Eur J Clin Pharmacol 16:183–187, 1979.

15. M Eichelbaum, L Bertilsson, J Säwe, C Zekorn. Polymorphic oxidation of sparteine and debrisoquine. Related pharmacogenetic entities. Clin Pharmacol Ther 31:184–186, 1982.

16. G Alván, P Bechtel, L Iselius, U Gundert-Remy. Hydroxylation polymorphisms of debrisoquine and mephenytoin in European populations. Eur J Clin Pharmacol 39:533–537, 1990.

17. M Eichelbaum, AS Gross. The genetic polymorphism of debrisoquine/sparteine metabolism—clinical aspects. In: W Kalow, ed. Pharmacogenetics of Drug Metabolism. New York: Pergamon Press, 1992, pp 625–648.

18. L Bertilsson, YQ Lou, YL Du, Y Liu, T-Y Kuang, XM Liao, KY Wang, J Reviriego, L Iselius, F Sjöqvist. Pronounced differences between native Chinese and Swedish populations in the polymorphic hydroxylations of debrisoquine and S-mephenytoin. Clin Pharmacol Ther 51:388–397, 1992.

19. K Nakamura, F Goto, WA Ray, CB McAllister, E Jacqz, GB Wilkinson, RA Branch. Interethnic differences in genetic polymorphism of debrisoquin and mephenytoin hydroxylation between Japanese and Caucasian populations. Clin Pharmacol Ther 38:402–408, 1985.

20. D-R Sohn, S-G Shin, C-W Park, M Kusaka, K Chiba, T Ishizaki. Metoprolol oxidation polymorphism in a Korean population: comparison with native Japanese and Chinese populations. Br J Clin Pharmacol 32:504–507, 1991.

21. M Eichelbaum, MP Baur, HJ Dengler, BO Osikowska-Evers, G Tieves, C Zekorn,

C Rittner. Chromosomal assignment of human cytochrome P450 (debrisoquine/ sparteine type) to chromosome 22. Br J Clin Pharmacol 23:455–458, 1987.

22. RC Skoda, FJ Gonzalez, A Demierre, UA Meyer. Two mutant alleles of the human cytochrome P450 db1 gene (P450 II D1) associated with genetically deficient metabolism of debrisoquine and other drugs. Proc Natl Acad Sci USA 85:5240–5243, 1988.

23. A Gaedigk, M Blum, R Gaedigk, M Eichelbaum, UA Meyer. Deletion of the entire cytochrome P450 CYP2D6 gene as a cause of impaired drug metabolism in poor metabolizers of the debrisoquine/sparteine polymorphism. Am J Hum Genet 48: 943–950, 1991.

24. HM Heim, UA Meyer. Genotyping of poor metabolisers of debrisoquine by allele-specific PCR amplification. Lancet 336:529–532, 1990.

25. HM Heim, UA Meyer. Evolution of a high polymorphic human cytochrome P450 gene cluster: CYP2D6. Genomics 14:49–58, 1992.

26. AK Daly, J Brockmöller, F Broly, M Eichelbaum, WE Evans, FJ Gonzalez, J-D Huang, JR Idle, M Ingelman-Sundberg, T Ishizaki, E Jacqz-Aigrain, UA Meyer, DW Nebert, VM Steen, CR Wolf, UM Zanger. Nomenclature for human CYP2D6 alleles. Pharmacogenetics 6:193–201, 1996.

27. M-L Dahl, I Johansson, M Porsmyr Palmertz, M Ingelman-Sundberg, F Sjöqvist. Analysis of the CYP2D6 gene in relation to debrisoquin and desipramine hydroxylation in a Swedish population. Clin Pharmacol Ther 51:12–17, 1992.

28. SL Wang, JD Huang, MD Lai, B-H Liu, M-L Lai. Molecular basis of genetic variation in debrisoquine hydroxylation in Chinese subjects: polymorphism in RFLP and DNA sequence of CYP2D6. Clin Pharmacol Ther 53:410–418, 1993.

29. I Johansson, M Oscarsson, Q-Y Yue, L Bertilsson, F Sjöqvist, M Ingelman-Sundberg. Genetic analysis of the Chinese CYP2D locus. Characterization of variant CYP2D6 genes present in subjects with diminished capacity for debrisoquine hydroxylation. Mol Pharmacol 46:452–459, 1994.

30. H-K Roh, M-L Dahl, I Johansson, M Ingelman-Sundberg, Y-N Cha, L Bertilsson. Debrisoquine and S-mephenytoin hydroxylation phenotypes and genotype in a Korean population. Pharmacogenetics 6:441–447, 1996.

31. C Masimirembwa, I Persson, L Bertilsson, J Hasler, M Ingelman-Sundberg. A novel mutant variant of the CYP2D6 gene (CYP2D6*17) common in a black African population: association with diminished debrisoquine hydroxylase activity. Br J Clin Pharmacol 42:713–719, 1996.

32. A Wennerholm, I Johansson, AY Massele, M Jande, C Alm, Y Aden Abdi, M-L Dahl, M Ingelman-Sundberg, L Bertilsson, LL Gustafsson. Decreased capacity for debrisoquine metabolism among black Tanzanians: analyses of the CYP2D6 genotype and phenotype. Pharmacogenetics 9:707–714, 1999.

33. E-U Griese, S Asante-Poku, D Ofori-Adjei, G Mikus, M Eichelbaum. Analysis of the CYP2D6 gene mutations and their consequences for enzyme function in a West African population. Pharmacogenetics 9:715–723, 1999.

34. E Aklillu, I Persson, L Bertilsson, I Johansson, F Rodriguez, M Ingelman-Sundberg. Frequent distribution of ultrarapid metabolizers of debrisoquine in an Ethiopian population carrying duplicated and multiduplicated functional CYP2D6 alleles. J Pharmacol Exp Ther 278:441–446, 1996.

35. L Bertilsson, A Åberg-Wistedt, LL Gustafsson, C Nordin. Extremely rapid hydroxylation of debrisoquine—a case report with implication for treatment with nortriptyline and other tricyclic antidepressants. Ther Drug Monit 7:478–480, 1985.

36. L Bertilsson, M-L Dahl, F Sjöqvist, A Åberg-Wistedt, M Humble, I Johansson, E Lundqvist, M Ingelman-Sundberg. Molecular basis for rational megaprescribing in ultrarapid hydroxylators of debrisoquine. Lancet 341:63, 1993.

37. I Johansson, E Lundqvist, L Bertilsson, M-L Dahl, F Sjöqvist, M Ingelman-Sundberg. Inherited amplification of an active gene in the cytochrome P450 CYP2D-locus as a cause of ultrarapid metabolism of debrisoquine. Proc Natl Acad Sci USA 90:11825–11829, 1993. .

38. ML Bernal, B Sinues, I Johansson, RA McLellan, A Wennerholm, M-L Dahl, M Ingelman-Sundberg, L Bertilsson. Ten percent of North Spanish individuals carry duplicated or triplicated CYP2D6 genes associated with ultrarapid metabolism of debrisoquine. Pharmacogenetics 9:657–660, 1999.

39. M-L Dahl, I Johansson, L Bertilsson, M Ingelman-Sundberg, F Sjöqvist. Ultrarapid hydroxylation of debrisoquine in a Swedish population. Analysis of the molecular genetic basis. J Pharmacol Exp Ther 274:516–520, 1995.

40. C Sachse, J Brockmöller, S Bauer, I Roots. Cytochrome P450 2D6 variants in a Caucasian population: allele frequencies and phenotypic consequences. Am J Hum Genet 60:284–295, 1997.

41. JAG Agúndez, MC Ledesma, JM Ladero, J Benitez. Prevalence of CYP2D6 gene duplication and its repercussion on the oxidative phenotype in a white population. Clin Pharmacol Ther 57:265–269, 1995.

42. MG Scordo, E Spina, G Facciolá, A Avenoso, I Johansson, M-L Dahl. Cytochrome P450 2D6 genotype and steady state plasma levels of risperidone and 9-hydroxy risperidone. Psychopharmacology 147:300–305, 1999.

43. RA McLellan, M Oscarson, JE Seidegård, DAP Evans, M Ingelman-Sundberg. Frequent occurrence of CYP2D6 gene duplication in Saudi Arabians. Pharmacogenetics 7:187–191, 1997.

44. L Bertilsson, M Eichelbaum, B Mellström, J Säwe, HU Schulz, F Sjöqvist. Nortriptyline and antipyrine clearance in relation to debrisoquine hydroxylation in man. Life Sci 27:1673–1677, 1980.

45. B Mellström, L Bertilsson, J Säwe, HU Schulz, F Sjöqvist. E- and Z-hydroxylation of nortriptyline in man—relationship to polymorphic hydroxylation of debrisoquine. Clin Pharmacol Ther 30:189–193, 1981.

46. P Dalén, M-L Dahl, ML Bernal Ruiz, J Nordin, L Bertilsson. 10-Hydroxylation of nortriptyline in Caucasians with 0, 1, 2, 3 and 13 functional CYP2D6 genes. Clin Pharmacol Ther 63:444–452, 1998.

47. M-L Dahl, L Bertilsson, C Nordin. Steady-state plasma levels of nortriptyline and its 10-hydroxy metabolite: relationship to the CYP2D6 genotype. Psychopharmacology 123:315–319, 1996.

48. Q-Y Yue, Z-H Zhong, G Tybring, P Dalén, M-L Dahl, L Bertilsson, F Sjöqvist. Pharmacokinetics of nortriptyline and its 10-hydroxy metabolite in Chinese subjects of different CYP2D6 genotypes. Clin Pharmacol Ther 64:384–390, 1998.

49. S Morita, K Shimoda, T Someya, Y Yoshimura, K Kamijima, N Kato. Steady-state

plasma levels of nortriptyline and its hydroxylated metabolites in Japanese patients: impact of CYP2D6 genotype on the hydroxylation of nortriptyline. J Clin Psychopharmacol 20:141–149, 2000.

50. A Llerena, C Alm, M-L Dahl, B Ekqvist, L Bertilsson. Haloperidol disposition is dependent of debrisoquine hydroxylation phenotype. Ther Drug Monit 14:92–97, 1992.

51. S Nyberg, L Farde, C Halldin, M-L Dahl, L Bertilsson. D2 dopamine receptor occupancy during low-dose treatment with haloperidol decanoate. Am J Psychiatry 152: 173–178, 1995.

52. A Suzuki, K Otani, K Mihara, N Yasui, S Kaneko, Y Inoue, K Hayashi. Effects of the CYP2D6 genotype on the steady-state plasma concentrations of haloperidol and reduced haloperidol in Japanese schizophrenic patients. Pharmacogenetics 7:415–418, 1997.

53. K Mihara, A Suzuki, T Kondo, N Yasui, H Furukori, U Nagashima, K Otani, S Kaneko, Y Inoue. Effects of the CYP2D6*10 allele on the steady-state plasma concentrations of haloperidol and reduced haloperidol in Japanese patients with schizophrenia. Clin Pharmacol Ther 65:291–294, 1999.

54. LC Woodson, MM Ames, CD Selassie, C Hansch, RM Weinshilboum. Thiopurine methyltransferase: aromatic thiol substrates and inhibition by benzoic acid derivatives. Mol Pharmacol 24:471–478, 1983.

55. RM Weinshilboum, SL Sladek. Mercaptopurine pharmacogenetics: monogenic inheritance of erythrocyte thiopurine methyltransferase activity. Am J Hum Genet 32: 651–662, 1980.

56. L Lennard. Clinical implications of thiopurine methyltransferase—optimization of drug dosage and potential drug interactions. Ther Drug Monit 20:527–531, 1998.

57. L Lennard, JA van Loon, JS Lilleyman, RM Weinshilboum. Thiopurine pharmacogenetics in leukemia: correlation of erythrocyte thiopurine methyltransferase activity and 6-thioguanine nucleotide concentrations. Clin Pharmacol Ther 41:18–25, 1987.

58. C Szumlanski, D Otterness, C Her, D Lee, B Brandriff, D Kelsell. Thiopurine methyltransferase pharmacogenetics: human gene cloning and characterization of a common polymorphism. DNA Cell Biol 15:17–30, 1996.

59. J Aarbakke, G Janka-Schaub, GB Elion. Thiopurine biology and pharmacology. Trends Pharmacol Sci 18:3–7, 1997.

60. D Otterness, C Szumlanski, L Lennard, B Klemetsdal, J Aarbakke, JO Park-Hah, H Iven, K Schmeigelow, E Branum, J O'Brien, R Weinshilboum. Human thiopurine methyltransferase pharmacogenetics: gene sequence polymorphisms. Clin Pharmacol Ther 62:60–73, 1997.

61. N Brynne, P Dalén, G Alván, L Bertilsson, J Gabrielsson. The influence of CYP2D6 polymorphism on the pharmacokinetics and dynamics of tolterodine. Clin Pharmacol Ther 63:529–539, 1998.

62. N Brynne. Consequences of CYP2D6 polymorphism for the disposition and dynamics of tolterodine. Ph.D. dissertation, Karolinska Institutet, Stockholm, 1998.

63. N Brynne. Y Böttiger, B Hallén, L Bertilsson. Tolterodine does not affect the human in vivo metabolism of the probe drugs caffeine, debrisoquine and omeprazole. Br J Clin Pharmacol 47:145–150, 1999.

64. J Lazarou, BH Pomeranz, PN Corey. Incidence of adverse drug reactions in hospital-ized patients. JAMA 279:1200–1205, 1998.
65. J de Leon, J Barnhill, T Rogers, J Boyle, W-H Chou, PJ Wedlund. Pilot study of the cytochrome P450-2D6 genotype in a psychiatric state hospital. Am J Psychiatry 155:1278–1280, 1998.

4

Pharmacogenetics—Receptors

Wendell W. Weber
University of Michigan, Ann Arbor, Michigan

1 INTRODUCTION

Most biological responses of higher organisms to drugs and other exogenous chemicals are receptor related. Information about the pharmacology and genetics of receptor proteins is thus central to our understanding of human sensitivity to these environmental substances. Hereditary changes in drug metabolizing enzymes rank first and foremost in pharmacogenetics, but the origin of traits such as malignant hyperthemia and insulin resistance has long been attributed to changes in receptors. Recent reports have led to a better documentation and understanding of these disorders and of additional receptor-related disorders such as the long QT syndrome, androgen insensitivity and prostate cancer, and the retinoic acid receptor in acute promyelocytic leukemia. Our objective in this chapter is to tell of recent advances in the pharmacogenetics of receptors by giving examples. A complete listing of known information is not intended.

1.1 Historical Perspective

The structural diversity emerging from the flood of cloning and sequencing of naturally occurring protein variants, including receptor variants, is immense [1]. Evidence for this diversity was first recognized by Ahlquist [2], who reported in 1948 that different adrenergic agonists imparted two distinct patterns of response within a given tissue. By probing with type-selective antagonists such as phen-oxybenzamine and phentolamine and dichloroisoproterenol and propranolol, Ahlquist deduced the existence of α- and β-adrenergic receptors to explain these unusual findings. Subsequently, experimental refinements stemming from differences of specificity and affinity of agonists and antagonists for receptors led investigators to deduce the presence of more than one subtype of receptors in tissues, such as the β_1 receptor located in cardiac muscle and the β_2 receptor located in bronchial smooth muscle.

Until the 1980s, pharmacologists had to rely on such properties to identify receptors and to distinguish between receptors of different types and subtypes, but such evidence was inadequate to give a detailed picture of the molecular basis of the heterogeneity of receptor proteins. With the advent of molecular biology, a field that has come to include restriction analysis, polymerase chain reaction and other techniques for manipulating DNA and RNA molecules, the cloning, sequencing and site-directed mutagenesis of genes became the norm in many laboratories in the 1980s, and the structural and functional analysis of receptors advanced rapidly.

1.2 Literature Searches

To get a better view of how the emphasis on receptor genetics and receptor polymorphisms may have shifted with the application of these new methods to pharmacogenetics, literature citations were searched on the Medline computerized database from 1987 to 1998 (Table 1). A total of 7825 citations for genetic studies

TABLE 1 Literature Citations on Receptor Genetics and Receptor Polymorphisms from 1987 to 1998

| | Medline Textwords (tw) Searched* | | | |
| | Receptor genetics | | Receptor polymorphisms | |
Citations	All species	Human	All species	Human
1987–89	833	460	321	249
1990–92	1420	868	498	412
1993–95	2200	1393	906	812
1996–98	3372	2235	1581	1453
Total citations 1987–98	7825	4956	3306	2926

* The combinations of (receptor$ and genetic$).tw. and (receptor$ and poly-morphi$).tw. were searched on the Medline database from 1987 to 1998 in 3-year intervals. At the time of these searches (11/8/99), 1998 was the last available full year of information.

of receptors and 3306 citations for receptor polymorphisms were found. The record for the entire period shows that human genetic receptor citations (4956) comprise almost two-thirds of all genetic receptor citations (7825), and that the proportion of human studies increases gradually from about 55% (460/833) in 1987–89 to about 66% (2235/3372) in 1996–98. The citations that deal with human receptor polymorphisms (2926) compared with those for receptor polymorphisms from all species (3306) make up a much higher proportion (88.5%) of total citations for 1987–1998. The number of investigations of human receptor polymorphisms increases by almost sixfold (1453/249) from 1987 to 1998, and the proportion of human polymorphisms studied increases from about 78% (249/321) in 1987–89 to about 92% (1453/1581) in 1996–98.

A chronology of receptor pharmacogenetics is presented in Table 2 [3–34]. The record leaves no doubt that recombinant DNA technology has facilitated the identification of receptors and receptor subtypes and has greatly refined their structural and functional analysis.

1.3 Classification of Receptors

Based on their cellular location and mechanistic features, receptors are grouped into those that reside within the cell and move to the nucleus (*nuclear receptors*), and those that insert into the cell surface and span the membrane (*cell surface receptors*). The two groups of receptors are considered separately in the following discussion.

2 NUCLEAR RECEPTORS

Nuclear receptors are best represented by the superfamily of regulatory proteins that interact with hormones such as cortisol, the sex steroids estradiol and testosterone, and thyroxine, and with drugs such as dexamethasone, the steroidal contraceptives, certain vitamins, and tri-iodothyronine. The Ah receptor, a receptor that interacts with exogenous planar aromatic toxins and carcinogens such as dioxin (2,3,7,8-tetrachlorobezon-p-dioxin; TCDD) and benzo[a]pyrene, though distinct from the steroid receptor, is another member of this superfamily. The nuclear receptor protein consists of a C-terminal domain that binds the ligand; a well-conserved, central DNA binding domain; and a variable N-terminal *trans*-activating domain whose function is less well understood. Nuclear receptors are direct signal transduction systems that in their ligand-bound form, bind to hormone response and enhancer elements of the genome to alter transcription rates of quiescent genes.

Numerous disorders of pharmacogenetic interest are associated with aberrant forms of these receptors (Table 3) [35–61]. Those we consider below are attributed to the receptors for glucocorticoids, androgens, estrogens, retinoic acid,

TABLE 2 A Chronology of Receptor Pharmacogenetics

Year	Event	Reference
1960	Malignant hyperthermia identified in a human kindred	3
1964	Coumarin anticoagulant resistance identified in a human kindred	4
1977	APL* attributed to balanced translocation t(15;17)	5
1985	Insulin receptor cloned	6
1986	Estrogen receptor cloned and mapped	7, 8
1987	β_2-Adrenoceptor cloned, sequenced and mapped	9
1988	Vitamin D resistant rickets associated with mutant Vitamin D receptor	10
1988	Androgen insensitivity associated with mutant androgen receptor	11, 12
1988	Severe insulin resistance associated with mutant insulin receptor	13, 14
1991	Malignant hyperthermia associated with mutant ryanodine receptor	15, 16
1991	Glucocorticoid resistance associated with mutant glucocorticoid receptor	17
1991	LQT1 (Romano-Ward) syndrome associated with mutant potassium channel alleles	18
1991	APL associated with ATRA-responsive chimeric PML-RARα gene[a]	19, 20
1992	Vasopressin resistance due to mutant AVPR2 receptor on X chromosome	21
1993	Mutation of the $\beta_2$adrenergic receptor first characterized	22
1994	Human AH receptor localized to chromosome 7p21-15	23
1994	Paradoxical response to antiandrogens tied to CAG repeats in androgen receptor	24
1994	Estrogen resistance identified with mutant estrogen receptor	25
1995	Nocturnal asthmatic phenotype associated with β_2AR polymorphism	26
1995	Sulfonylurea receptor cloned, and associated with hyperinsulin secretion	27, 28
1996	Asthmatic phenotype associated with FcεRIβ subunit mutation	29
1996	Resistance to HIV-induced infection due to CCR5Δ32 allele	30–32
1998	High CYP1A1 activity associated with AH receptor polymorphism	33
1998	Gram-negative (LPS) shock associated with mutant *Tlr4* receptor	34

* APL = acute promyelocytic leukemia; ATRA = all-trans-retinoic acid; RARα = retinoic acid receptor, subtype α.

TABLE 3 Nuclear Receptors of Pharmacogenetic Interest

Receptor (chromosome)	Ligand(s)	Response	Molecular basis	Reference
Glucocorticoid (5q-q32) [35]	Dexamethasone	Glucocorticoid resistance	Agr641Val missense mutation creates receptor with decreased affinity for dexamethasone	17
	Generalized compensated glucocorticoid resistance	Increased cortisol secretion	Splice site deletion creates reduced receptor abundance	36
	Dexamethasone	Decreased dexamethasone potency	Ile729Val missense mutation creates receptor with decreased affinity for dexamethasone	37
	Endogenous cortisol; dexamethasone	Cushing's syndrome	Ile559Asp missense mutation creates an aberrant receptor with reduced abundance, an inability to bind dexamethasone, and a dominant negative effect on gene transcription	38
	Dexamethasone	Increased cortisol suppression and insulin sensitivity	Asp363Ser missense mutation creates higher sensitivity to dexamethasone	39
Androgen (Xq11–q13) [12]	Endogenous testosterone and dihydrotestosterone	Androgen insensitivity syndromes. Impaired response to exogenous testosterone	Missense mutations, large deletions, and frameshift mutations create receptors with absent or reduced hormone binding, increased lability, and failure of upregulation	40,41
	Hormonal therapy	Hormone refractory prostate tumors	Somatic missense mutations (e.g., Thr877Ala in exon 1) create tumors refractory to hormonal therapy	41–44

TABLE 3 Continued

Receptor (chromosome)	Ligand(s)	Response	Molecular basis	Reference
	Antiandrogens (Cyproterone acetate, andronon, hydroxyflutamide)	Paradoxical response to antiandrogens	Thr868Ala missense mutation in the ligand binding domain creates a receptor that responds to low doses of estrogens and progestens, and has an increased affinity for antiandrogenic drugs	45,46
	Flutamide	Paradoxical response to flutamide	Hypothesize that polymorphism in glutamine (CAG) repeat length creates a receptor that affects prostate tumor response to anticancer agents.	24,47
Estrogen (6q25.1) [8]	Transdermal ethinyl estradiol	Estrogen insensitivity. Impaired response to exogenous estrogen	Replacement of Arg 157 (CGA) codon with a premature stop codon (TGA) creates receptor lacking both the DNA binding and hormone binding domains	25,48
	4-hydroxytamoxifen (4OHT); ICI 164,384	Reduced estrogen-dependent transcriptional activation	Substitution of L543A/L544A or M547A/L548A creates a receptor less responsive to estradiol but strongly stimulated by 4OHT and ICI 164,384.	49
	None	Occurs in cell line (MCF-7.2A) that developed estrogen independent growth	Creates cell with 4–5 copies of the wild-type receptor; acts as dominant negative receptor	50
	Estradiol; ICI 164,384; RU 54,876; *trans*-hydroxytamoxifen	Inverted ligand activity	Leu540Gln mutant creates a receptor that interprets antiestrogens as estrogens and *vice versa*	51

Receptor	Ligand	Clinical	Description	Ref
	Estradiol; tamoxifen, ICI 164,384	Constitutive transactivation	Tyr537Asn creates a receptor that displays constitutive transactivation	52
	Estradiol; raloxifene; keoxifene; ICI 182,780	Antiestrogen keoxifene increase estrogenic activity but antiestrogen 182,780 maintains antagonistic activity	Asp351Tyr mutation occurs in tamoxifen-stimulated breast tumor; changes pharmacology of non-steroidal antiestrogen (keoxifene)	53,54
Retinoic acid (t 15;17) [5]	All-*trans*-retinoic acid (ATRA)	ATRA induces remission of newly diagnosed acute promyelocytic leukemia	Chimeric receptor (PML-RARα) blocks differentiation of APL cells by complexing with corepressors. ATRA promotes complex dissociation of this complex to relieve the block.	55
Vitamin D (nuclear) (12cen-q12) [56]	1,25-Dihydroxyvitamin D$_3$ (calcitriol)	Vitamin D–resistant rickets; osteoporosis	A variety of mutations, mainly in the DNA-binding domain and to a lesser extent in the ligand-binding domain, create a receptor that is non-functional or hyporesponsive to the vitamin D$_3$.	57
Vitamin D (cell membrane) (not established)	1,25 Dihydroxyvitamin D$_3$ (calcitriol)	Definitive studies on human cells not yet performed	Activation of signal transduction pathways by an unknown mechanism.	58,59
Arylhydrocarbon (AH) (7p15 [23,60])	Halogenated and polyaromatic hydrocarbons	Metabolic activation of chemicals to genotoxins, teratogens and carcinogens as well as detoxification of toxic and carcinogenic xenobiotics	Ligand activates a battery of genes coding for enzymes involved in drug and toxicant metabolism. Arg554Lys polymorphism creates a receptor associated with high inducible CYP1A1.	33,60,61

vitamin D, and environmental pollutants such as the halogenated and polycyclic aromatic hydrocarbons.

2.1 Glucocorticoid Receptors and Glucocorticoid Resistance

The actions of endogenous glucocorticoids and analogous drugs such as dexamethasone are mediated by the glucocorticoid receptor. In humans, complete absence of the glucocorticoid receptor has not been observed, but in knockout mice, its absence is lethal shortly after birth [62]. Mutations in the hormone binding domain of the glucocorticoid receptor gene create receptors with reduced affinity for exogenous steroids [17,37,39], or a reduced abundance of receptors [36] (Table 3). In one case, a mutation in the hormone-binding domain created a dominant negative inhibition of the wild-type receptor [38].

The symptoms of partial glucocorticoid resistance are attributed primarily to increased cortisol production by the adrenal glands that compensates for reduced feedback inhibition of the hypothalamic-pituitary axis by the aberrant receptor. Increased adrenal activity results in increased production of adrenal androgens and mineralocorticoids. Overproduction of other adrenal steroids leads to the primary symptoms accompanying glucocorticoid resistance such as hirsutism, menstrual irregularities and fertility problems in women and precocious puberty in boys. Hypertension and hypokalemia attributed to increased mineralocorticoids also occur. Even though partial resistance to glucocorticoids among humans is rather frequent in otherwise healthy persons, it is not usually associated with mutations or polymorphisms in the glucocorticoid receptor gene [63].

2.2 Androgen Receptors, Androgen Insensitivity, and Prostate Cancer

The androgen receptor mediates the actions of testosterone and dihydrotestosterone. Mutations of the androgen receptor gene have been reported since 1988 when the androgen receptor gene was cloned [11,12]. Missense mutations, large deletions, and frameshift mutations of the androgen receptor gene create receptors whose ability to bind testosterone or dihydrotestosterone is absent or reduced, whose thermolability is increased, or whose ability to upregulate is impaired (Table 3). These are germline mutations that impair to varying degrees the development of male sexual differentiation.

Since 1995, a disproportionate increase in reporting of somatic mutations in the androgen receptor associated with prostate cancer has occurred [41] (Table 3). The occurrence of multiple mutations within individual patients is noteworthy. A large part of these occur in exon 1 and among these the Thr877Ala mutation is prevalent, but the pathogenicity of relatively few prostatic mutations has been proven. There also appears to be a strong association between CpG sites and the occurrence of the same mutation within families. That some mutant receptors can be activated by weak androgens or nonandrogens is a property of pharmacogenetic interest [45,46,64].

Mutations in other parts of the androgen receptor gene capable of affecting drug response have also been reported. Interestingly, the frequency of androgen receptor alleles with different CAG repeat lengths in the general population varies in different racial groups [65]. The most common androgen receptor allele among Caucasians has 21 CAGs, and the most common allele among Africans, who have a significantly higher prostate cancer incidence associated with a higher mortality rate, has 18 CAGs. Barrack has proposed that this polymorphism of glutamine repeat length may cause genomic instability that in turn affects androgen receptor activity in prostate cancer as well as in certain other androgen-mediated processes. The hypothesis that receptors with shorter glutamine repeats may have more activity and the effect in prostate cancer may be greater in individuals with such alleles is currently being tested [47].

2.3 Estrogen Receptors, Estrogen Resistance, and Antiestrogen Responses

Estrogens are key regulators of many physiological functions, particularly those associated with reproduction and mammary gland development. The estrogen receptor is the principal pathway by which responses to steroidal and nonsteroidal estrogens and antiestrogens are mediated in either normal or cancerous target cells. Disturbances of this pathway are believed to contribute to aberrant growth and development, and to influence tumor progression, particularly in breast cancer and the development of a hormone-independent, more aggressive, cancerous phenotype. Alterations in the structure of the estrogen receptor itself could be responsible for these disturbances.

The estrogen receptor was cloned in 1986 [7] and localized to chromosome 6q25.1 [8]. An intact estrogen receptor is important for normal skeletal growth and development but mutations are not necessarily lethal. A tall masculine male patient with decreased bone age and open epiphyses, low bone density and increased serum gonadotrophins and estrogen levels is a unique case in point of this statement (Table 3). His condition is explained by a point mutation that results in a severely truncated, functionally inert receptor lacking both the DNA- and hormone-binding domains. Estrogen therapy failed to suppress gonadotrophins, alter bone age or induce gynecomastia. Continued lack of response to treatment with exogenous estrogen indicates he is completely insensitive to estrogen.

A large and rapidly growing body of molecular evidence exists about naturally occurring variant and mutant estrogen receptors [66,67]. Several different patterns of estrogen receptor-like mRNA transcripts are associated with unusual responses to estrogens and antiestrogens. Several of these are of pharmacogenetic interest (Table 3). For example, Mahfoudi et al. [49] have found that substitution of certain hydrophobic residues of the ligand binding domain (AF-2) dramatically alters the pharmacology of estrogen antagonists in a manner that may explain the insensitivity of some breast cancers to tamoxifen. Pink and colleagues [50] have identified an estrogen receptor variant that contains an in-frame duplication of exons 6 and 7. This variant has four to five copies of the wild-type estrogen receptor gene instead of the usual two copies. It was discovered in a cell line that developed estrogen independent growth, and is the first variant expressing multiple copies of the receptor to be identified.

Montano et al. [51] describe a point mutant receptor (Leu540Gln) with "inverted" properties; i.e., it interprets antiestrogens as estrogens. It is activated by several antiestrogens but not by estradiol, and is capable of discriminating among different antiestrogens. Zhang et al. [52] identified three naturally occurring missense mutations among tumors from patients with metastatic breast cancer. One of these (Tyr537Asn) possesses a potent, constitutive transcriptional activity compared to the wild-type estrogen receptor. This constitutive receptor was unaffected by tamoxifen, or the pure antiestrogen, ICI 164,384. The authors believe this amino acid substitution induces conformational changes in the receptor that confer constitutive activity on the receptor without affecting the ability of the receptor to dimerize. Another mutation in the receptor at Asp351Tyr exhibits a gene-specific effect that converts raloxifene (synonym keoxifene) from an antiestrogen to an estrogen [53,54].

The occurrence of two forms (ERα and ERβ) not heretofore recognized [68] may help explain the broad spectrum of estrogen pharmacology and some of the paradoxical effects of estrogenlike drugs. The two forms are genetically distinct, and can differ in their distribution in normal and cancerous tissue. For example the ratio of α:β is higher, and different β isoform patterns occur in breast cancer compared to adjacent normal tissue [69]. Functionally, their transcriptional activity differs; e.g. ERα activates while ERβ inhibits the activity at AP-1 sites, and their interactions with antiestrogens differ; e.g., tamoxifen has greater antagonist activity through ERβ than ERα, but this relationship is reversed for raloxifene.

2.4   Retinoic Acid Receptors and Acute Promyelocytic Leukemia

The dramatic effect of retinoic acid on remission of acute promyelocytic leukemia (APL) and the subsequent discovery that mutant forms of the retinoic acid receptor associated with APL yield a splendid example of how molecular studies may translate into a stunning advance in the pharmacotherapy of cancer [55,70,71]. Retinoic acid belongs to a family of molecules capable of profound effects on many biologic functions including growth, vision, reproduction, epithelial cell differentiation, and immune function. Vitamin A and its analogs, natural and synthetic, belong to this family.

APL is a common form of acute myeloid leukemia that affects some 10% of adult patients. In 1977, Rowley and colleagues [5] found that a balanced translocation between chromosomes 15 and 17 was pathognomonic of APL. The RARα gene maps to the long arm of chromosome 17q21 [72]. In 1981, Breitman and colleagues [73] observed that all-*trans*-retinoic acid (ATRA) induced APL blasts in primary cultures to differentiate into mature granulocytes. ATRA is a natural retinol metabolite formed by enterocytes from dietary sources such as β-carotene and from tissue metabolites of retinol and retinaldehyde. Clinical scientists in Shanghai [74] and the United States [19,20] found that ATRA induced complete remission with trivial morbidity in a very high proportion of the patients with newly diagnosed APL.

In patients who contract APL, the 15:17 translocation disrupts the RARα gene resulting in a head-to-tail fusion of the promyelocytic leukemia (PML) locus with the RARα locus to form a chimeric PML-RARα receptor gene that remains under the transcriptional control of the PML promoter. Similarly, patients with the t(11;17) results in the PLZF-RARα chimera. These chimeras are believed to cause leukemias by interfering with the function of RARs [55]. RARs heterodimerize with RXRs on DNA to form ligand-inducible transcriptional units. In the absence of ATRA, they recruit corepressors that suppress terminal granulocyte differentiation, but pharmacological concentrations of ATRA induce the dissociation of this complex from PML-RARα to promote gene transcription, and bring about the production of normal granulocytes. The fact that ATRA does not release corepressors from PLZF-RARα, affords a molecular explanation of clinical ATRA resistance of patients who carry t(11;17) APLs [75].

2.5 Vitamin D Receptors, Vitamin D–Resistant Rickets, and Osteoporosis

The vitamin D receptor mediates the actions of dietary vitamin D, the active form of which is 1,25-dihydroxyvitamin D (vitamin D_3). Disruptions of the vitamin D receptor may lead to generalized resistance to D_3 as occurs in children with hereditary vitamin D–resistant rickets, and to impaired mineralization of newly formed bone as occurs in older persons with osteoporosis.

Clinical, cellular, and molecular discoveries have all been exceedingly valuable in understanding the physiological mechanism of vitamin D_3 and the receptor's role in hereditary vitamin D–resistant rickets. Point mutations of the receptor described by Hughes and colleagues in 1988 [10] were among the first natural occurring disease-causing mutations to be identified in the nuclear receptor gene superfamily (see Table 2). Since this initial report appeared many additional missense, splice site, and deletion mutations have been identified in association with this disorder [57], most commonly in the receptor's DNA-binding domain. They interfere with the high affinity binding of the receptor to DNA, and prevent the receptor from activating transcription even in the presence of very high concentrations of hormone.

Mutations of the ligand-binding domain are next most common. They cause reduced or complete hormone insensitivity either by decreasing hormone affinity and/or interfering with heterodimerization with RXR. Numerous mutations that produce premature stop codons have also been identified. They truncate the receptor to a variable extent and usually lead to complete hormone resistance. The major cellular defect caused by these variant receptors is to decrease absorption of intestinal calcium and phosphate that leads to decreased bone mineralization and rickets [57].

Whereas hereditary vitamin D–resistant rickets is a rare disorder of children, osteoporosis is commonly seen in older women and large numbers of men. Recently, a study of one Australian community indicated that the remaining lifetime risk of thinning bones for a 60-year-old woman was almost 60% and nearly 30% for a man of the same age [76]. It is reasonable to expect polymorphisms of the vitamin D receptor gene that cause variations in the absorption of dietary calcium and bone mineral density may in turn alter the susceptibility of individuals to osteoporosis. Several recent epidemiological studies have been conducted to test whether the vitamin D receptor genotype may influence the absorption of dietary calcium and the density of bone mineral [77–81]. The strength of these associations varies from one study to another and is stronger at low calcium intakes (<800 mg/day) and more apparent in younger than older subjects; the issue is subject to continuing controversy because other studies have not found such an association [82,83].

One other study compared persons with or without polymorphism at the *Bsm*I restriction site of the vitamin D receptor gene [84]. The *Bsm*I polymorphism occurs at a commonly studied restriction site that exerts an effect on bone mineral density among individuals with the BB genotype (who lack the site) having lower bone density than bb individuals (who possess the site) [57]. This study failed to detect significant differences between BB and bb genotypes in receptor abundance and receptor mRNA levels, or in the affinity of the receptor for vitamin D_3. Consequently, the investigators concluded that the *Bsm*I polymorphism does not affect receptor function and proposed instead that it might be a marker for a nearby gene that is responsible for the association of vitamin D receptor genotype and osteoporosis. Many studies indicate that hormonal and environmental factors may affect the risk to osteoporosis, but further investigation is required to clarify the mechanism by which vitamin D receptor alleles determine calcium and bone homeostasis, and to assess the role of vitamin D receptor allelic variation in the genetics of osteoporosis.

During the last decade, observations have shown that vitamin D_3 can bring about rapid signal transduction pathways. These observations support the hypothesis that a membrane-bound receptor similar to cell surface receptors exists. The recent report of Nemeri et al. [58] is the first to provide evidence for such a vitamin D receptor, but as yet little is known about the properties of this new receptor and its effects on cellular responsiveness to vitamin D_3.

2.6 Arylhydrocarbon Hydroxylase Receptors and Toxicity to Halogenated and Polycyclic Hydrocarbons

Studies in animal models have demonstrated the Ah receptor is a transcription factor whose activity is regulated by halogenated and polycyclic aromatic hydrocarbons. The Ah receptor is of pharmacogenetic interest because halogenated hydrocarbons such as TCDD (2,3,7,8,-tetrachlorodibenzo-p-dioxin, dioxin), a by-product of the synthesis of agent orange, and benzo[a]pyrene, a polycyclic hydrocarbon of cigarette smoke, are high on the list of injurious environmental pollutants. Exposure to TCDD, for example, results in the activation of a diverse battery of genes, the best characterized of which are involved in drug and toxicant metabolism such as the P450-mediated CYP1A1 enzyme. Exposure to these substances produces a variety of effects including tumor promotion; immuno- and skin toxicity; and alterations in endocrine homeostasis, teratogenesis, and lethality [60,61].

Most of the research to prove that the Ah locus encodes a receptor and to define the biochemical and molecular mechanisms of Ah receptor action were performed in mice. Efforts to define the biological effects of TCDD and related toxicants have focused on the induction of arylhydrocarbon hydroxylase activity, now renamed CYP1A1 activity [85] (see Table 1). These studies indicate that the Ah receptor gene is located on mouse chromosome 12, is constitutively expressed in many cell types, and that its expression is regulated in a tissue-cell, developmental- and chemical-specific manner [61].

In humans, the locus of the AH receptor has been localized to 7p15 [23,60]. Data from a number of laboratories suggest that human responsiveness to halogenated and polycyclic arylhydrocarbon ligands could be determined by polymorphism at a single regulatory locus as has been demonstrated for the differences in response of C57BL6 and DBA2 mice [85,86]. However, such a relationship between AH receptor-dependent differences in response and susceptibility to cancer or chemical toxicity has not been demonstrated in humans. Recently a polymorphism in the AH receptor gene (Arg554Lys) was detected in Japanese subjects, but it was not associated with a change in arylhydrocarbon hydroxylase activity, nor with susceptibility to lung cancer [87]. Subsequently, other investigators showed that this mutation imparts a high transactivating activity in the mouse [88]. Regulatory genes such as those encoding transcription factors, including the Ah receptor gene, are generally highly conserved throughout evolution, and it is not unreasonable to expect the mechanisms that account for CYP1A1 inducibility in the mouse and in humans may be similar. More recently, Daly et al. [33] have confirmed the presence of the Arg554Lys polymorphism in Caucasians, and have shown it is associated with highly inducible CYP1A1 activity. The frequencies of the Arg-coded and Lys-coded alleles were 0.57 and 0.43, respectively, in Japanese, whereas they were 0.12 and 0.88, respectively, in Caucasians. This allele may account in part for the variation observed in human CYP1A1 activity, but further studies are necessary to examine its presence in other human populations and determine its significance in disease.

3   CELL SURFACE RECEPTORS

Cell surface receptors account for the actions of the great majority of biological responses to chemicals because of their capacity to bind biogenic amines, protein and polypeptide hormones, autocoids, neurotransmitters, and environmental chemicals. The receptors for these substances are divided into three subgroups: the ion channels and ion transporters; those that act by an enzymatic cascade involving a second messenger such as the adenylyl cyclase cascade or the phosphoinositol cascade; and those whose action depends on an integral enzyme activity.

In the discussions of receptor pharmacogenetics that follow, the ion channel group is represented by several receptors associated with the long QT syndrome, and the ion transporter group is represented by the sulfonylurea receptor that is associated with infantile hyperinsulinism and non-insulin-dependent diabetes mellitus (NIDDM). The second group is represented by the β_2-adrenergic receptor and by the CCR5 receptor. The insulin receptor is prototypical of the third group of receptors; but we have not discussed this receptor here because the pharmacogenetics of this receptor has been considered at length elsewhere recently [1]. In addition, the *Tlr4* receptor (see Sect. 3.5) and the putative vitamin D cell surface receptor (see Sect. 2.5) are discussed, but these receptors are not assigned to any of the three groups of cell surface receptors because the mechanism of transmembrane signaling has not been reported for either one.

3.1   The Long-QT Syndrome (LQTS) and Ion Channel Receptors

In the late 1980s, reports of syncope, prolonged QT, episodic ventricular arrhythmias, and sudden death appeared in the literature associated with the administration of antiarrhythmic agents such as quinidine, macrolide antibiotics such as clathromycin (combined with conazoles), and H1 antihistamines such as terfenadine and astemizole (Table 4) [1,103]. The familial nature of these cardiac syndromes has been known since the 1960s and two inherited forms of LQTS have been described [104–106]. The Romano-Ward syndrome is the most common inherited form of the LQTS. It is transmitted as an autosomal dominant trait whereas the Jervell and Lange-Nielsen syndrome is uncommon and is an autosomal-recessive disorder.

Cardiologists have a much better understanding of the molecular bases and heterogeneous mechanisms that cause these syndromes since Keating [18] and succeeding investigators have cloned and characterized the ion channel receptors responsible for them [90]. A total of six LQTS genes, designated *LQT1-LQT6*, have been identified and their chromosomal positions mapped (see Table 4). *LQT1*, which is designated *KCNQ1* (formerly *KVQT1*), and *LQT2* also designated *HERG*, are potassium channels. *LQT3* also designated as *SCN5A*, is a sodium channel gene. The candidate area designated as *LQT4* maps to chromosome 4q25-27, and does not contain an ion channel gene motif, but from data in a rat model, a Ca^{2+}/calmodulin-dependent protein has been proposed as a candidate to explain LQT4. *LQT5*, also designated as *minK*, encodes a short protein that cannot form a functional channel but apparently achieves its effect by physically interacting with *KVLQT1*. *LQT6*, designated as *MiRP1*, is a potassium channel [89,93,94].

Genetic and physiological studies of affected families indicate that in general, heterozygous mutations in *KVLQT1* cause Romano-Ward syndrome (LQTS alone) [107], whereas homozygous mutations in *KVLQT1* cause Jervell Lange-Nielsen syndrome (LQTS with deafness). A plausible explanation suggests that heterozygous mutations act by a dominant-negative mechanism leaving some functional *KVLQT1* channels in the ear, thereby averting deafness in Romano-Ward syndrome, while homozygous *KVLQT1* mutations prevent the formation of any functional *KVLQT1* channels, which results in deafness.

Knowledge of the LQTS genotype that results in a specific phenotype may enable prediction of a specific clinical outcome [108]. For example, *LQT1* and *LQT2* result in a higher frequency of cardiac events (e.g., syncope) associated with stress or exercise but a lower risk of sudden death. In contrast, *LQT3* is of lower frequency and is more likely to be associated with sleep [109] but a higher risk of sudden death [92]. Knowledge of the genotype also provides a basis for effective therapeutic strategies to avoid LQTS. Thus, potassium supplementation or potassium channel openers may be useful as pharmacotherapy in patients with potassium channel defects while sodium channel blockers (e.g., mexilitene) may be more effective in patients with *LQT3*.

3.2 The Sulfonylurea Receptor and Impaired Insulin Responses

An intact sulfonylurea receptor is necessary for the normal regulation of insulin secretion by the pancreatic β-cells. The sulfonylurea receptor has multiple membrane-spanning domains and is classed as a member of the ATP-binding cassette

TABLE 4 Cell Surface Receptors of Pharmacogenetic Interest

Receptor (chromosome)	Response	Associated with	Molecular basis	Reference
Potassium channel KVLQT1 α-subunit (1p155) [89]	LQT1 syndrome	Spontaneous and drug-induced ventricular arrhythmias. Induced by antiarrhythmics (quinidine), antipsychotics (chlorpromazine), Psychotropics (tricylic antidepressants), macrolide antibiotics (clathromycin), H1 antihistamines (terfenadine, astemizole) [1]	At least eleven different heterozygous (Romano-Ward) and homozygous (JL-N) missense and deletions mutations create defective ion channel receptors	90
Potassium channel HERG α-subunit (7q35–36) [89]	LQT2 syndrome		At least six missense, intragenic and splicing mutations create defective ion channel receptors	91
Sodium channel SCN5A (3p21–24) [89]	LQT3 syndrome; Brugada variant of LQT3 syndrome		At least three missense and intragenic activating mutations create defective ion channel receptors	92
Potassium channel minK KVLQT1 β-subunit (21q22.1) [93]	LQT5 syndrome		At least two missense mutations create defective ion channel receptors	93
Potassium channel MiRP1 (KCNE2) β-subunit (21q22.1) [94]	LQT6 syndrome		At least three missense mutations create defective ion channel receptors	94

Receptor		Disease		References
Sulfonylurea (11p15.1) [27,28]	Decreased secretion of insulin and tolbutamide stimulated insulin	Familial hyperinsulinisma nd hypoglycemia of infancy, and NIDDM	Splice site and missense mutations in non-coding and coding regions create defective receptors	28,95
β_2-Adrenergic (5q31–32) [9]	Bronchial hyperresponsiveness. Patients with the Gly 16 and Arg 16 polymorphism exhibit different responses to albuterol	Asthma	Two common polymorphisms (Arg16Gly; Gln27Glu); and one rare polymorphism (Thr164Ile) in the coding region whose receptors whose abundance and function are altered in persons homozygous for the polymorphism	96,97
FcεRI beta (11q13) [98]	FcεRI receptor is located on mast cells and other effector cells. Exposure to allergen causes formation of IgE receptor complex which degranulates mast cells and initiates inflammation	Atopic individuals that produce excess amounts of IgE are predisposed to asthma, hay fever and eczema	A missense mutation (Glu237Gly) of the β-subunit of the receptor creates a receptor associated with bronchial hyper-responsiveness. The mechanism of this response is not clear.	99–101
CCR5Δ32 (3p21) [30–32]	HIV-induced infection	Resistance to HIV-induced infection	32 basepair deletion of the coding region creates a severely truncated, nonfunctional receptor incapable of binding HIV-suppressive β-chemokines	30–32
Toll-like (not determined)	Gram-negative shock	Susceptibility to endotoxic (LPS) shock from gram-negative bacteria	Human variants not known; missense and null variants known in C3H/HeJ and C57BL/10ScCr mice	34,102

superfamily of receptors because of the presence of two nucleotide-binding folds in its consensus sequence [95,110].

Various naturally occurring deletions and splice site and missense mutations (Table 4) occur in the second nucleotide-binding fold of the β-cell ATP-dependent potassium channel. These mutations give rise to severely truncated, nonfunctional forms of the receptor gene that cause familial hyperinsulinemic hypoglycemia of infancy, a syndrome defined by elevations of serum insulin, profound hypoglycemia, brain damage, and death [28,95,111]. Mapping this disorder to chromosome 11p15.1 [27,112] excluded the insulin receptor gene, which maps to 19p13.2-13.3 [6], and several other previously mapped genes involved in β cell function [28]. More recently, mutations in the region of the first nucleotide binding fold that lead to this disorder have been described. One introduces a missense mutation that leads to an amino acid substitution while two others affect RNA processing of the receptor transcript [95]. These findings indicate that disruption of either of the two nucleotide binding fold regions of the sulfonyl receptor gene may lead to unregulated insulin secretion.

Mutational analysis in a Danish Caucasian population has revealed additional missense and silent mutations of the coding region, and four intron mutations of the sulfonylurea gene [113]. A silent C/T mutation at exon 18 is associated with NIDDM. Of 386 NIDDM subjects, 17 had a combined variant comprising the mutation at exon 18 and at intron 3c/-3t. Subjects with the combined variant exhibited a 50% reduction in serum insulin secretion on tolbutamide injection, but normal serum C-peptide and insulin responses on glucose injection. Young healthy carriers of the intragenic combined variant were also found to have reduced serum C-peptide and insulin responses to tolbutamide, that was even more highly associated with NIDDM than the single silent polymorphism at exon 18 [113].

3.3 Receptor Genes and Asthma

Genetic analysis in families indicates that asthma is likely to be influenced by only a few genes each with a moderately strong effect, rather than many genes of small effect [114]. Several receptor genes appear to be essential components of the asthmatic phenotype. Two of these receptors, the beta-adrenergic receptor and the high affinity receptor for IgE (FcεRI-β), have been studied extensively, and they will be considered here. An effect of the Il-4 receptor (on chromosome 16) on atopy and serum IgE levels is also known. Quite recently, a gain-of-function mutation in the α-subunit of this receptor has been identified, but its effect on the predisposition of persons to asthma has not yet been reported [115].

The β_2 adrenergic receptor has been the target of investigation since the beta-adrenergic receptor theory of atopy was set forth some 30 years ago. It has also been extensively studied as a prototype of the G-protein-coupled receptor.

In the initial molecular studies, a total of nine naturally occurring polymorphisms were identified in the coding region of the receptor [98]. Four resulted in changes in the amino acid sequence of the receptor, and three of these (Arg16Gly, Gln27Glu, Thr164Ile) altered the abundance and function of the receptor [116]. Ethnic differences in allelic frequencies were also significant—for instance, in Caucasians, blacks, and Asians Gly16 = 0.61, 0.50, and 0.40. At position 27, the allelic frequencies for Gln27 = 0.57, 0.73, and 0.80. The Ile164 polymorphism is rare, occurring in the heterozygous state in ≈6% of the population, and persons homozygous for this polymorphism have not been identified.

Several studies have been performed to examine the effect of polymorphism on the asthmatic phenotype. The frequencies of each polymorphism are the same for normal adults and asthmatics, so that these primary variations in the structure of the receptor are not considered a major cause of asthma. However, the Gly16 form of the receptor undergoes agonist-promoted downregulation while Glu27 displays resistance to such downregulation. Additionally, a clustering of the Gly16 polymorphism was noted in more severe asthmatics [96]. Subsequently, Gly16 was found to be associated with nocturnal asthma [26]. Still further the Glu27 form of the receptor was found to protect against bronchial hyperactivity [117]. These observations imply that the Gly16Arg and Gln27Glu polymorphisms may act as modifiers of the asthmatic phenotype. However, these polymorphisms appear to be linked, and larger population studies (not available at this writing) will be necessary to determine the importance of each one [116,118].

The effect of polymorphic variation on the clinical response of asthmatic patients to β-adrenergic agonists and corticosteroids has also been studied [119–123]. The studies are not easily compared because different drugs were tested under different circumstances, and the measures of therapeutic effect achieved varied from one study to another. Several studies find that asthmatic patients who are homozygous for the Arg16 form of the receptor are more likely to respond favorably to albuterol (salbutamol) than patients who are homozygous for the Gly16 form [119,120,122]. For instance, Martinez et al. [120] found that homozygotes for Arg16 were 5.3 times and heterozygotes for Arg16 were 2.3 times more likely to respond to albuterol than homozygotes for Gly16. In contrast, Lipworth et al. [123] found that neither of the polymorphisms at position 16 or at position 27 influenced the response to isoproterenol or to formerterol protection against methacholine. Additionally, two studies of the effect of these polymorphisms on the response of asthmatic patients to inhaled corticosteroids (used on demand) showed that this mode of treatment afforded equal protection of patients regardless of the β_2-receptor polymorphism [121,123].

Receptors with Ile at position 164 which is located in the region of agonist binding do not couple efficiently to the G protein. The change in the primary structure at position 164 causes the receptor to exhibit sustained, markedly dysfunctional properties [22,116], but the rarity of this polymorphism has so far precluded its study in the homozygous state or in situations of clinical interest.

The high-affinity receptor for IgE, FcεRI, has a central role in mast cell degranulation and IgE-mediated atopic asthma. A few coding changes have been identified within the receptor [114]. A missense mutation of the receptor's β-subunit (Glu237Gly) [99] (Table 4) was found to increase the relative risk of individuals with the Gly form of the receptor having asthma by 2.3-fold, suggesting that variants of the FcεRI receptor may predispose individuals to atopic asthma [100,101]. The position of this polymorphism adjacent to the tyrosine activation motif of the receptor also suggests a means whereby this variation may modify the function of FcεRI. Further study of heterozygotes versus that in homozygotes is needed to understand more fully the effect of this polymorphism on the asthmatic phenotype.

3.4 AIDS Susceptibility and the CCR5 Receptor

Evidence has recently emerged for the requirement of CCR5 (also designated CC-CKR-5 and CKR5) for HIV-induced infection. The CCR5 gene encodes a 7-transmembrane, G-protein coupled, cell surface receptor that binds several HIV-suppressive β-chemokines [124]. Mutations of this receptor gene may alter expression or function of the receptor protein, and thereby alter chemokine binding/signaling of HIV infection. Identification of a naturally occurring 32-bp deletion (Δ32 allele) in the CCR5 gene in several laboratories [30–32] has explained the genetic basis for resistance to HIV-induced disease. The defective gene is severely truncated and not expressed at the cell surface. Survival analysis of HIV high-risk cohorts shows that homozygous persons for the defective allele are highly protected from HIV infection. Additionally, the progression of AIDS is slower in individuals who are heterozygous for the deletion than in individuals homozygous for the normal CCR5 gene [32].

The CCR5Δ32 allele has been identified in Caucasian populations and in populations of Western Europe with a frequency of approximately 0.10, reaching approximately 0.20 in some populations. Numerous CCR5 codon-altering alleles have been identified, but the Δ32 allele dominates sequence variations observed in Caucasian Americans [125]. A study of the population distribution of the Δ32 allele indicates its presence throughout Europe, the Middle East, and the Indian subcontinent [126]. An extensive genotype survey revealed a cline of CCR5Δ32 allele frequencies of 0–14% across Eurasia, whereas the variant was absent among native African, American Indian, and East Indian ethnic groups. The geographic cline frequencies of CCR5Δ32 and its recent emergence (estimated at 700–2000 years ago) are consistent with a strong selective event such as an epidemic of a pathogen that, like HIV-1, uses CCR5, driving its frequency upward in ancestral Caucasian populations [127].

An allele of the neighboring CCR2 gene (V641) is also independently associated with slower AIDS progression, although the frequency of occurrence of this allele and the mechanism for CCR2 resistance have not been ascertained.

3.5 The *Tlr4* Receptor and Endotoxic Shock

Endotoxin refers to an abundant component of gram-negative bacteria that evokes fever, shock, and other disturbances in mammals [128]. The endotoxic principle is a lipopolysaccharide (LPS) comprising a toxic lipid A moiety and several other nontoxic moieties of highly variable structure. LPS is of great interest because gram-negative infection annually claims tens of thousands of lives in the United States alone, and genetic studies suggest that recognition of this toxin is important to permit containment and eradication of a gram-negative infection.

Some 30 years ago, identification of LPS-resistant mice [129] suggested the existence of a single pathway for responses to LPS because mutation of a single gene entirely ablated LPS responses. The mouse gene was cloned from mice that exhibited defective *Lps* signaling [102]. Although these mice were overly susceptible to infection by gram-negative bacteria, they were resistant to endotoxin. C3H/HeJ mice were found to have a missense mutation in a Toll-like receptor-4 (*Tlr4*), and C57BL/10ScCr mice were found to have a null allele. The identification of these two mutations at once confirmed that *Lps* and *Tlr4* were the same gene [34].

Tlr4 represents an ancient self-defense immune response, and it appears to be the only gene in the *Lps* critical region. Mice with *Tlr4* mutations, fruitflies with Toll defects, and perhaps humans with Tlr-related problems are all susceptible to gram-negative infections, and the mammals develop gram-negative shock. Interestingly, an immunodeficient human patient with coresistance to LPS and interleukin-1 (IL-1) has been described [130], suggesting that both inflammatory pathways utilize a common signaling pathway.

The total number of Tlr proteins has not yet been determined, although *Tlr4* has emerged as a specific conduit for the LPS response. Among humans and mice, many relatively uncommon variants have been observed, but a single *Tlr4* allele predominates. In addition to their role against endotoxic shock, such receptors may also play a developmental role. The mutational deletion of Tlr genes, alone and in combination, may help establish the functions of each member of this new family of proteins.

4 SUMMARY

A wealth of new nuclear and cell surface receptors have been identified and characterized within the last decade. Among them are receptors that determine the responses of healthy individuals and patients to therapeutic agents, to components of the diet, and to infectious disease. The naturally occurring hereditary and genetically determined changes that occur in these molecules can, in many instances, explain the ineffectiveness of therapeutic agents, adverse or paradoxical drug responses, sensitivity to various foodstuffs, and susceptibility to infectious disease, and suggest new strategies of therapy and prevention.

REFERENCES

1. WW Weber. Pharmacogenetics. Oxford: Oxford University Press, 1997, pp 240–278.
2. RP Ahlquist. A study of the adrenotropic receptors. Am J Physiol 153:586–600, 1948.
3. MA Denborough, JFA Forster, RRH Lovell, PA Maplestone, JD Villiers. Anaesthetic deaths in family. Br J Anaesth 34:395–396, 1962.
4. RA O'Reilly, PM Aggler, S Hoag, LS Leong, ML Kropatkin. Hereditary transmission of exceptional resistance to coumarin anticoagulant drugs. N Engl J Med 271: 809–813, 1964.
5. J Rowley, HM Golomb, C Dougherty. 15/17 translocation, a consistent chromosomal change in acute promyelocytic leukemia. Lancet i:549–550, 1977.
6. TL Yang-Feng, U Francke, A Ullrich. Gene for human insulin receptor: localization to site on chromosome 19 involved in pre-B-cell leukemia. Science 228:728–731, 1985.
7. S Green, P Walter, V Kumar, A Krust, J-M Bornert, P Argos, P Chambon. Human oestrogen receptor cDNA sequence, expression and homology to v-erb-A. Nature 320:134–139, 1986.
8. LP Menasche, GRM White, CJ Harrison, JM Boyle. Localization of the estrogen receptor locus (ESR) to chromosome 6q25.1 by FISH and a simple post-FSH banding technique. Genomics 17:263–265, 1993.
9. BK Kobilka, RAF Dixon, T Frielle, HG Dohlman, MA Bolanowski, IS Sigal, TL Yang-Feng, U Francke MG Caron, RJ Lefokowitz. cDNA for the human β_2-adrenergic receptor: a protein with multiple membrane-spanning domains and encoded by a gene whose chromosomal location is shared with that of the receptor for platelet-derived growth factor. Proc Natl Acad Sci USA 84:46–50, 1987.
10. MR Hughes, PJ Malloy, DG Kieback, RA Kesterson, JW Pike, D Feldman, BW O'Malley. Point mutations in the human vitamin D receptor gene associated with hypocalcemic rickets. Science 242:1702–1705, 1988.
11. C Chang, J Kokontis, S Liao. Structural analysis of complementary DNA and amino acid sequences of human and rat androgen receptors. Proc Natl Acad Sci USA 85: 7211–7215, 1988.
12. DB Lubahn, DR Joseph, M Sar, J Tan, HN Higgs, RE Larson, FS French, EM Wilson. The human androgen receptor: complementary deooxyribonucleic acid cloning, sequence analysis and gene expression in prostate. Mol Endocrinol 2: 1265–1275, 1988.
13. T Kodawaki, CL Bevins, A Cama, K Ojamaa, B Marcus-Samuels, H Kodawaki,

L Beitz, C McKeon, SI Taylor. Two mutant alleles of the insulin receptor gene in a patient with extreme insulin resistance. Science 240:787–790, 1988.

14. Y Yoshimasa, S Seino, J Whittaker, T Kakehi, A Kosaki, H Kuzuya, H Imura, GI Bell, DF Steiner. Insulin-resistant diabetes due to a point mutation that prevents insulin propreceptor processing. Science 240:784–787, 1988.

15. EF Gillard, K Otsu, J Fujii, VK Khanna, S De Leon, J Derdemezi Jr, BA Britt, CL Duff, RG Worton, DH MacLennan. A substitution of cysteine for arginine 614 in the ryanodine receptor is potentially causative of human malignant hyperthermia. Genomics 11:751–755, 1991.

16. K Otsu, VK Khanna, AL Archibald, DH MacLennan. Cosegregation of porcine malignant hyperthermia and a probable causal mutation in the skeletal muscle ryanodine receptor gene in backcross families. Genomics 11:744–750, 1991.

17. DM Hurley, D Accili, CA Stratakis, M Karl, N Vamvakopoulos, E Rorer, K Constantine, SI Taylor, GP Chrousos. Point mutation causing a single amino acid substitution in the hormone binding domain of the glucocorticoid receptor in familial glucocorticoid resistance. J Clin Invest 87:680–686, 1991.

18. M Keating, C Dunn, D Atkinson, K Timothy, GM Vincent, M Leppert. Consistent linkage of the long QT syndrome to the Harvey *Ras-1* locus on chromosome 11. Am J Hum Genet 49:1335–1339, 1991.

19. H de Thé, C Lavau, A Marchi, C Chomienne, L Degos, A Dejean. The PML-RARα fusion mRNA generated by the t(15;17) translocation in acute promyelocytic leukemia encodes a functionally altered RAR. Cell 66:675–684, 1991.

20. A Kazizuka, WH Miller Jr, K Umesons, RP Warrell Jr, SR Frankel, VVVS Murty, E Dmitrovsky, RM Evans. Chromosomal translocation t(15;17) in human acute promyelocytic leukemia fuses RARα with a novel putative transcription factor, PML. Cell 66:663–674, 1991.

21. M Birnbaumer, A Seibold, S Gilbert, M Ishido, C Barberia, A Antaramian, P Brabet, W Rosenthal. Molecular cloning of the receptor for human antidiuretic hormone. Nature 357:333–335, 1992.

22. SA Green, G Cole, M Jacinto, M Innis, SB Liggett. A polymorphism of the human β_2-adrenergic receptor within the fourth transmembrane domain alters ligand binding and functional properties of the receptor. J Biol Chem 268:23116–23121, 1993.

23. MM LeBeau, LA Carver, R espinosa III, JV Schmidt, CA Bradfield. Chromosomal localization of the human AHR locus encoding the structural gene for the Ah receptor to 7p21-15. Cytogenet Cell Genet 66:172–176, 1994.

24. MP Schoenberg, JM Rakimi, S Wang, GS Bova, JI Epstein, KH Fishbeck, WB Isaacs, PC Walsh, ER Barrack. Microsatellite mutation ($CAG_{24\to18}$) in the androgen receptor gene in human prostate cancer. Biochem Biophys Res Commun 198:74–80, 1994.

25. EP Smith, J Boyd, GR Frank, H Takahashi, RM Cohen, B Specker, TC Williams, DB Lubahn, KS Korach. Estrogen resistance caused by a mutation in the estrogen-receptor gene in a man. N Engl J Med 331:1056–1061, 1994.

26. J Turki, J Pak, SA Green, RJ Martin, SB Liggett. Genetic polymorphisms of the β_2-adrenergic receptor in nocturnal and nonnocturnal asthma. J Clin Invest 95:1635–1641, 1995.

27. B Glaser, KC Chiu, L Liu, R Anker, A Nestorowicz, NJ Cox, H Landau, N Kaiser, PS Thornton, CA Stanley. Recombinant mapping of the familial hyperinsulinism gene to an 0.8 cM region on chromosome 11p15.1 and demonstration of a founder effect in Ashkenzi Jews. Hum Mol Genet 5:879–886, 1995.

28. PM Thomas, GC Cote, N Wohlik, B Hassad, PM Mathew, W Rabi, L Aguilar-Bryan, RF Gagel, J Bryan. Mutations in the sulfonylurea receptor gene in familial persistent hyperinsulinemia of infancy. Science 268:426–429, 1995.

29. MR Hill, WO Cookson. A new variant of the beta subunit of the high affinity receptor for immunoglobulin E (Fc episoln RI-beta E237G): associations with measures of atopy and bronchial hyper-responsiveness. Hum Mol Genet 5:959–962, 1996.

30. R Liu, WA Paxton, S Choe, D Ceradini, SR Martin, R Horuk, ME MacDonald, H Stuhlmann, RA Koup, NR Landau. Homozygous defect in HIV-1 coreceptor accounts for resistance of some multipy-exposed individuals to HIV-1 infection. Cell 86:367–377, 1996.

31. M Samson, F Libert, BJ Doranz, J Rucker, C Liesnard C-M Farber, S Saragosti, C Lapoumeroulie, J Cognaux, C Forceille, G Muyldermans, C Verhofstede, G Burtoboy, M Georges, T Imai, S Rana, Y Yi, RJ Smyth, RG Collman, RW Doms, G Vassart, M Parmentier. Resistance to HIV-1 infection in Caucasian individual bearing mutant alleles of the CCR-5 chemokine receptor gene. Nature 382:722–725, 1996.

32. M Dean, M Carrington, C Winkler, GA Huttley, MW Smith, R Allikmets, JJ Goedert, SP Buchbinder, E Vittinghoff, E Gomperts, S Donfield, D Vlahov, R Kaslow, A Saah, C Rinaldo, R Detels, SJ O'Brien. Genetic restriction of HIV-1 infection and progression to AIDS by a deletion allele of the CKR5 structural gene. Science 273:1856–1862, 1996.

33. AK Daly, KS Fairbrother, J Smart. Recent advance in understanding the molecular basis of polymorphisms in genes encoding cytochrome P450 enzymes. Toxicol Lett 102–103:143–147, 1998.

34. A Poltorak, X He, I Smirnova, M-Y Liu, C Van Huffel, X Du, D Birdwell, E Alejos, M Silva, C Galanos, MA Freudenberg, P Riccardi-Castagnoli, B Layton, B Beutler. Defective LPS signaling in C3H/HeJ and C57BL/10ScCr mice: mutations in Tlr4 gene. Science 282:2085–2088, 1998.

35. U Francke, BE Foellmer. The glucocorticoid receptor gene is in 5q-q32. Genomics 4:610–612, 1989.

36. M Karl, SW Lamberts, SD Detera-Wadleigh, IJ Encio, CA Strtakis, DM Hurley, D Accili, GP Chrousos. Developmental glucocorticoid resistance caused by a splice site deletion in the human glucocorticoid receptor gene. J Clin Endocrinol Metab 76:683–689, 1993.

37. DM Malchoff, A Brufsky, G Reardon, P McDermott, EC Javier, C-H Bergh, D Rowe, CD Malchoff. A mutation of the glucocorticoid receptor in primary cortisol resistance. J Clin Invest 91:1918–1925, 1993.

38. M Karl, SWJ Lamberts, JW Koper, DA Katz, NE Huizenga, T Kino, BR Haddad, MR Hughes, GP Chrousos. Cushing's disease preceded by generalized glucocorticoid resistance: clinical consequences of a novel, dominant-negative glucocorticoid receptor mutation. Proc Assoc Am Phys 108:296–307, 1996.

39. NATM Huizenga, JW Koper, P De Lange, HAP Pols, RP Stolk, H Burger, DE Grobbee, AO Brinkmann, FH de Jong, SWJ Lamberts. A polymorphism in the glucocorticoid receptor gene may be associated with an increased sensitivity to glucocortiocids in vivo. J Clin Endocrinol Metab 83:144–151, 1998.

40. DG Tincello, PTK Saunders, MB Hodgins, NB Simpson, CRW Edwards, TB Hargreaves, FCW Wu. Correlation of clinical, endocrine and molecular abnormalities with in vivo responses to high-dose testosterone in patients with partial androgen insensitivity syndrome. Clin Endocrinol 46:497–506, 1997.

41. B Gottlieb, M Trifiro, R Lumbroso, L Pinsky. The androgen receptor gene mutations database. Nucleic Acids Res 25:158–162, 1997.

42. M-E Taplin, GJ Bubley, TD Shuster, ME Frantz, AE Spooner, GK Ogata, HN Keer, SP Balk. Mutation of the androgen-receptor gene in metastatic androgen-independent prostate cancer. N Engl J Med 332:1393–1398, 1995.

43. WD Tilley, G Buchanan, TE Hickey, JM Bentel. Mutations in the androgen receptor gene are associated with progression of human prostate cancer to androgen independence. Clin Cancer Res 2:277–285, 1996.

44. C-P Chen, S-R Chen, T-Y Wang, MS Wayseen, Y-M Hwu. Fertil Steril 72:170–173, 1999.

45. Veldscholte, C Ris-Staplers GGJM Kuiper, G Jenster, C Berrevoets, E Klassen, HCJ van Rooij, J Trapman, AO Brinkmann, E Mulder. A mutation in the ligand binding domain of the androgen receptor of human LNCaP cells affects steroid binding characteristics and response to antiandrogens. Biochem Biophys Res Commun 173:534–540, 1990.

46. Veldscholte, C Berrevoets, AO Brinkmann, JA Grootegoed, E Mulder. Antiandrogens and the mutated androgen receptor of LNCaP cells: differential effects on binding affinity, heat-shock protein interaction and transcription activation. Biochemistry 31:2393–2399, 1992.

47. ER Barrack. Androgen receptor mutations in prostate cancer. Mt Sinai J Med 63:403–412, 1996.

48. K Sudhir, TM Chou, K Chatterjee, EP Smith, TC Willimas, JP Kane, MJ Malloy, KS Korach, GM Rubanyi. Premature coronary artery disease associated with a disruptive mutation in the estrogen receptor gene in a man. Circulation 96:3774–3777, 1997.

49. A Mahfoudi, E Roulet, S Dauvois, MG Parker, W Wahli. Specific mutations in the estrogen receptor change the properties of antiestrogens to full agonists. Proc Natl Acad Sci USA 92:4206–4210, 1995.

50. JJ Pink, S-Q Wu, DM Wolf, MM Bilimoria, VC Jordan. A novel 80 kDa human estrogen receptor containing a duplication of exons 6 and 7. Nucleic Acids Res 24:962–969, 1996.

51. MM Montano, K Ekena, AL Keller, BS Katzenellenbogen. Human estrogen receptor ligand activity inversion mutants: receptors that interpret antiestrogens as estrogens and estrogens as antiestrogens and discriminate among different antiestrogens. Mol Endocrinol 10:230–242, 1996.

52. Q-X Zhang, Å Borg, DM Wolf, S Oesterreich, SAW Fuqua. An estrogen receptor mutant with strong hormone-independent activity from a metastatic breast cancer. Cancer Res 52:1244–1249, 1997.

53. AS Levenson, WH Catherino, VC Jordan. Estrogenic activity is increased for an antiestrogen by a natural mutation of the estrogen receptor. J Steroid Biochem Mol Biol 60:261–268, 1997.

54. AS Gevesnon, VC Jordan. The key to the antiestrogenic mechanismof raloxifene is amino acid 351 (aspartate) in the estrogen receptor. Cancer Res 58:1872–1875, 1998.

55. RJ Lin, DA Egan, RM Evans. Molecular genetic of acute promyelocytic leukemia. Trends Genet 15:179–184, 1999.

56. SE Taymans, S Pack, E Pak, Z Orban, J Barsony, Z Zhuang, CA Stratakis. The human vitamin D receptor gene (VDR) is localized to region 12cen-q12 by fluorescent in situ hybridization and radiation hybrid mapping: genetic and physical VDR map. J Bone Miner Res 14:1163–1166, 1999.

57. PJ Malloy, JW Pike, D Feldman. The vitamin D receptor and the syndrome of hereditary 1,25-dihydroxy vitamin D–resistant rickets. Endocr Rev 20:156–188, 1999.

58. I Nemeri, Z Schwartz, H Pedrozo, VL Sylvia, DD Dean, BD Boyan. Identification of a membrane receptor for 1,25-dihydroxyvitamin D3 which mediates rapid activation of protein kinase C. J Bone Miner Res 13:1353–1359, 1998.

59. JC Fleet. Vitamin D receptors: not just in the nucleus anymore. Nutr Rev 57:60–62, 1999.

60. J Micka, A Milatovitch, A Menon, GA Brabowski, A Puga, DW Nebert. Human Ah receptor (AHR) gene: localization to 7p15 and suggestive correlation of polymorphism with CYP1A1 inducibility. Pharmacogenetics 7:85–101, 1997.

61. PM Garrison, MS Denison. Analysis of the murine AhR gene promoter. J Biochem Mol Toxicol 14:1–10, 2000.

62. T Cole, J Blendy, A Monaghan, K Kriegstein, W Schmid, A Aguzzi, G Fantuzzi, E Hummler, K Unsicker, G Schütz. Targeted disruption of the glucocorticoid receptor gene blocks adrenergic chromaffin cell development and severely retards lung maturation. Genes Dev 9:1606–1621, 1995.

63. JW Korper, RP Stolk, P de lange, NATM Huizenga, G-J Molijn, HAP Pols, DE Grobbee. M Karl. FH de Long, AO Brinkmann, SWJ Lamberts. Lack of association between five polymorphisms in the human glucocorticoid receptor gene and glucocorticoid resistance. Hum Genet 99:663–668, 1997.

64. JD Wilson. The promiscuous receptor. Prostate cancer comes of age. N Engl J Med 332:1440–1441, 1995.

65. A Edwards, HA Hammond, L Jin, CT Caskey, R Chakraborty. Genetic variation at five trimeric and tetrameric tandem repeat loci in four human population groups. Genomics 12:241–253, 1992.

66. KS Korach, JF Couse, SW Curtis, TF Washburn, J Lindzey, KS Kimbro, EM Eddy, S Migliaccio, SM Snedeker, DB Lubahn, DW Schomberg, EP Smith. Estrogen gene disruption: Molecular characterization and experimental and clinical phenotypes. Recent Prog Horm Res 51:159–186, 1996.

67. LC Murphy, H Dotzlaw, E Leygue, D Douglas, A Coutts, PH Watson. Estrogen receptor variants and mutations. J Steroid Biochem Mol Biol 62:363–372, 1997.

68. K Paech, P Webb, GGJM Kuiper, S Nilsson, J-Å Gustafsson, PJ Kushner, TS Scanlan. Differential ligand activation of estrogen receptors ERα and ERβ at AP1 sites. Science 277:1508–1510, 1997.

69. SM Lippman, PH Brown. Tamoxifen prevention of breast cancer: an instance of the fingerpost. J Natl Cancer Inst 91:1809–1819, 1999.

70. MS Tallman, JW Andersen, CA Schiffer, FR Appelbaum, JH Feusner, A Ogden, L Shepherd, C Willman, CD Bloomfield, JM Rowe, PH Wiernik. All-*trans*-retinoic acid in acute promyelocytic leukemia. N Engl J Med 337:1021–1028, 1997.

71. P Fenaux, L Degos. Differentiation therapy for acute promyelocytic leukemia. N Engl J Med 337:1076–1077, 1997.

72. MG Mattei, M Petkovich, JF Mattei, N Brand, P Chambon. Mapping of the human retinoic acid receptor to the q21 band of chromosome 17. Hum Genet 80:186–188, 1988.

73. T Breitman, SJ Collins, BR Keene. Terminal differentiation of promyelocytic leukemic cells in primary cultures in response to retinoic acid. Blood 57:1000–1004, 1981.

74. M-E Huang, Y-C Ye, S-R Chen, J-R Chai, J-X Lu, L Zhuto, L-G Gu, ZY Wang, Use of all-trans retionic acid in treatment of acute promyelocytic leukemia. Blood 72:567–572, 1988.

75. L-Z He, F Guidez, C Triboli, D Peruzzi, M Ruthardt, A Zelent, PP Pandolfi. Distinct interactions of PML-RARα with co-repressors determine differential responses to RA in APL. Nat Genet 18:126–135, 1998.

76. G Jones, T Nguyen, PN Sambrook, PJ Kelly, C Gilbert, JA Eisman. Symptomatic fracture incidence in elderly men and women. Osteoporosis Int 4:277–282, 1994.

77. B Dawson-Hughes, SS Harris, S Finneran. Calcium absorption on high and low calcium intakes in relation to vitamin D. J Clin Endocrinol Metab 80:3657–3661, 1995

78. DP Kiel, RH Myers, LA Cupples, XF Kong, XH Zhu, J Orddovas, EJ Schaefer, DT Felson, D Rush, PW Wilson, JA Eisman, MF Holick. The BsmI vitamin D receptor restriction fragment length polymorphism (bb) influences the effect of calcium intake on bone mineral density. J Bone Miner Res 12:1049–1057, 1997.

79. JM Wishart, M Horowitz, AG Need, F Scopacasa, HA Morris, PM Clifton, BE Nordin. Relations between calcium intake, calcitriol, polymorphisms of the vitamin D receptor gene, and calcium absorption in premenopausal women. Am J Clin Nutr 65:798–802, 1997.

80. SK Ames, KJ Ellis, SK Gunn, KC Copeland, SA Abrams. Vitamin D receptor gene FokI polymorphism predicts calcium absorption and bone mineral density in children. J Bone Miner Res 14:740–746, 1999.

81. G Gong, HS Stern, SC Cheng, N Fong, J Mordeson, HW Deng, RR Recker. The association of bone mineral density with vitamin D receptor gene polymorphisms. Osteoporosis Int 9:55–64, 1999.

82. RM Francis, F Harrington, E Turner, SS Papiha, HK Datta. Vitamin D receptor polymorphism in men and its effect on bone density and calcium absorption. Clin Endocrinol 46:83–86, 1997.

83. M Gunnes, JP Berg, J Halse, EH Lehmann. Lack of relationship between vitamin

D receptor genotype and forearm bone gain in healthy children, adolescents, and young adults. J Clin Endocrinol Metab 82:851–855, 1997.

84. C Gross, IM Musiol, TR Eccleshall, PJ Malloy, D Feldman. Vitamin D receptor gene polymorphisms: analysis of ligand binding and hormone responsiveness in cultured skin fibroblasts. Biochem Biophys Res Commun 242:467–473, 1998.

85. DW Nebert, DD Petersen, A Puga. Human AH locus polymorphism and cancer: inducibility of CYP1A1 and other genes by combustion products and dioxin. Pharmacogenetics 1:68–78, 1991.

86. HI Swanson, CA Bradfield. The AH-receptor: genetics, structure and function. Pharmacogenetics 3:213–230, 1993.

87. K Kawajiri, J Watanabe, H Egchi, K Nakachi, C Kiyohara, S Hayashi. Polymorphisms of human Ah receptor gene are not involved in lung cancer. Pharmacogenetics 5:151–158, 1995.

88. HP Ko, ST Okino, Q Ma, JP Whitlock Jr. Translation domains facilitate promoter occupancy for dioxin-inducible CYP1A1 gene in vivo. Mol Cell Biol 17:3497–3507, 1997.

89. I Splawski, KW Timothy, GM Vincent, DL Atkinson, MT Keating. Molecular basis of the long-QT syndrome associated with deafness. N Engl J Med 336:1562–1567, 1997.

90. SG Priori, J Barhanin, RNW Hauer, W Haverkamp, HJ Jongsman, AG Kleber, WJ McKenna, DM Roden, Y Rudy, K Schwartz, PJ Schwartz, JA Towbin, AM Wilde. Genetic and molecular basis of cardiac arrhythmias: impact on clinical management. Part III. Circulation 99:674–681, 1999.

91. ME Curran, I Splawski, KW Timothy, GM Vincent, ED Green, MT Keating. A molecular basis for cardiac arrhythmia: HERG mutations cause long QT syndrome. Cell 80:795–803, 1995

92. Q Chen, GE Kirsch, D Zhang, R Brugada, J Brugada, P Brugada, D Potenza, A Moya, M Borggrefe, G Breithardt, R Ortiz-Lopez, Z Wang, C Antzelevitch, RE O'Brien, E Schulz-Bahr, MT Keating, JA Towbin, Q Wang. Genetic basis and molecular mechanism for idiopathic ventricular fibrillation. Nature 392:293–296, 1998.

93. L Bianchi, Z Shen, AT Dennis, SG priori, C Napolitano, E Ronchetti, R Bryskin, PJ Schwartz, AM Brown. Cellular dysfunction of LQT5-minK mutants: abnormalities of I_{Ks}, I_{Kr}, and trafficking in long QT syndrome. Hum Mol Genet 8:1499–1507, 1999.

94. GW Abbott, F Sesti, I Splawski, ME Buck, MH Lehmann, KW Timothy, MT Keating, SA Goldstein. MiRP1 forms IKr potassium channels with HERG and is associated with cardiac arrhythmia. Cell 97:175–187, 1999.

95. PM Thomas, N Wohlik, E Huang, U Kuhnle, W Rabl, RF Gagel, GJ Cote. Inactivation of the first nucleotide-binding fold of the sulfonylurea receptor, and familial persistent hyperinsulinemic hypoglycemia of infancy. Am J Hum Genet 59:510–518, 1996.

96. E Riehsaus, M Innis, N MacIntyre, SB Liggett. Mutations in the gene encoding for the β_2-adrenergic receptor in normal and asthmatic subjects. Am J Respir Cell Mol Biol 8:334–339, 1993.

97. SA Green, J Turki, M Innis, SB Liggett. Amino-terminal polymorphisms of the

human β_2-adrenergic receptor impart distinct agonist-promoted regulatory properties. Biochemistry 33:9414–9419, 1994.

98. AJ Sandford, T Shirakawa, MF Moffatt, SE Daniels, C Ra, JA Faux, RP Young, Y Nakamura, GM Lathrop, WOCM Cookson, JM Hopkin. Localisation of atopy and beta subunit of high-affinity IgE receptor (FCepisilonRI) on chromosome 11q. Lancet 341:332–334, 1993.

99. MR Hill, WO Cookson. A new variant of the beta subunit of the high-affinity receptor for immunoglobulin E (Fc epsilon RI-beat E237G): associations with measure of atopy and bronchial hyper-responsiveness. Hum Mol Genet 5:959–962, 1996.

100. T Shirakawa, XQ Mao, S Sasaki, T Enomoto, M Kawai, K Morimoto, J Hopkin. Association between atopic asthma and a coding variant of Fc epsilon RI beta in a Japanese population. Hum Mol Genet 5:1129–1130, 1996.

101. L van Herwerden, SB Harrap, ZYH Wong, MJ Abramson, JJ Kutin, AB Forbes, J Raven, A Lanigan, E Haydn. Linkage of high-affinity IgE receptor gene with bronchial hyperreactivity, even in absence of atopy. Lancet 346:1262–1265, 1995.

102. A Poltorak, I Smirnova, X he, MY Liu, C Van Huffel, O McNally, D Birdwell, E Alejos, M Silva, X Du, P Thompson. EK Chan, J Ledesma, B Roe, S Clifton, SN Vogel, B Beutler. Genetic and physical mapping of the Lps locus: identification of the toll-4 receptor as a candidate gene in the critical region. Blood Cells Mol Dis 24:340–355, 1998.

103. M-L Roy, R Dumaine, AM Brown. HERG, a primary human ventricular target of the nonsedating antihistamine terfenadine. Circulation 94:817–823, 1996.

104. A Jervell, F Lange-Nielsen. Congenital deaf-mutism, functional heart disease, with prolongation of the QT interval and sudden death. Am Heart J 54:59–68, 1957.

105. C Roman, G Gemme, R Pongiglione. Artimie cardiache rare dell'eta pediatrica. Clin Pediatr 45:658–683, 1963.

106. OC Ward. New familial cardiac syndrome in children. J Irish Med Assoc 54:103–106, 1964.

107. N Neyroud, F Tesson, I Dennoy, M Leibovici, C Donger, J Barhanin, S Faure, F Gary, P Coumel, C petit, K Schwartz, P Guicheney. A novel mutation on the potassium channel gene KVLQT1 causes the Jervell and Lange-Nielsen cardioauditory syndrome. Nat Genet 15:186–189, 1997.

108. W Zareba, AJ Moss, PJ Schwartz, M Vincent, JL Robinson, SG Priori, J Benhorin, EH Locati, JA Towbin, MT Keating, MH Lehmann, WJ Hall. Influence of the genotype on the clinical course of the long-QT syndrome. N Engl J Med 339:960–965, 1998.

109. MJ Ackerman. The long QT syndrome: ion channel diseases of the heart. Mayo Clin Proc 73:250–269, 1998.

110. LH Philipson, DF Steiner. Pas de deux or more: the sulfonylurea receptor and K^+ channels. Science 268:372–373, 1995.

111. B Glaser, F Ryan, M Donath, H Landau, CA Stanley, L Baker, DE Barton, PS Thornton. Hyperinsulinism caused by paternal-specific inheritance of a recessive mutation in the sulfonylurea-receptor gene. Diabetes 48:1652–1657, 1999.

112. PM Thomas, GJ Cote, DM Hallman, PM Mathew. Homozygosity to chromosmome 11p, of the gene for familial persistent hyperinsulinemic hypoglycemia of infancy. Am J Hum Genet 56:416–421, 1995.

113. T Hansen, SM Echwald, L Hansen, AM Moller, K Almind, JO Clausen, SA Urhammer, H Inoue, J Ferrer, J Bryan, L Aguilar-Bryan, MA Permutt, O Pedersen. Decreased tolbutamide-stimulated insulin secretion in healthy subjects with sequence variants in the high-affinity sulfonylurea receptor gene. Diabetes 47:598–605, 1998.

114. W Cookson. The alliance of genes and environment in asthma and allergy. Nature 402(suppl):B5–B11, 1999.

115. GK Khurana Hershey, MF Friedrich, LA Esswein, ML Thomas, TA Chatila. The association of atopy with a gain-of-function mutation in the α subunit of the interleukin-4 receptor. N Engl J Med 337:1720–1725, 1997.

116. TD Weir, N Mallek, AJ Sandford, TR Bai, N Awadh, JM Fitzgerald, D Cockcroft, A James, SB Liggett, PD Paré. β_2-Adrenergic receptor haplotypes in mild, moderate and fatal/near fatal asthma. Am J Respir Crit Care Med 158:787–791, 1998.

117. IP Hall, A Wheatley, P Wilding, SB Liggett. Association of Glu 27 β_2-adrenoceptor with lower airway reactivity in asthmatic subjects. Lancet 345:1213–1214, 1995.

118. IP Hall. Beta$_2$ adrenoceptor polymorphisms: are they clinically important? Thorax 51:351–353, 1996.

119. S Tan, IP Hall, J Dewar, E Dow, B Lipworth. Association between beta$_2$ adrenoceptor polymorphism and susceptibility to bronchodilator desensitisation in moderately severe stable asthmatics. Lancet 350:995–999, 1997.

120. FD Martinez, PE Graves, M Baldini, S Solomon, R Erickson. Association between genetic polymorphisms of the β_2 adrenoceptor and response to albuterol in children with and without a history of wheezing. J Clin Invest 100:3184–3188, 1997.

121. RJ Hancox, MR Sears, DR Taylor. Polymorphism of the β_2 adrenoceptor and the response to long-term β_2-agonist therapy in asthma. Eur Respir J 11:589–593, 1998.

122. JJ Lima, DB Thomason, MHN Mohamed, LV Eberle, TH Self, JA Johnson. Impact of genetic polymorphisms of the β_2-adrenergic receptor on albuterol bronchodilator pharmacodynamics. Clin Ther Pharmacol 65:519–525, 1999.

123. BJ Lipworth, IP Hall, S Tan, I Aziz, W Couty. Effects of genetic polymorphism in ex vivo and in vivo function of beta$_2$ adrenoceptors in asthmatic patients. Chest 115:324–328, 1999.

124. AS Fauci. Host factors and the pathogenesis of HIV-induced disease. Nature 384:529–534, 1996.

125. M Carrington, T Kissner, B Gerrard, S Ivanov, SJ O'Brien, M Dean. Novel alleles of the chemokine-receptor gene CCR5. Am J Hum Genet 61:1261–1267, 1997.

126. MA Ansari-Lari, X-M Liu, ML Metzker, AR Rut, RA Gibbs. The extent of genetic variation in the CCR5 gene. Nat Genet 16:221–222, 1997.

127. JC Stephens, DE Reich, DB Goldstein, et al. Dating the origin of the CCR5-Δ32 AIDS-resistance allele by the coalescence of haplotypes. Am J Hum Genet 62:1507–1515, 1998.

128. J Parnas. Peter Ludwig Panum: great Danish pathologist and discoverer of endotoxin. Dan Med Bull 23:143–146, 1976.

129. G Heppner, DW Weiss. High susceptibility of strain A mice to endotoxin and endotoxin–red blood cell mixtures. J Bacteriol 90:696–703, 1965.

130. DB Kuhns, PD Long, JI Gallin. Endotoxin and IL-1 hyporesponsiveness in a patient with recurrent bacterial infections. J Immunol 158:3959–3864, 1997.

5

Pharmacogenetics of Drug Transporters

Richard B. Kim and Grant R. Wilkinson
Vanderbilt University, Nashville, Tennessee

1 INTRODUCTION

The translocation of solutes across biological membranes has, for many years, been recognized to involve other processes besides passive diffusion, and this led to the concept of carrier-mediated transport. However, it is only recently that insights have been obtained about the specific transporter genes/proteins, their molecular characteristics and, to a more limited extent, factors involved in their regulation. Moreover, the area is still evolving with new information becoming rapidly available. A major reason for such interest has been the recognition of the critical and evolutionary conserved role that transporters have in the essential cellular functioning of archaebacteria, prokaryotes, and eukaryotes [1]. In fact, it has been suggested that about 5–15% of the genome may be related to membrane transporter function [2], and a general classification scheme has been developed (http://www.biology.ucsd.edu/~msaier/transport/titlepage.html).

Some carrier-type transporters mediate the unidirectional translocation of a single substrate (uniporters), while other function as antiporters where two substrates are transported in opposite directions in a tightly coupled process, and still others involve the linked co-transport of two separate substrates in the same direction (symporters). It is also apparent that transporters are often expressed within the cell membrane in a domain-specific fashion such that they mediate either solute uptake or efflux, and often such an arrangement facilitates vectorial translocation across cells, e.g., from the blood through the hepatocyte and into bile.

The ever-increasing number of identified transporters with diverse function precludes a comprehensive overview of the whole area. Accordingly, this review focuses on a limited number of transporters, with an emphasis on those identified in humans and which appear to be importantly involved in the disposition of xenobiotics including drugs. That is, transporter genes/proteins which are predominantly expressed in either the liver, intestine or kidney, but may also be present in other organs of interest—for example, the brain (Table 1). Such proteins can mediate the uptake and efflux of a wide range of anionic and cationic amphipathic xenobiotics, and may be important determinants of a drug's absorption, distribution, and excretion. At the present time, information on such transporters is mainly descriptive with respect to function; however, initial insights

TABLE 1   Localization and Expression Domain of Human Membrane Transporters in Organs of Importance in Drug Disposition

	Apical	Basolateral	Unknown
Intestinal tract	MDR1* BCRP* MRP2* OCT2†	MRP3*	MRP1* MRP4* MRP5* OATP-B OCT3†
Liver	MDR1* BCRP* MRP2* BSEP*	MRP3* LST1† OCT2† MRP6*	MRP5* MRP6* OATP-B OCT1† MRP6*
Kidney	MDR1* BRCP* MRP2* OAT-K1 OCT2† OCTN2†	MRP3* OATP-B	MRP1* MRP4* MRP5* MRP6*
Brain	MDR1* BCRP* OATP-A†	MRP1* OCT2†	MRP3* MRP5* OATP-B OCT3†

* Mediates efflux from cell.
† Mediates uptake into cell.

into their pharmacogenomics are beginning to be revealed and this aspect will, undoubtedly, receive increased attention in the next few years.

2 ABC TRANSPORTERS

The ATP-binding (ABC) superfamily is part of an even larger group, termed the major facilitator superfamily (MFS), of membrane-associated transporter and includes a diverse group of proteins present in a wide variety of organisms and cell types. Currently, about 250 ABC transporters, also termed traffic ATPases, have been identified—about 50 in humans—and further genome mapping will undoubtedly increase this number [3,4]. The function of some of the identified transporters is currently unknown but, in general, the ABC superfamily members transport a diverse array of substrates, which include ions, sugars, amino acids, glycans, peptides, proteins, phospholipids, toxins, antibiotics, and hydrophobic drugs. The characteristic ABC unit is a 200–250 amino acid sequence containing two conserved peptide motifs (Walker A and Walker B), both of which are involved in ATP binding and hydrolysis [3,4]. A third conserved sequence or Walker C motif is located between the Walker A and B motifs and is termed the ABC signature. The minimal functional transport unit appears to consist of two membrane-associated domains each consisting of six putative transmembrane helices and two ATP binding sites [3,4]. Depending on the particular organism, this unit may be constructed from a single polypeptide chain, by homo- or heterodimers, or from multi-subunit systems, all of which include the required membrane and ATP domains [3,4]. ATP-hydrolysis provides the energy required for transport, which involves positive cooperativity between the two ABC binding/ utilization domains and a tight molecular coupling of the transmembrane domains to these. Such a coupling ensures the transmission of the necessary conformational changes caused by substrate binding and ATP hydrolysis.

A regularly updated and informative website provides an excellent source of information on ABC- and other transporters (http://www.med.rug.nl/mdl/humanabc.htm) and provides information on an evolving nomenclature for transporter genes proposed by the Human Genome Nomenclature Committee (http://www.gene.ucl.ac.uk/users/hester/abc.html). However, at the present time, the common trivial names of the transporters are generally used and this convention will be followed in this review.

Amino acid sequence similarities of ABC-transporter proteins indicate several distinct subfamilies, each containing a number of individual members (Fig. 1). In humans, for examples, four large subfamilies are present—MRP/CFTR (10 members), MDR/TAP (11 members), ALD (4 members), and ABC1 (11 members); and four smaller groups exist—White (7 members), ANSA (2 members), ABC50 (1 member) and RNAI (1 member). However, proteins of the

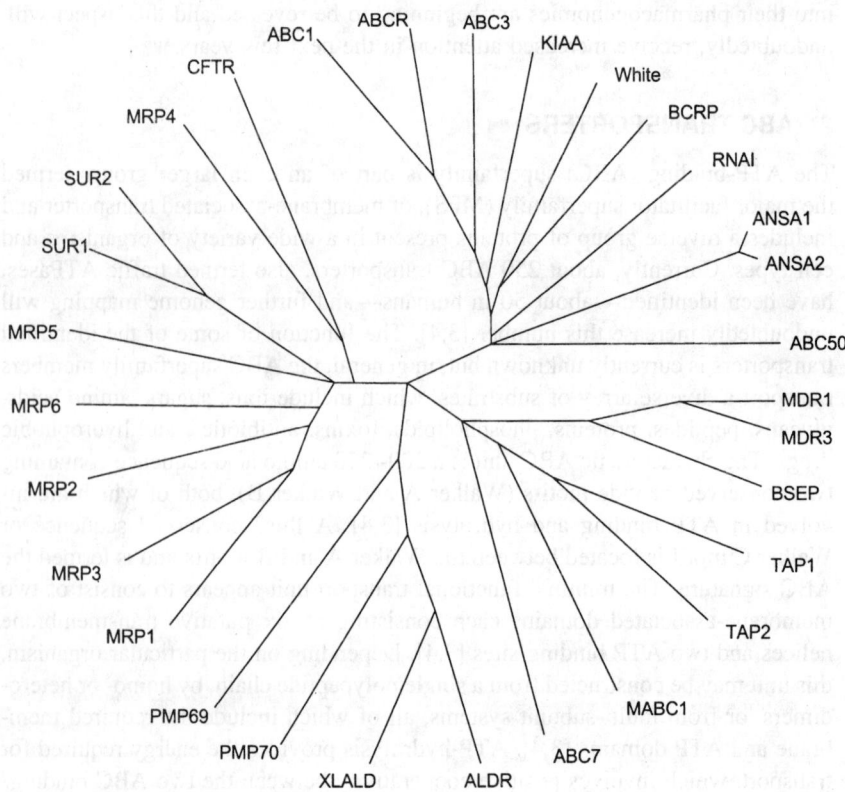

Figure 1 Dendogram illustrating the similarity between amino acid sequences of 30 human ABC proteins and their classification into four major subfamilies. From Ref. 4.

MRP/CFTR and MDR/TAP subfamilies appear to be primarily involved in the transport of xenobiotics.

2.1 Multidrug Resistance Proteins (MDR), Subfamily B

1.1 Transporter Associated with Antigen Processing (TAP)

TAP1 and TAP2 are half-transporters located in the endoplasmic reticulum membrane and form heterodimers which transport peptides from the cytosol into the lumen of the endoplasmic reticulum [5]. There, in concert with the proteasome and MHC class I glycoproteins, they are involved in antigen presentation on the cell surface for T-cell recognition. Drugs are not known substrates of TAP transporters.

2.1.2 MDR1 (P-glycoprotein)

The apparent molecular weights of mature P-glycoproteins ranges from about 130 to 180 kDa, depending on the species and cell type in which they are expressed. Such proteins function as efflux pumps, i.e., translocating a substrate from the inner leaflet side of the membrane to the outer leaflet side; thus, they are visualized as flippases or membrane vacuum cleaners. It is also possible the P-glycoproteins function as membrane pores to export intracellularly located substrates. In humans, P-glycoprotein transporters are encoded by two genes *MDR1* (*PGY1*) and *MDR3* (also named *MDR2* and *PGY3*) adjacently located at chromosomal region 7q21 [6,7]. By contrast, three genes are present in rodents: *mdr1a* (referred to in earlier works as *mdr3*), *mdr1b* (*mdr1*), and *mdr2*. In the mouse, the genes are clustered on chromosome 5 whereas they are located at chromosomal region 4q11–12 in the rat. All mammalian P-glycoproteins display a high level of amino acid identity (>76%), with the ATP binding region and the first and second intracytosolic loops of each half of the protein exhibiting the greatest homology [6,7]. *MDR1* encodes a drug transporter with a very promiscuous substrate specificity and this function is mimicked by both Mdr1a and Mdr1b in rodents. A plethora of compounds with diverse chemical structures and properties are effectively transported; these include many natural products, semisynthetic analogs of such products, and synthetic organic compounds such as drugs and other xenobiotics. Attempts to define a common pharmacophore in these substrates have not been particularly successful other than the fact that the compounds tend to be hydrophobic and amphipathic [6]. Of particular interest from the drug disposition standpoint, is an overlap in substrate and inhibitor specificity for P-glycoprotein and that for cytochrome P450 3A4/5 isoforms importantly involved in the metabolism of many xenobiotics [8]. However, such an overlap is not absolute, but probably reflects the broad and independent substrate specificities of the two proteins; in fact, essentially selective substrates do exist [9]. This phenomenon of substrate overlap is of importance because P-glycoprotein and cytochrome P4503A4/5 are frequently expressed in the same cells. Thus, in the enterocyte and hepatocyte their separate functions complement each other in eliminating substrate from the cell thereby reducing its intracellular concentration [8]. Moreover, drug-drug interactions previously thought to solely reflect reduced cytochrome P4503A4/5 activity through inhibition may, in fact, also involve inhibition of MDR1-mediated transport at these tissue sites [10].

 MDR1 contains 28 exons encoding for a 1280 amino acid transporter consisting of two homologous halves. The protein's membrane topology is thought to reflect 12 transmembrane domains, six at the NH_2- and six at the COOH terminus; two ATP binding/utilization sites, and a linker region. *MDR1* encoded

P-glycoprotein undergoes considerable posttranslational modification, in particular, N-glycosylation at sites located in the first putative extracellular loop [7,11]. However, several studies indicate that the multidrug transport function of MDR1 does not depend on glycosylation. Phosphorylation of the many serine and threonine residues also occurs and involves multiple kinases, and it has been speculated that a phosphorylation/dephosphorylation mechanism may be involved in the regulation of P-glycoprotein's transporter activity [7,12]. However, definitive evidence in support of this hypothesis has yet to be reported.

The 5'-flanking regions of human and rodent P-glycoproteins have been sequenced and, interestingly, there is not a lot of sequence conservation [7]. This is consistent with the differential expression of Mdr1a and Mdr1b, and differences in expression between human and rodent cells in response to induction. Transcription of *MDR1* appears to be regulated by multiple factors. For example, the proximal promoter region has a GC-rich region, at approximately -100 to -120 bp from the transcriptional start codon, that contains a site responsible for the repression of transcription. Also, basal transcription appears to involve a consensus site that binds NF-Y transcription factors at a Y-box (inverted CCAAT box) between -70 and -80 bp. In addition, a binding site for SP-1 and members of the early growth response (EGR) family of transcriptional factors is present which overlaps with the NF-Y consensus site. A 13-bp region around the initiation site (INR) involved in accurate initiation of the transcription has also been identified [7,13].

A variety of stimuli have been found to increase *MDR1* RNA in different cells and tissues, including partial hepatectomy and treatment with xenobiotics [7]. Whether such factors involve transcriptional activation is unclear. However, strong evidence suggests that certain steroids, such as progesterone and estrogen during pregnancy, and in the midsecretory phase of the menstrual cycle can increase MDR1 expression in the uterus. Moreover, one of the tissues that expresses very high levels of MDR1 is the adrenal cortex, consistent with induction by steroids in this tissue. MDR1 is also expressed at a high frequency by tumor cells and both c-H-Ras and mutant forms of p53 have been shown to activate the *MDR1* promoter. On the other hand, c- and N-Myc expression is apparently inversely correlated with Mdr1 expression. Collectively, such data suggest that MDR1 levels are highly regulated at the transcriptional level. However, as with the transporter's posttranslational modifications, the mechanism of regulation is complex and not well understood at the present time.

In order to elucidate the transport mechanism and structure:function relationships of MDR1, mutational analysis has been widely investigated using either site-directed mutagenesis or by the use of drug selection [6,7]. A relatively large number of mutants alter the transporter's substrate specificity in particular those in transmembrane domains 5, 6, 11, and 12. Along with photo-affinity labeling studies, these findings indicate that such domains probably are of major importance in substrate binding. Other domains, however, may also be directly or indirectly involved because mutations in the intra- and extracellular loops and ATP-binding/utilization domains have been found to alter substrate specificity. Mutations in the ATP binding/utilization domain invariably result in the expression of a non-functional transporter; moreover, both nucleotide binding domains are essential for proper functioning. Lack of function also results from mutations that lead to mis-processing of the gene transcript. An important questions, therefore, is whether genetic variability is present in MDR1 which affects its physiological function. In mice there is supportive evidence that this can occur, since a subpopulation of CF-1 outbred mice exist which does not express Mdr1a, and this trait is inherited in a Mendelian, autosomal-recessive fashion [14]. The molecular genetic mechanism of this null model, which is analogous to a knockout mouse resulting from experimental targeted genetic disruption (see later), appears to involve the deletion of exon 23, secondary to the insertion of the murine leukemia virus gene into intron 22 [15]. This presumably results in mRNA mis-splicing and no functional protein is synthesized. A strain of collie dogs also may be genetically deficient in P-glycoprotein based on the fact that they are unusually sensitive to the CNS effects of ivermectin [16], which is usually prevented from entering the brain by P-glycoprotein (see later). Whether similar allelic variability exists with respect to humans is, however, largely unknown. Initial studies suggest that mutations are present in both the 5'-regulatory and coding regions [17,18]. Some of these are sporadic but others are more stable; in the latter case, the allelic frequencies appear to be dependent upon race. Whether such allelic variabilities have functional consequences are obviously important, and recent reports suggest this possibility [17,18].

Human MDR1 was initially identified because of its overexpression in cultured tumor cells associated with an acquired cross-resistance to multiple cytotoxic anticancer agents. It, therefore, provided a mechanistic explanation for the multiple drug resistance phenomenon, which is observed clinically when cancer patients are treated with cancer chemotherapeutic drugs for a prolonged period. This aspect of MDR1's function has been extensively investigated for obvious reasons, and several recent reviews are available [6,7,19]. However, subsequent to the initial characterization of *MDR1* and its gene product, the transporter was also recognized to be expressed in many normal tissues, suggestive of a physiological function [20]. For example, P-glycoprotein is located in the apical domain of the enterocyte of the lower gastrointestinal tract (jejunum, duodenum, ileum, and colon), suggesting that the transporter functions to facilitate excretion of substrates from the systemic circulation into the gastrointestinal tract. Similarly, P-glycoprotein expressed in the canalicular domain of the hepatocyte (Fig. 2) and the brush border of the proximal renal tubule is consistent with a role for the transporter in the biliary and urinary excretion of xenobiotics and endogenous substrates, respectively. The localization of MDR1 in other tissues suggests, however, an additional physiological function, namely that of a transport barrier.

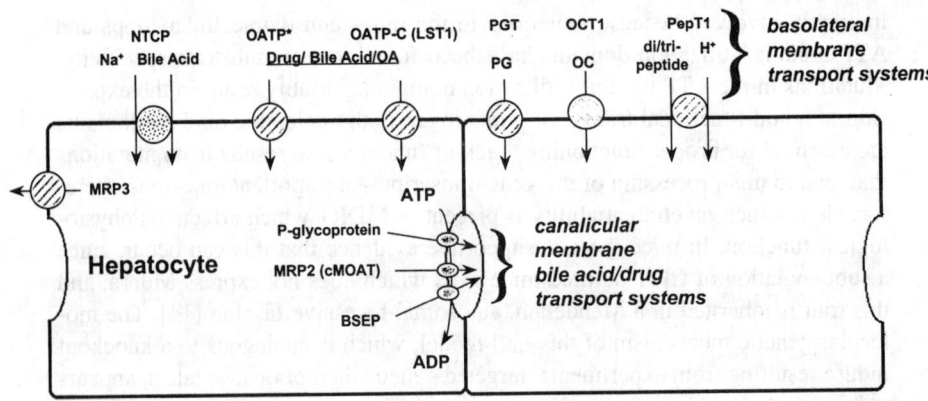

FIGURE 2 Localization of uptake and efflux transporters involved in the translocation of endogenous compounds and xenobiotics across the hepatocyte (*several OATPs including OATP-B and the recently reported OAT-8 [20a] are likely to be involved in hepatic organic anion transport in addition to OATP-C).

Thus, MDR1 expression, especially in the jejunum and duodenum, limits the uptake and absorption of drugs and other substrates from the intestine into the systemic circulation [21]. Likewise, the presence of the transporter on the lumenal membrane of capillary endothelial cells of the brain is consistent with a role for MDR1 in the blood:brain barrier, which restricts drug distribution into the central nervous system [22]. A similar protective role to limit the distribution of potentially toxic xenobiotic into tissues could explain the presence of P-glycoprotein in the placenta and also the testes. The functional significance of the transporter in other cell types and tissues such as the adrenal, pancreas and certain hematopoietic cells is less clear.

Supportive evidence for such physiological functions has been primarily provided by investigations with CF-1 mice deficient in Mdr1a and knockout mice in which *mdr1a, mdr1b*, or both genes have been disrupted leading to null alleles and loss of transporter function [14,23,24]. Such mice appear to be completely healthy and fertile indicative that the encoded transporters have no essential physiologic function [24]. However, when challenged by exposure to xenobiotics that are MDR1 substrates, Mdr1a-deficient mice respond differently than syngeneic animals [15,25,26]. In particular, the extent of oral drug absorption is increased and the rate of drug elimination, whether by biliary or urinary excretion, is impaired [25]. Accordingly, systemic exposure is substantially higher and more prolonged. In addition, drug uptake into the brain is markedly enhanced by up to about 10- to 100-fold [14,23,27,28]. The combination of increased systemic exposure and enhanced penetration into the brain results in relatively innocuous drugs, like ivermectin, which have a wide therapeutic ratio in wild-type mice, being lethal to Mdr1a-deficient CF-1 and *mdr1a* (−/−) mice [23,26]. Also, in pregnant mice, fetal drug exposure is significantly increased [29,30]. For example, the teratological effects of avermectin when maternally administered are markedly more frequent in Mdr1a-deficient CF-1 mice than in wild-type animals [29]. Interestingly, the genotype of the fetus determines the level of placental Mdr1a rather than that of the mother. Comparative studies in *mdr1a* (−/−) and *mdr1a/1b* (−/−) mice have also shown that *mdr1a* is the major mouse P-glyco-protein and the only form of the transporter in the brain capillaries, intestinal tract and placenta *i.e.*, its tissue localization is the same as MDR1 in humans. In contrast, *mdr1b* is found only in the liver and kidney [24].

Because of the importance of MDR1 in multidrug resistance, considerable effort has been expended to identify compounds which inhibit P-glycoprotein function and would, therefore, reverse the phenomenon [31]. It has also become recently appreciated that such reversing agents or chemosensitizers could also be useful in altering a drug's disposition; for example, increasing drug absorption, reducing drug elimination and modulating tissue distribution, particularly to the brain. While many such agents have been identified and shown to be effective in vitro using cultured cells, the development of clinically successful P-glycoprotein inhibitors has been disappointing [32]. This has been primarily related to the difficulty of attaining and maintaining adequate concentrations of the agents in vivo and/or the lack of specificity of inhibition such that the function of other proteins is also affected. For example, PSC-833 (Valspodar) is a relatively potent inhibitor of cytochrome P4503A as well as P-glycoprotein; hence, its use is often complicated by metabolic interactions with co-administered drugs that are bio-transformed by this isoform [33]. More selective and potent P-glycoprotein inhibitors are under development and have the ability to inhibit MDR1 without affecting drug metabolism [34], but clinical evaluations are still in early stages.

Another active area of investigation with regard to altering P-glycoprotein function is gene therapy, i.e., the delivery of cDNA encoding MDR1 into specific target cells and tissues, e.g., bone marrow and other drug-sensitive sites, to protect them against the toxic effects of cancer chemotherapy. The feasibility of this concept has been demonstrated in transgenic mice and gene transfer experiment, and clinical trials to test the hypothesis in humans are ongoing [7].

2.1.3 MDR3

Despite its close amino acid sequence similarity with MDR1 (75%), MDR3 does not appear to encode a multidrug transporter. Instead, MDR3 is a phospholipid (phosphatidylcholine) translocator that is highly expressed in the canalicular membrane of the hepatocyte [35]. Studies with a knockout mouse model support this notion since phospholipid secretion into bile is severely impaired and this may be reversed by transgenic expression of MDR3 [36]. Significantly, such animals develop severe liver disease with symptoms similar to progressive familial intrahepatic cholestasis type 3 (PFIC3). This genetic disease has been mapped to chromosomal region 7q21.3 and studies of patients with PFIC3 indicated a complete loss of MDR3 protein from the canalicular membrane [37]. A 7-bp deletion in one patient and a nonsense mutation in a second were identified as the molecular bases for the null phenotype. A family has also been identified in whom PFIC3 and intrahepatic cholestasis of pregnancy exists [38]. In the affected women, a single nucleotide deletion starting at codon 571 of *MDR3* results in a frameshift and introduction of a downstream stop codon [39]. It has also been speculated that individuals homozygous for such *MDR3* mutations, i.e., complete congenital defects, may be predisposed to severe liver disease early in life rather than a more latent disease in adulthood associated with a partial congenital impairment [40].

2.2 Bile Salt Export Pump (Sister P-Glycoprotein)

The vectorial transport of bile salts from the systemic circulation into bile is a critically important aspect of liver function. Recently, the transporter at the canalicular membrane of the hepatocyte responsible for bile acid secretion into the bile has been identified. This is the bile salt export pump (BSEP), also known as sister-P-glycoprotein (sisPGP, SPGP) whose gene, in humans, is located in chromosomal region 2q24. Mutations at 10 or more different sites in the 1321 amino acid protein result in another subtype of progressive familial intrahepatic cholestasis, (PFIC2), characterized by persistent neonatal cholestasis [41]. This disease appears to be associated with significantly impaired expression of BSEP. It is also likely that downregulation of BSEP may be involved in the pathophysiological defect in acquired forms of cholestasis produced by endotoxin and certain drugs (ethinylestradiol and cyclosporin A) [40]. Future studies will, undoubtedly, provide further characterization of this physiologically important transporter, but it is unlikely that it is involved in the biliary secretion of drugs.

2.3 Multiple Drug Resistance–Associated Proteins (MRP), Subfamily C

Initially, overexpression of MDR1 was thought to be the major mechanism by which multidrug resistance developed to cytotoxic cancer chemotherapeutic agents. However, this proved not to be the case and another transporter, the multidrug resistance–associated protein (MRP1), was identified as a major contributor [42]. When sequenced, the most closely related member of the ABC superfamily to MRP1 (30% identity) was the cystic fibrosis transmembrane conductance regulator (CFTR). Subsequently, the sulfonylurea receptors (SUR1 and SUR2) were also found to be members of the same subfamily, as were additional MRPs.

2.3.1 MRP1

Human *MRP1*, located at chromosomal region 16q13.1 and spanning at least 200 kb, has 31 exons that encode a 1531 amino acid protein which, in its mature glycosylated form, has a molecular weight of 190 kDa [43,44]. Two features distinguish MRP1 and related transporters from other ABC-superfamily members [44–46]. First, in comparison with P-glycoproteins, there is an absence of 13 amino acids located between the Walker A and B motifs in the proximal nucleoside binding domain (NBD1), these corresponding amino acids are, however, present in the COOH-proximal NBD2. This account for the low sequence identity (~30%) between the two domains (cf., the close similarity in P-glycoproteins) and the deletion affects the folding and activity of the protein.

A second distinguishing feature is that MRP1-related transporters are typically larger than other full-length ABC proteins—up to 250 additional amino acids at the NH$_2$-terminus for which there is no comparable region in other ABC transporters. This forms an additional transmembrane domain that characterizes MRPs from other ABC-transporters and is critical for transport activity. In contrast to MDR1 in which the transmembrane domains contain six membrane spanning helices, the topology of MRP transporter has not yet been fully defined. However, determinants located between amino acids 204 and 229 in the third intracellular loop connecting membrane spanning domain MSD1 to MSD2 appear to be essential for transport. Also, MRP1 lacking the glycosylated extracytosolic NH$_2$-terminus and the first transmembrane α-helix (amino acids 1–66) is inactive.

The regulatory mechanisms determining the expression of MRP1 have only been partly characterized. For example, a number of putative transcription factor motifs have been identified such as the activator proteins AP1 and AP2 (Sp1), a glucocorticoid response element (GRE), and also ERE and CRE [47]. Furthermore, reporter gene transfection studies showed an element residing within the −91 to +103 bp region of the *MRP1* promoter that was suppressed by wild-type p53 [48]. Conversely, an Sp1 expression vector increased promoter activity up to 200-fold and this was attenuated by wild-type p53. Thus, the loss of wild-type p53 function and/or an increase in Sp1 activity, at least in tumor cells, upregulates the *MRP1* gene. In addition, endotoxin-induced cholestasis, which produces marked downregulation of BSEP (Sect. 2.2) and MRP2 (Sect. 2.3.2) in rat liver, also increases Mrp2 in this situation and enhances excretion of organic anions from the hepatocyte into sinusoidal blood [40]. There is also evidence that changes in the degree of phosphorylation of serine residues in MRP1 are involved in the short-term regulation of the transporter's activity [49].

MRP1 is expressed in various tissues throughout the body; with highest levels being found in the testes, skeletal muscle, heart, kidney, and lung [44–46]. MRP1 is also expressed in the brain and spleen but, significantly, only low levels are present in the liver and intestine. A substantial fraction of MRP1 in these tissues appears to be located in intracellular vesicles rather than the plasma membrane. Moreover, MRP1 is localized to the basolateral side of epithelial cells; accordingly, it tends to pump drugs into the body rather than into the bile, urine or intestinal tract for elimination, in contrast to MDR1. Possibly, such a basolateral transporter is valuable in providing protection of certain cells and organs. For example, MRP1 may be important in the blood:CSF barrier since the choroid plexus contains a high level of the transporter that could function to remove xenobiotics from the CSF [50,51]. Similarly, MRP1 in the basal membrane of Sertoli cells may protect germ cells by pumping out xenobiotics from the testicular tubule [52]. *MRP1* knockout mice do not exhibit any obvious phenotype other than a modest increase in drug resistance to certain anticancer agents such as etoposide [53]. Given the extent of MRP1 expression in various tissues and the overlapping substrate specificities of MRP family members, this finding is not too surprising.

MRP1 is involved in a number of glutathione-related cellular processes [44–46]. Its major physiological function appears to be the transport of leukotriene C_4 (LTC$_4$), which is formed from arachidonic acid through a series of metabolic steps culminating in conjugation with glutathione (GSH). LTC$_4$ is the highest affinity substrate for MRP1 ($K_m \sim 100$ nM) but other endogenous anionic compounds are also transported, including glutathione disulfide (GSSG), bilirubin glucuronide, conjugated bile salts, 17β-estradiol glucuronide, and the GSH conjugate of prostaglandin A2. In addition, a number of conjugated metabolites of xenobiotics also have been shown to be substrates. Interestingly, from the teleological standpoint, the GSH conjugate of aflatoxin B_1—a potent mutagen and carcinogen—is the highest affinity exogenous substrate identified to date ($K_m \sim 200$ nM). Also, MRP1 transports GSH and glucuronide metabolites of a number of cytotoxic chemotherapeutics agents, like melphalan, chlorambucil and etoposide [44–46].

2.3.2 MRP2/cMOAT

The ability of the liver to secrete amphipathic anionic compounds into bile led to the identification of a carrier-mediated transporter at the canalicular membrane that was termed cMOAT (canalicular multiple organic anion transporter). When cloned, this was found to be an ABC transporter of the MRP subfamily, namely Mrp2 [54]. In humans, this full transporter is a 1545 amino acid protein whose 32 exon gene is located in chromosomal region 10q23–24 [46]. Although there is limited sequence similarity between MRP2 and MRP1 (49%), the primary structural features and membrane topology of the two proteins are thought to be similar. The two transporters also have similar substrate characteristics, i.e., conjugates, especially with GSH, of endogenous and exogenous compounds [46]. However, in contrast to MRP1, cMOAT/MRP2 is localized in the apical membrane of epithelial cells found in such tissues as the liver, kidney, and intestine [45]. MRP2 is therefore importantly involved in the excretion of metabolites of xenobiotics and endogenous compounds with an anionic nature. Emerging evidence suggests that MRP2 is possibly involved in the multidrug resistance phenomenon [45].

The Dubin-Johnson syndrome is an autosomal, recessively inherited disorder in the excretion of amphipathic anionic conjugates from hepatocytes into bile and is predominantly characterized by conjugated hyperbilirubinemia. In patients with this syndrome, MRP2 is not present in the hepatic canalicular membrane [55]. The responsible mutations, currently seven, are scattered preferentially over the 3'-proximal half of the mRNA, including exons encoding both nucleotide-binding domains [46,56,57]. A nonsense mutation leads to a premature termination codon, another missense mutation affects the first nucleotide-binding domain, and a deletion mutation results in the loss of two amino acids in the second nucleotide-binding domain. Other established mutations involving splice junctions lead to exon deletions and premature termination codons. Two well-characterized hyperbilirubinemic rat strains have been considered as animal models of the human Dubin-Johnson syndrome. These are the GY/TR⁻ mutant rat and the Eisai hyperbilirubinemic rat (EHBR), and mRNA for *mrp2* is not detectable in the livers of these animals. Mutations in *mrp2* have been identified in such animals which introduce premature termination codons that presumably lead to a functionally deficient transporter [46,54].

2.3.3 MRP3–6

Additional members of the MRP subfamily have been identified, recently; however, available information on these transporters, which are also termed MOATs, is still limited. The human *MRP3* gene is located in chromosomal region 17q21.3 and encodes a 1527 amino acid protein that has 58% and 48% sequence similarity to MRP1 and MRP2, respectively [45,46]. Currently available evidence indicates that MRP3 is a basolateral export pump which is predominantly localized in the liver (cholangiocytes), small intestine, colon and kidney. Other tissues in which *MRP3* mRNA has been detected include the pancreas and prostate [58]. Alternative transcription splice variants of *MRP3* have been reported [58]. This transporter also appears to be upregulated by cholestasis and phenobarbital pretreatment, but the molecular mechanism(s) of these changes is unknown [59].

Human MRP4 is a 1325 amino acid protein coded by a gene located in chromosomal region 13q31–32, and is widely distributed throughout the body [45,46]. However, whether it is expressed apically or basolaterally is not yet established. Interestingly, particularly high levels of MRP4 are found in the prostate, but it is barely detectable in liver. Preliminary evidence suggests that MRP4 may be involved in the efflux of the monophosphate metabolites of nucleoside analogs, such as HIV reverse transcriptase inhibitors, from cells [60]. The 1503 amino acid protein MRP5 is encoded by a gene in chromosomal region 3q27 and its polarized location in the cell is also unknown [45,46]. Only low MRP5 levels are found in the liver, however, intermediate expression occurs in kidney, testis, heart, and brain, and the highest level of MRP5 is in skeletal muscle. Like MRP4, MRP5 lacks a first NH_2-terminal membrane-spanning domain, indicating that the topologies of these transporters are distinct from those of MRP1 and MRP2. Finally, it appears that MRP6—a 1503 amino acid protein encoded by a gene at chromosomal region 16p13—is specifically expressed in the liver and kidney [45,46]. MRP6 is most closely related to MRP1 (46%), MRP2 (39%), and MRP3 (44%).

All of these recently identified MRPs appear to have about 30–45% sequence identity to the well-characterized MRP1 and MRP2 transporters. Moreover, available data, although limited at this time, suggest that they have very similar substrate specificities as other MRPs; i.e., they are GS-X pumps that transport multiple amphipathic anionic compounds, particularly glutathione conjugates of endogenous and exogenous compounds. However, the physiological function of MRP3-6 are not known.

2.3.4 CFTR and SUR

The CFTR and sulfonylurea receptors (SUR) are also members of the MRP subfamily even though they do not transport anionic amphipathic compounds. SUR1 and SUR2 are receptors that appear to function as sensors of ATP and ADP concentrations and are important in modulating insulin release [61]. Mutations in SUR1 have been found to cause a rare genetic disease, persistent hyperinsulinemic hypoglycemia of infancy (PHHI), that is inherited in an autosomal recessive fashion [62]. By contrast, cystic fibrosis, associated with an alteration in CFTR's ion-channel function, is one of the most frequent inherited human diseases with a prevalence of 1 in 25,000 births within Caucasian populations [63]. While the major mutation—a single amino acid deletion (F508)—accounts for about 70% of disease alleles, over 800 disease-causing mutations have been identified (http://www.genet.sickkids.on.ca/cftr/).

2.4 Breast Cancer Resistance Protein (BCRP), Subfamily G

The role of MDR and MRPs in the clinical drug resistance exhibited by human breast cancer is unclear and studies to identify alternative mechanisms have led to the discovery of a breast cancer resistance protein [64]. Amino acid sequence similarities indicate that BCRP1 is identical to the placental-specific ATP-binding cassette protein (ABCP) that was simultaneously identified [65] which, in turn, is similar to a mitoxantrone-resistance (MXR1) transporter [66]. The BCRP1/MXR1/ABCP gene is located at chromosomal region 4q22 and encodes a 655 amino acid half-transporter protein that is a member of the White subfamily of ABC transporters. It is not known whether the functional transporter is a homodimer or whether it forms a heterodimer. In addition to very high level of expression in the placenta, BCRP1 is also found at lower levels in the brain, liver, kidney, testis, and small intestine where it appears to be localized to the apical membrane domain. The similarity between BCRP1 and MDR1 also appears to extend beyond their similar tissue localization since there appears to be considerable overlap in the substrate specificity of the two transporters; in particular, cancer chemotherapeutic agents such as topotecan, mitoxantrone, and doxorubicin [67,68]. On the other hand, vincristine and paclitaxel do not appear to be transported by BCRP, although they are both good MDR1 substrates. Because of these similarities, it is likely that for some drugs BRCP may be important in their absorption from the intestinal tract, distribution into tissues and hepatic, renal, and intestinal elimination, as with substrates of MDR1.

3 ORGANIC ANION TRANSPORTERS

The presence of carrier systems capable of transporting various anionic drugs in the liver and kidney was established by classical biochemical approaches, many years ago. However, it is only recently that molecular insights into the individual transporter genes/proteins have been obtained. Furthermore, this is currently still a developing area of knowledge and in certain cases present information is largely limited to rodents rather than humans. As a consequence, understanding of the genetics of regulation and expression of the involved genes is sparse. Nevertheless, it is highly likely that the activity of such transporters is important in the overall disposition profiles of many drugs, and inhibition of transport may be the basis of some drug-drug interactions.

3.1 Organic Anion Transporter Family (OATP)

The active uptake of bile acids from sinusoidal blood into the hepatocyte is a critical component in the secretion of bile [40,69]. A large proportion of such uptake is Na^+-dependent and mediated by the sodium taurocholate cotransporting polypeptide (NTCP), which is a member of the superfamily of sodium/solute symporters (solute carrier family 10). This transporter's substrate specificity is predominantly limited to conjugated bile acids rather than drugs/metabolites other than selected sulfated steroids [40,69]. In contrast, unconjugated bile salts such as cholate as well as multiple organic anions are taken up into hepatocytes by Na^+-independent transport. However, such transport does not reflect the function of a single transporter protein, rather a family of OATP transporters (solute family 21) appear to be present in the liver and other organs. It now appears that members of the OATP transporter family mediate the cellular uptake of many drugs, and that they have broad substrate specificities. Moreover, they are capable of transporting not only anionic drugs, as the family name implies, but also of neutral, zwitterionic, and positively charged drugs [70].

3.1.1 OATP-A and OATP-B

Human OATP-A, initially termed simply OATP, mediates the basolateral transport of a wide range of amphipathic substrates including bile salts, estrogen conjugates (e.g., estrone-3-sulfate and estradiol 17β-glucuronide), organic anions (e.g., bromosulfophthalein), and numerous xenobiotics ranging from neutral to even permanently charged bulky organic type II cations [71,72]. This substrate specificity is similar but not identical to that of rat Oatp1 (currently, the trivial nomenclature differentiates the various human subfamily members alphabetically whereas in the rat a numerical system is used), but it is highly likely that these two transporters, which have only 67% amino acid sequence identity, are not the products of orthologous genes [72]. Although OATP-A was originally identified in human liver, its level of expression in this organ is low and substantially higher mRNA levels are present in lung, kidney, and testis, and are especially high in the brain [73]. In fact, the latter localization is probably the major site for OATP-A's physiological function, i.e., removal of drug substrates from the CSF. Such function would be consistent with the expression of rat Oatp1 on the apical surface of the choroid plexus. By contrast, rat Oatp1 is basolaterally expressed in the liver. OATP-A is a 670 amino acid protein whose gene is localized to the 12p12 chromosomal region [74]. Eight potential N-glycosylation sites are present in the protein of which three to four may actually be conjugated, and 10 to 12 putative transmembrane domains have been identified [70]. The *OATP-A* gene's 5'-promoter elements have been partially characterized and putative, transcriptional regulatory regions include HNF1, HNF3, HNF4, HNF5, AP1, AP2, c/EBP, and GRE motifs. In addition, a potential suppressor element in the −662 to −440 nucleotide region relative to the transcription initiation site is present [70]. Currently, however, the roles of such potential regulatory mechanisms are unknown.

More recently, a related transporter, OATP-B has been identified in human brain tissue (GenBank accession numbers AF085224 and AL117465). This is 709 amino acid protein whose functional characteristics have yet to be described. Northern analysis revealed highest expression in the liver, and readily detectable expression in the kidney, heart, placenta, in addition to brain. Expression of the rat ortholog (Oatp2) in the brain is localized to the basolateral membrane of the capillary endothelial cells that make up the blood-brain and blood-CSF barrier [75]. At present, it is not clear what the endogenous role for such transporters are in tissues such as the brain, although, one function may be to transport hormones such as T3 and T4.

3.1.2   OATP-C (LST-1)

Because of the low level of expression of OATP-A in human liver, the presence of other basolateral, polyspecific organic anion transporters was suspected. The search for these resulted in the isolation of a 691 amino acid transporter, OATP-C, also termed liver-specific transporter (LST-1) because of its essentially exclusive expression in the liver [73]. OATP-C is a 691 amino acid protein with 42% sequence identity to OATP-A. Like the latter, OATP-C has broad substrate specificity and transports conjugated steroids, cardiac glycosides, thyroid hormones, and many xenobiotics [73]. In fact, OATP-C now appears to be the predominant Na^+-independent uptake transporter responsible for the hepatic uptake of several anionic drugs, including HMG-CoA inhibitors like pravastatin [76]. Hydrophobicity analysis suggests that OATP-C is a 12 transmembrane domain transporter, and there are seven putative NH_2-glycosylation sites in the predicted extracellular loops [73]. A potential phosphorylation site for cAMP-dependent protein kinase and another for protein kinase C are also present in the third cytosolic loop. However, other topological insights or determinants in OATP-C's regulation and expression are unknown. Interestingly, the rat ortholog, rLst-1, transports a much narrower spectrum of xenobiotic substrates relative to its human counterpart and apparently lacks approximately 80 bp of sequence encoding one of the transmembrane spanning domains [77]. Whether this is the result of alternative splicing and how this relates to rLst-1's more restrictive substrate specificity is not clear.

3.1.3   Other OATP Transporters

A number of additional OATP transporter family members have been identified from human kidney; however, their role and function to drug disposition have not been defined. These include OAT-K1, and OATP-D, and OATP-E. OAT-K1 is apically expressed and appears to have a relatively narrow spectrum of drug substrates, in that only methotrexate is currently known to be transported [78]. Furthermore, another member of the OATP transporter family is the prostaglandin transporter (PGT) [79]. This 643 amino acid protein shares ~40% similarity with OATP-A, but transports only eicosanoids.

4   ORGANIC CATION TRANSPORTERS (OCT)

Classical biochemical transport studies established, many years ago, the presence of carrier systems capable of transporting organic cations in a number of epithelial tissues including the intestine, liver, and kidney. Such systems were considered to be important in the transport of both endogenous amines and various xenobiotics. Moreover, in the liver, the involved transporters could be classified into two types on the basis of their specificity—type I carriers mediated the cellular uptake of small monovalent organic cations such as choline, tetraethylammonium *N*-

methylnicotinamide and 1-methyl-4-phenylpyridinum (MPP), whereas larger, bi-valent cations, like vecuronium, pancuronium, and quinine, were transported by a type II carrier [80]. In many instances transport was linked to a proton antiporter process. Efforts to identify and characterize the molecular aspects of organic cation transporters are only just beginning to provide useful insights [81,82]. From a classification standpoint, such transporters belong to solute carrier family 22 which, in turn, is a member of the MFS superfamily.

4.1 OCT1

The first organic cation transporter (rOct1) was cloned from a rat kidney cDNA library and the 556 amino acid protein was initially found to have functional characteristics of the biochemical type I carrier system, i.e., a polyspecific, small organic cation transporter [83]. However, it was later found that rOct1 is also capable of mediating the uptake of bulkier, type II cations and polyamines like spermidine [81]. In addition to the proximal renal tubule and collecting duct of the kidney, rOct1A is also basolaterally expressed in the hepatocyte and all regions of the intestine. A splice variant of rOct1, termed rOct1A, has also been identified, but this does not appear to affect the substrate specificity of the translated protein [81].

Recently a human ortholog (hOCT1) has been identified as a 554 amino acid transporter with 78% identity to rOct1, and the *hOCT1* gene has a 6q26 chromosomal location [84,85]. However, hOCT1 exhibits significant differences in tissue distribution and functional characteristics from rOct1. For example, hOCT1 is expressed essentially only in the liver in contrast to the additional intestinal and renal distribution of rOCT1. Moreover, hOct1 appears to be more specific for type I organic cations [86].

Based on rOct1, it has been suggested that the transporter's topology in-volves 12 transmembrane spanning α-helices with both the NH_2- and $COOH-$ termini being intracellularly located. An extracellular loop between transmem-brane regions 1 and 2 has two potential glycosylation sites and a number of phosphorylation sites are present on the intracellular loops [82].

4.2 OCT2

Another organic cation in the rat kidney is rOct2 which has 67% amino acid similar-ity to rOct1 [81,82]. In addition to its high level of expression in the basolateral membrane of S2 and S3 segments of the renal proximal tubule, rOct2 is also local-ized to brain tissue, with higher levels in the medulla than cortex. Again, however, the human ortholog, hOCT2—a 554 amino acid encoded by a gene chromosomally located at 6q26—differs in some respects from the rat transporter despite being 81% identical at the amino acid level. In particular, hOCT2 appears to expressed on the apical membrane domain of the distal renal tubule rather than basolateral, suggesting a functional role in the reabsorption of some types of cations. It has also been speculated that neuronal hOCT2 may reduce the background concentration of basic neurotransmitters and their metabolites in the brain [82].

4.3 Other Multispecific Organic Cation Transporters

Other genes capable of transporting organic cations have recently been described [81]. For example, *rOct3* and *hOCT3* have been identified and, in the rat, found to be expressed at high levels in the placenta, intestine, and brain [87]. This transporter appears to be identical to the extra neuronal monoamine transporter (uptake$_2$) that transports norepinephrine and dopamine [88]. Rabbit and murine Oct1s with 81% and 95% amino acid similarity to rOct1 have also been cloned, but, again, interspecies differences appear to be present with respect to tissue expression. A porcine Oct2 has also been cloned from a kidney cell line (LLCPK) cDNA library. NKT is also a kidney-specific gene product with 30% identity to rOct1. In addition, genes homologous to rOct1 have been reported from nonmammalian species such as *Caenorhabditis elegans* and *Drosophila melanogaster*.

A separate OCTN subfamily of organic cation transporters with only ~30% amino acid sequence similarily to the OCTs, has also been recently described. In the rat, rOctn appears to be expressed at the apical surface of the cell and is localized to the kidney, liver, and colon, where it is presumably involved in the cellular reabsorption of organic cations [89]. By contrast, the human orthologs (OCTN1/2) are widely expressed in many tissues. Little is known regarding the functional characteristics of OCTN1 other than it can transport organic cations [90,91]. This Na^+-independent characteristic is also apparently present with OCTN2; uniquely, however, OCTN2 also mediates the transport of carnitine but only in the presence of Na^+ [89,91]. This latter function in the kidney is important in the reabsorption of carnitine across the brush-border membrane of renal tubular cells. Importantly, mutations in OCTN2, primarily resulting in premature stop codons in mRNA and formation of truncated proteins, are associated with primary systemic carnitine deficiency [92–96]. On the other hand, certain of these mutations do not affect the transport of carnitine and organic cations, suggesting that the ability of mutant OCTN2s to reabsorb organic cations in the kidney, for example, may vary between patients depending on the individual mutation [89]. However, the potential pharmacologial and therapeutic relevance of OCTNs other than carnitine transport remains to be determined.

Clearly, multiple transporters capable of mediating the uptake of organic cations exist and presumably have separate physiological functions in different tissues. Some of these may be important in drug disposition, especially uptake and excretion by the liver and kidney. However, knowledge of such roles is limited.

5 FUTURE PERSPECTIVES

Over the past 5–10 years, membrane transporters have developed from a model concept to, in several instances, a fundamental understanding of the involved genes and the proteins themselves. This knowledge is not limited to the transporters described above. Other systems of pharmacological significance such as those involved in the transport of neurotransmitter amines [97,98], nucleosides [99–102], and small peptides [103] have also been identified, functionally characterized, and further defined. Such information along with the recent description of the human genome will provide a unique opportunity to define the specific roles, if any, of individual transporters in the absorption, distribution and excretion of drugs and metabolites. A similar situation followed the characterization of the individual human isoforms of the various families of xenobiotic metabolizing enzymes, like cytochrome P450s, glucuronosyltransferases, and glutathione-S-transferases. As a result of such understanding, a paradigm shift occurred in the study of human xenobiotic metabolism both in vitro and in vivo. It is probable that an analogous change will also occur with further understanding of the role and importance of transporters in drug disposition.

In addition to defining the involvement of individual transporters in the disposition of specific drugs, it will also be important to investigate whether allelic variation occurs in the transporter gene that is associated with a functional consequence. Such genetic variability already exists, for example, with MDR1, MDR3, BSEP, and MRP2 (Sects. 2.1.2, 2.1.3, 2.2, and 2.3.2), and the possibility that similar situations occur with other transporters needs to be addressed. Information is also limited with respect to the molecular determinants of the regulation and expression of essentially all proteins that transport drugs. The sequences of the 5′-promoter regions of several transporter genes indicate the presence of several putative transcription factor motifs that could be involved in up- and down-regulation, as well as tissue specific expression. However, the roles of such elements are unclear as is the possibility of modulation of transporter activity by other mechanisms such as phosphorylation/dephosphorylation. Another molecular mechanistic question that needs to be addressed relates to the substrate specificity and species-related differences in drug transporter structure and function. Similarly, factors responsible for the trafficking of transporter proteins to a specific membrane domain (e.g., basolateral vs. apical) need to be determined.

It will also be important to better understand the functional interactions between different transporters. This is particularly relevant to the situation where, for example, a drug is a substrate for multiple transporters several of which may be expressed in the same cell and mediate transport in a vectorial fashion or in the same membrane domain and have different directional properties, i.e., uptake versus efflux.

Finally, there is the likelihood that these and other advances in the understanding of transporters will result in the improved design and development of new drugs or strategies to exploit such knowledge in order to improve therapeutics. Efforts to modulate MDR1 activity in order to enhance absorption, or to alter distribution to target sites like, for example, tumor cells and the brain, or to reduce exposure and protect critical tissues from toxic drug effects, such as hematopoetic, cells indicate the potential for application of this type of understanding. Undoubtedly drug transporters will remain an exciting and important area of research for many additional years.

REFRENCES

1. RA Clayton, O White, KA Ketchum, JC Venter. The first genome from the third domain of life. Nature 387:459–462, 1997.
2. J Griffith, C Sansom. The Transporter FactBook. New York: Academic Press, 1997.
3. SV Ambudkar, MM Gottesman, eds. ABC Transporters: Biochemical, Cellular and Molecular Aspects. Methods in Enzymology, Vol. 292. London: Academic Press, 1998.
4. I Klein, B Sarkadi, A Váradi. An inventory of the human ABC proteins. Biochim Biophys Acta 1461:237–262, 1999.
5. R Abele, R Tampé. Function of the transport complex TAP in cellular immune recognition. Biochim Biophys Acta 1461:405–419, 1999.
6. SV Ambudkar, S Dey, CA Hrycyna, M Ramachandra, I Pastan, MM Gottesman. Biochemical, cellular, and pharmacological aspects of the multidrug transporter. Annu Rev Pharmacol Toxicol 39:361–398, 1999.
7. MM Gottesman, CA Hrycyna, PV Schoenlein, UA Germann, I Pastan. Genetic analysis of the multidrug transporter. Annu Rev Genet 29:607–649, 1995.
8. VJ Wacher, C-Y Wu, LZ Benet. Overlapping substrate specificities and tissue distribution of cytochrome P4503A and P-glycoprotein: implications for drug delivery and activity in cancer chemotherapy. Mol Carcinogen 13:129–134, 1995.
9. RB Kim, C Wandel, B Leake, M Cvetkovic, MF Fromm, PJ Dempsey, MM Roden, F Belas, AK Chaudhary, DM Roden, AJ Wood, GR Wilkinson Interrelationship between substrates and inhibitors of human CYP3A and P-glycoprotein. Pharm Res 16:408–414, 1999.
10. EG Schuetz, WT Beck, and JD Schuetz. Modulators and substrates of P-glycoprotein and cytochrome P4503A coordinately up-regulate these proteins in human colon carcinoma cells. Mol Pharmacol 49:311–318, 1996.
11. R Preiss. P-glycoprotein and related transporters. Int J Clin Pharmacol Ther 36: 3–8, 1998.
12. UA Germann, TC Chambers, SV Ambudkar, T Licht, CO Cardarelli, I Pastan, MM Gottesman. Characterization of phosphorylation-defective mutants of human P-glycoprotein expressed in mammalian cells. J Biol Chem 271:1708–1716, 1996.

13. MM Gottesman, SV Ambudkar, MM Cornwell, I Pastan, UA Germann. Multidrug resistance transporter. In: SG Schultz, TE Andreoli, A Brown, D Fambrugh, J Hoffman, MJ Welsh, eds. Molecular Biology of Membrane Transporter Disorders. New York: Plenum Press, 1996, pp 243–257.

14. DR Umbenhauer, GR Lankas, TR Pippert, LD Wise, ME Cartwright, SJ Hall, CM Beare. Identification of a P-glycoprotein-deficient subpopulation in the CF-1 mouse strain using a restriction fragment length polymorphism. Toxicol Appl Pharmacol 146:88–94, 1997.

15. TR Pippert, DR Umbenhauer. The subpopulation of CF-1 mice deficient in P-glycoprotein contains a murine retroviral insertion in the *mdr1a* gene. J Biochem Mol Toxicol, in press.

16. AJ Paul, WJ Tranquilli, RL Seward, KS Todd, JA DiPietro. Clinical observations in collies given ivermectin orally. Am J Vet Res 48:684–685, 1987.

17. S Hoffmeyer, O Burk, O von Richter, HP Arnold, J Bröckmoller, A Johne, I Cascorbi, T Gerloff, I Roots, M Eichelbaum, U Brinkmann. Functional polymorphisms of the human multidrug-resistance gene: multiple sequence variations and correlation of one allele with P-glycoprotein expression and activity in vivo. Proc Natl Acad Sci USA 97:3473–3478, 2000.

18. RB Kim, B Leake, E Choo, GK Dresser, SV Kubba, U Schwarz, A Taylor, H-G Xie, CM Stein, AJJ Wood, J McKinsey, EG Schuetz, JD Schuetz, GR Wilkinson. Identification of functionally important MDR1 variant alleles among African-American and Caucasian subjects. Drug Metab Rev 32:199, 2000.

19. MM Gottesman, I Pastan. Biochemistry of multidrug resistance mediated by the multidrug transporter. Annu Rev Biochem 62:385–427, 1993.

20. F Thiebaut, T Tsuruo, H Hamada, MM Gottesman, I Pastan, MC Willingham. Cellular localization of the multidrug-resistance gene product P-glycoprotein in normal human tissues. Proc Natl Acad Sci USA 84:7735–7738, 1987.

20a. J Konig, Y Cui, AT Nies, D Keppler. Localization and genomic organization of a new hepatocellular organic anion transporting polypeptide. J Biol Chem 275: 23161–23168, 2000.

21. VJ Wacher, L Salphati, LZ Benet. Active secretion and enterocytic drug metabolism barriers to drug absorption. Adv Drug Del Rev 20:99–112, 1996.

22. AH Schinkel. P-glycoprotein, a gatekeeper in the blood-brain barrier. Adv Drug Del Rev 36:179–194, 1999.

23. AH Schinkel, JJM Smit, O van Tellingen, JH Beijnen, E Wagenaar, L van Deemter, CAAM Mol, MA van der Valk, EC Robanus-Maandag, HPJ Riele, AJM Berns, P Borst. Disruption of the mouse mdr1a P-glycoprotein gene leads to a deficiency in the blood-brain barrier and to increased sensitivity to drugs. Cell 77:491–502, 1994.

24. AH Schinkel, U Mayer, E Wagenaar, CAAM Mol, L van Deemter, JJM Smit, MA van der Valk, AC Voordouw, H Spits, O van Tellingen, JMJM Zijlmans, WE Fibbe, P Borst. Normal viability and altered pharmacokinetics in mice lacking mdr1-type (drug-transporting) P-glycoproteins. Proc Natl Acad Sci USA 94:4028–4033, 1997.

25. AH Schinkel, E Wagenaar, L van Deemter, CAAM Mol, P Borst. Absence of the mdr1a P-glycoprotein in mice affects tissue distribution and pharmacokinet-

ics of dexamethasone, digoxin, and cyclosporin A. J Clin Invest 96:1698–1705, 1995.

26. GY Kwei, RF Alvaro, Q Chen, HJ Jenkins, CEAC Hop, CA Keohane, VT Ly, JR Strauss, RW Wang, Z Wang, TR Pippert, DR Umbenhauer. Disposition of ivermectin and cyclosporin A in CF-1 mice deficient in mdr1a P-glycoprotein. Drug Metab Dispos 27:581–587, 1999.

27. RB Kim, MF Fromm, C Wandel, B Leake, AJJ Wood, DM Roden, GR Wilkinson. The drug transporter P-glycoprotein limits oral absorption and brain entry of HIV-1 protease inhibitors. J Clin Invest 101:289–294, 1998.

28. AH Schinkel, E Wagenaar, CAAM Mol, L van Deemter. P-glycoprotein in the blood-brain barrier of mice influences the brain penetration and pharmacological activity of many drugs. J Clin Invest 97:2517–2524, 1996.

29. GR Lankas, LD Wise, ME Cartwright, T Pippert, DR Umbenhauer. Placental P-glycoprotein deficiency enhances susceptibility to chemically induced birth defects in mice. Reprod Toxicol 12:457–463, 1998.

30. JW Smit, MT Huisman, O van Tellingen, HR Wiltshire, AH Schinkel. Absence or pharmacological blocking of placental P-glycoprotein profoundly increases fetal drug exposure. J Clin Invest 104:1441–1447, 1999.

31. JM Ford. Experimental reversal of P-glycoprotein-mediated multidrug resistance by pharmacological chemosensitisers. Eur J Cancer 32A:991–1001, 1996.

32. DR Ferry. Testing the role of P-glycoprotein expression in clinical trials–applying pharmacological principles and best methods for detection together with good clinical trials methodology. Int J Clin Pharmacol Ther 36:29–40, 1998.

33. V Fischer, A Rodriguez-Gascon, F Heitz, R Tynes, C Hauck, D Cohen, AE Vickers. The multidrug resistance modulator valspodar (PSC 833) is metabolized by human cytochrome P4503A. Implications for drug-drug interactions and pharmacological activity of the main metabolite. Drug Metab Dispos 26:802–811, 1998.

34. EF Choo, B Leake, C Wandel, H Imamura, AJJ Wood, GR Wilkinson, RB Kim. Pharmacological inhibition of P-glycoprotein transport enhances the distribution of HIV-1 protease inhibitors into brain and testes. Drug Metab Dispos 28:665–670, 2000.

35. A van Helvoort, AJ Smith, H Sprong, I Fritzsche, AH Schinkel, P Borst, G van Meer. MDR1 P-glycoprotein is a lipid translocase of broad specificity, while MDR3 P-glycoprotein specifically translocates phosphatidylcholine. Cell 87:507–517, 1996.

36. JJ Smit, AH Schinkel, RPJ Oude Elferink, AK Groen, E Wagenaar, L van Deemter, CAAM Mol, R Ottenhoff, NMT van der Lugt, MA van Roon, MA van der Valk, GJA Offerhaus, AJM Berns, P Borst. Homozygous disrupting of the murine mdr2 P-glycoprotein gene leads to a complete absence of phospholipid from bile and to liver disease. Cell 75:451–462, 1993.

37. JF Deleuze, E Jacquemin, C Dubuisson, D Cresteil, M Dumont, S Erlinger, O Bernard, M Hadchouel. Defect of multidrug-resistance 3 gene expression in a subtype of progressive familial intrahepatic cholestasis. Hepatology 23:904–908, 1996.

38. JM de Vree, E Jacquemin, E Sturm, D Cresteil, PJ Bosma, J Aten, JF Deleuze, M Desrochers, M Burdelski, O Bernard, RPJ Oude Elferink, M Hadchouel. Mutations

in the MDR3 gene cause progressive familial intrahepatic cholestasis. Proc Natl Acad Sci USA 95:282–287, 1998.

39. E Jacquemin, D Cresteil, S Manouvrier, O Boute, M Hadchouel. Heterozygous nonsense mutation of the *MDR3* gene in familial intrahepatic cholestasis of pregnancy. Lancet 353:210–211, 1999.

40. M Trauner, PJ Meier, JL Boyer. Molecular regulation of hepatocellular transport systems in cholestasis. J Hepatol 31:165–178, 1999.

41. SS Strautnieks, LN Bull, AS Knisely, SA Kocoshis, N Dahl, H Arnell, E Sokal, K Dahan, S Childs, V Ling, MS Tanner, AF Kagalwalla, A Nemeth, J Pawlowska, A Baker, G Mieli-Vergani, NB Freimer, RM Gardiner, RJ Thompson. A gene encoding a liver-specific ABC transporter is mutated in progressive familial intrahepatic cholestasis. Nat Genet 20:233–238, 1998.

42. SPC Cole, G Bhardwaj, J Gerlach, J Mackie, C Grant, K Almquist, A Stewart, E Kurz, A Duncan, R Deeley. Overexpression of a transporter gene in a multidrug-resistant human lung cancer cell line. Science 258:1650–1654, 1992.

43. ML Slovak, JP Ho, G Bhardwaj, EU Kurz, RG Deeley, SP Cole. Localization of a novel multidrug resistance-associated gene in the HT1080/DR4 and H69AR human tumor cell lines. Cancer Res 53:3221–3225, 1993.

44. DR Hipfner, RG Deeley, SP Cole. Structural, mechanistic and clinical aspects of MRP1. Biochim Biophys Acta 1461:359–376, 1999.

45. P Borst, R Evers, M Kool, J Wijnholds. The multidrug resistance protein family. Biochim Biophys Acta 1461:347–357, 1999.

46. J König, AT Nies, Y Cui, I Leier, D Keppler. Conjugate export pumps of the multidrug resistance protein (MRP) family: localization, substrate specificity, and MRP2-mediated drug resistance. Biochim Biophys Acta 1461:377–394, 1999.

47. Q Zhu, MS Center. Cloning and sequence analysis of the promoter region of the MRP gene of HL60 cells isolated for resistance to adriamycin. Cancer Res 54:4488–4492, 1994.

48. Q Wang, WT Beck. Transcriptional suppression of multidrug resistance-associated protein (MRP) gene expression by wild-type p53. Cancer Res 58:5762–5769, 1998.

49. L Ma, N Krishnamachary, MS Center. Phosphorylation of the multidrug resistance associated protein gene encoded protein P190. Biochemistry 34:3338–3343, 1995.

50. VV Rao, JL Dahlheimer, ME Bardgett, AZ Snyder, RA Finch, AC Sartorelli, D Piwnica-Worms. Choroid plexus epithelial expression of MDR1 P glycoprotein and multidrug resistance-associated protein contribute to the blood-cerebrospinal-fluid drug-permeability barrier. Proc Natl Acad Sci USA 96:3900–3905, 1999.

51. J Wijnholds, EC deLange, GL Scheffer, DJ van den Berg, CAAM Mol, M van der Valk, AH Schinkel, RJ Scheper, DD Breimer, P Borst. Multidrug resistance protein 1 protects the choroid plexus epithelium and contributes to the blood-cerebrospinal fluid barrier. J Clin Invest 105:279–285, 2000.

52. J Wijnholds, GL Scheffer, M van der Valk, P van der Valk, JH Beijnen, RJ Scheper, P Borst. Multidrug resistance protein 1 protects the oropharyngeal mucosal layer and the testicular tubules against drug-induced damage. J Exp Med 188:797–808, 1998.

53. J Wijnholds, R Evers, MR Van Leusden, CAAM Mol, GJR Zaman, U Mayer, JH

Beijnen, M Vandervalk, P Krimpenfort, P Borst. Increased sensitivity to anti-cancer drugs and decreased inflammatory response in mice lacking the multidrug resistance-associated protein. Nat Med 3:1275–1279, 1997.

54. CC Paulusma, PJ Bosma, GJR Zaman, CTM Bakker, M Otter, GL Scheffer, RJ Scheper, P Borst, RPJ Oude Elferink. Congenital jaundice in rats with a mutation in a multidrug resistance-associated protein gene. Science 271:1126–1128, 1996.

55. J Kartenbeck, U Leuschner, R Mayer, D Keppler. Absence of the canalicular iso-form of the MRP gene-encoded conjugate export pump from the hepatocytes in Dubin-Johnson syndrome. Hepatology 23:1061–1066, 1996.

56. M Wada, S Toh, K Taniguchi, T Nakamura, T Uchiumi, K Kohno, I Yoshida, A Kimura, S Sakisaka, Y Adachi, M Kuwano. Mutations in the canilicular multispe-cific organic anion transporter (cMOAT) gene, a novel ABC transporter, in patients with hyperbilirubinemia II/Dubin-Johnson syndrome. Hum Mol Genet 7:203–207, 1998.

57. S Kajihara, A Hisatomi, T Mizuta, T Hara, I Ozaki, I Wada, K Yamamoto. A splice mutation in the human canalicular multispecific organic anion transporter gene causes Dubin-Johnson syndrome. Biochem Biophys Res Commun 253:454–457, 1998.

58. MF Fromm, B Leake, DM Roden, GR Wilkinson, RB Kim. Human MRP3 trans-porter: identification of the 5′-flanking region, genomic organization and alternative splice variants. Biochim Biophys Acta 1415:369–374, 1999.

59. DF Ortiz, S Li, R Iyer, X Zhang, P Novikoff, IM Arias. MRP3, a new ATP-binding cassette protein localized to the canalicular domain of the hepatocyte. Am J Physiol 276:G1493–G1500, 1999.

60. JD Schuetz, MC Connelly, D Sun, SG Paibir, PM Flynn, RV Srinivas, A Kumar, A Fridland. MRP4: a previously unidentified factor in resistance to nucleoside-based antiviral drugs. Nat Med 5:1048–1051, 1999.

61. J Bryan, L Aguilar-Bryan. Sulfonylurea receptors: ABC transporters that regulate ATP-sensitive K(+) channels. Biochim Biophys Acta 1461:285–303, 1999.

62. PM Thomas, GJ Cote, N Wohllk, B Haddad, PM Mathew, W Rabl, L Aguilar-Bryan, RF Gagel, J Bryan. Mutations in the sulfonylurea receptor gene in fam-ilial persistent hyperinsulinemic hypoglycemia of infancy. Science 268:426–429, 1995.

63. T Jilling, KL Kirk. The biogenesis, traffic, and function of the cystic fibrosis trans-membrane conductance regulator. Int Rev Cytol 172:193–241, 1997.

64. LA Doyle, W Yang, LV Abruzzo, T Krogmann, Y Gao, AK Rishi, DD Ross. A multidrug resistance transporter from human MCF-7 breast cancer cells. Proc Natl Acad Sci USA 95:15665–15670, 1998.

65. R Allikmets, LM Schriml, A Hutchinson, V Romano-Spica, M Dean. A human placenta-specific ATP-binding cassette gene (*ABCP*) on chromosome 4q22 that is involved in multidrug resistance. Cancer Res 58:5337–5339, 1998.

66. K Miyake, L Mickley, T Litman, Z Zhan, R Robey, B Cristensen, M Brangi, L Greenberger, M Dean, T Fojo, SE Bates. Molecular cloning of cDNAs which are highly overexpressed in mitoxantrone-resistant cells: demonstration of homology to ABC transport genes. Cancer Res 59:8–13, 1999.

67. JD Allen, RF Brinkhuis, J Wijnholds, AH Schinkel. The mouse *Bcrp1/Mxr/Abcp* gene: amplification and overexpression in cell lines selected for resistance to topotecan, mitoxantrone, or doxorubicin. Cancer Res 59:4237–4241, 1999.

68. M Maliepaard, MA van Gastelen, LA de Jong, D Pluim, RC van Waardenburg, MC Ruevekamp-Helmers, BG Floot, JH Schellens. Overexpression of the *BCRP/MXR/ABCP* gene in a topotecan-selected ovarian tumor cell line. Cancer Res 59: 4559–4563, 1999.

69. M Müller, PLM Jansen. The secretory function of the liver—new aspects of hepatobiliary transport. J Hepatol 28:344–354, 1998.

70. GA Kullak-Ublick. Regulation of organic anion and drug transporters of the sinusoidal membrane. J Hepatol 31:563–573, 1999.

71. JE van Montfoort, B Hagenbuch, KE Fattinger, M Müller, GM Groothuis, DK Meijer, PJ Meier. Polyspecific organic anion transporting polypeptides mediate hepatic uptake of amphipathic type II organic cations. J Pharmacol Exp Ther 291: 147–152, 1999.

72. X Bossuyt, M Müller, B Hagenbuch, PJ Meier. Polyspecific drug and steroid clearance by an organic anion transporter of mammalian liver. J Pharmacol Exp Ther 276:891–896, 1996.

73. T Abe, M Kakyo, T Tokui, R Nakagomi, T Nishio, D Nakai, H Nomura, M Unno, M Suzuki, T Naitoh, S Matsuno, H Yawo. Identification of a novel gene family encoding human liver-specific organic anion transporter LST-1. J Biol Chem 274: 17159–17163, 1999.

74. GA Kullak-Ublick, U Beuers, PJ Meier, H Domdey, G Paumgartner. Assignment of the human organic anion transporting polypeptide (OATP) gene to chromosome 12p12 by fluorescence *in situ* hybridization. J Hepatol 25:985–987, 1996.

75. B Gao, B Stieger, B Noé, JM Fritschy, PJ Meier. Localization of the organic anion transporting polypeptide 2 (Oatp2) in capillary endothelium and choroid plexus epithelium of rat brain. J Histochem Cytochem 47:1255–1264, 1999.

76. B Hsiang, Y Zhu, Z Wang, Y Wu, V Sasseville, WP Yang, TG Kirchgessner. A novel human hepatic organic anion transporting polypeptide (OATP2). Identification of a liver-specific human organic anion transporting polypeptide and identification of rat and human hydroxymethylglutaryl-CoA reductase inhibitor transporters. J Biol Chem 274:37161–37168, 1999.

77. M Kakyo, M Unno, T Tokui, R Nakagomi, T Nishio, H Iwasashi, D Nakai, M Seki, M Suzuki, T Naitoh, S Matsuno, H Yawo, T Abe. Molecular characterization and functional regulation of a novel rat liver-specific organic anion transporter rlst-1. Gastroenterology 117:770–775, 1999.

78. H Saito, S Masuda, K Inui. Cloning and functional characterization of a novel rat organic anion transporter mediating basolateral uptake of methotrexate in the kidney. J Biol Chem 271:20719–20725, 1996.

79. N Kanai, R Lu, JA Satriano, Y Bao, AW Wolkoff, VL Schuster. Identification and characterization of a prostaglandin transporter. Science 268:866–869, 1995.

80. GMM Groothuis DKF Meijer. Drug traffic in the hepatobiliary system. J Hepatol 24(Suppl 1):3–28, 1996.

81. L Zhang, CM Brett, KM Giacomini. Role of organic cation transporters in drug absorption and elimination. Annu Rev Pharmacol Toxicol 38:431–460, 1998.

82. H Koepsell. Organic cation transporters in intestine, kidney, liver, and brain. Annu Rev Physiol 60:243–66:243–266, 1998.

83. D Gründemann, V Gorboulev, S Gambaryan, M Veyhl, H Koepsell. Drug excretion mediated by a new prototype of polyspecific transporter. Nature 372:549–552, 1994.

84. L Zhang, MJ Dresser, AT Gray, SC Yost, S Terashita, KM Giacomini. Cloning and functional expression of a human liver organic cation transporter. Mol Pharmacol 51:913–921, 1997.

85. V Gorboulev, JC Ulzheimer, A Akhoundova, I Ulzheimer-Teuber, U Karbach, S Quester, C Baumann, F Lang, AE Busch, H Koepsell. Cloning and characterization of two human polyspecific organic cation transporters. DNA Cell Biol 16:871–881, 1997.

86. MJ Dresser, AT Gray, KM Giacomini. Kinetic and selectivity differences between rodent, rabbit, and human organic cation transporters (OCT1). J Pharmacol Exp Ther 292:1146–1152, 2000.

87. R Kekuda, PD Prasad, X Wu, H Wang, YJ Fei, FH Leibach, V Ganapathy. Cloning and functional characterization of a potential-sensitive, polyspecific organic cation transporter (OCT3) most abundantly expressed in placenta. J Biol Chem 273: 15971–15979, 1998.

88. X Wu, R Kekuda, W Huang, YJ Fei, FH Leibach, J Chen, SJ Conway, V Ganapathy. Identity of the organic cation transporter OCT3 as the extraneuronal monoamine transporter (uptake$_2$) and evidence for the expression of the transporter in the brain. J Biol Chem 273:32776–32786, 1998.

89. X Wu, W Huang, PD Prasad, P Seth, DP Rajan, FH Leibach, J Chen, SJ Conway, V Ganapathy. Functional characteristics and tissue distribution pattern of organic cation transporter 2 (OCTN2), an organic cation/carnitine transporter. J Pharmacol Exp Ther 290:1482–1492, 1999.

90. H Yabuuchi, I Tamai, J Nezu, K Sakamoto, A Oku, M Shimane, Y Sai, A Tsuji. Novel membrane transporter OCTN1 mediates multispecific, bidirectional, and pH-dependent transport of organic cations. J Pharmacol Exp Ther 289:768–773, 1999.

91. I Tamai, H Yabuuchi, J Nezu, Y Sai, A Oku, M Shimane, A Tsuji. Cloning and characterization of a novel human pH-dependent organic cation transporter, OCTN1. FEBS Lett 419:107–111, 1997.

92. AM Lamhonwah, I Tein. Carnitine uptake defect: frameshift mutations in the human plasmalemmal carnitine transporter gene. Biochem Biophys Res Commun 252:396–401, 1998.

93. NL Tang, V Ganapathy, X Wu, J Hui, P Seth, PM Yuen, RJ Wanders, TF Fok, NM Hjelm. Mutatons of *OCTN2*, an organic cation/carnitine transporter, lead to deficient cellular carnitine uptake in primary carnitine deficiency [published erratum appears in Hum Mol Genet 8:943, 1999]. Hum Mol Genet 8:655–660, 1999.

94. Y Wang, J Ye, V Ganapathy, N Longo. Mutations in the organic cation/carnitine transporter OCTN2 in primary carnitine deficiency. Proc Natl Acad Sci USA 96: 2356–2360, 1999.

95. J Nezu, I Tamai, A Oku, R Ohashi, H Yabuuchi, N Hashimoto, H Nikaido, Y Sai, A Koizumi, Y Shoji, G Takada, T Matsuishi, M Yoshino, H Kato, T Ohura, G Tsujimoto, J Hayakawa, M Shimane, A Tsuji. Primary systemic carnitine defi-

ciency is caused by mutations in a gene encoding sodium ion-dependent carnitine transporter. Nat Genet 21:91–94, 1999.

96. K Lu, H Nishimori, Y Nakamura, K Shima, M Kuwajima. A missense mutation of mouse OCTN2, a sodium-dependent carnitine cotransporter, in the juvenile visceral steatosis mouse. Biochem Biophys Res Commun 252:590–594, 1998.

97. MEA Reith, ed. Neurotransmitter Transporters: Structure, Function, and Regulation. Totowa, NJ: Humana Press, 1997.

98. SG Amara, ed. Neurotransmitter Transporters. Methods in Enzymology, Vol. 296. London: Academic Press, 1998.

99. V Balimane, PJ Sinko. Involvement of multiple transporters in the oral absorption of nucleoside analogues. Adv Drug Del Rev 39:183–209, 1999.

100. ME Schaner, KM Gerstin, J Wang, KM Giacomini. Mechanisms of transport of nucleosides and nucleoside analogues in choroid plexus. Adv Drug Del Rev 39: 51–62, 1999.

101. CE Cass, JD Young, SA Baldwin, MA Cabrita, KA Graham, M Griffiths, LL Jennings, JR Mackey, AM Ng, MW Ritzel, MF Vickers, SY Yao. Nucleoside transporters of mammalian cells. Pharm Biotechnol 12:313–52:313–352, 1999.

102. CE Cass, JD Young, SA Baldwin. Recent advances in the molecular biology of nucleoside transporters of mammalian cells. Biochem Cell Biol 76:761–770, 1998.

103. CY Yang, AH Dantzig, C Pidgeon. Intestinal peptide transport systems and oral drug availability. Pharm Res 16:1331–1343, 1999.

6

Interethnic Differences in Drug Response

Werner Kalow
University of Toronto, Toronto, Ontario, Canada

1 INTRODUCTION

Attention to interethnic differences has become a major aspect of pharmacogenetics [1–8], stimulated by studies of drug response and toxicity in various human populations who differed in their response, even when taking usually well-tolerated doses of some common therapeutic chemicals. The purpose of this chapter is to indicate essential elements of this broad topic, and to provide examples of some of its important aspects.

When pharmacogenetic studies started, very little was known about the genes responsible for either intraindividual or interethnic differences. In fact, nobody knew for sure whether or not most of the interethnic differences had a genetic or a cultural basis; within a population, family or twin studies can easily show that a trait is genetic. However, the evidence that a trait is genetically controlled in one population does not prove that differences between populations are genetic. Many people did simply not believe that population differences were genetic; they did not want to be racists. They used words like ''cross-cultural'' or similar terms as an expression of their beliefs. It is only the rise of modern methods to study genes that established clearly the genetic basis of many interethnic differences of pharmacogenetics.

In short, differences in drug response between human populations first drew attention four or five decades ago. However, because of the initial methodological shortcomings, the science of interethnic pharmacogenetics is in a strict sense only 20–30 years old.

2 FUNDAMENTAL QUESTIONS

2.1 What Is Ethnicity?

Not too long ago, ethnic groups or races were defined by geography and appearance, most often simply by skin color, sometimes additionally by language. These factors are still considered by many people as main indicators, but at the present time, the scientifically defining factors are genetic differences between populations.

It is true that the majority of genes in different human populations are identical. Nevertheless, it would be wrong and inappropriate to take this overall similarity as an opportunity to disavow the medical importance of interethnic divisions of the human species.

A revolutionary book by Masatoshi Nei [9] entitled *Molecular Evolutionary Genetics* divided populations by their genetic diversities. More recently (1994), this work has been greatly extended, mostly confirmed but with some changes, by Cavalli-Sforza et al. [10] in a book entitled *The History and Geography of Human Genes*. These authors tested 120 allele frequencies in 42 human populations. They calculated from these measurements genetic distances between the populations and estimated the times of their separation. They summarized their data, and thus constructed nine population clusters (Fig. 1). The greatest differences were between African and all non-African populations, in support of the theory that all human beings derived from a wave of emigrants who left Africa ~100,000 years ago.

An interesting point in this figure is the indication that the separation between southeast and northeast Asians (~50,000 years ago) is older than that between northeast Asians and Europeans (~40,000 years ago). Most Chinese are northeast Asians while Japanese and Koreans are southeast Asians. Hence drug tests comparing Japanese and Koreans tend to be more similar than the equivalent comparisons between Japanese and Chinese.

It is largely a matter of economic and cultural factors that we know more about pharmacogenetic differences between Caucasian and Asian populations than between these and African populations. Data obtained with African-Americans must be interpreted as having a Caucasian admixture of approximately 30%; African populations are not a uniform group and often differ substantially from one another.

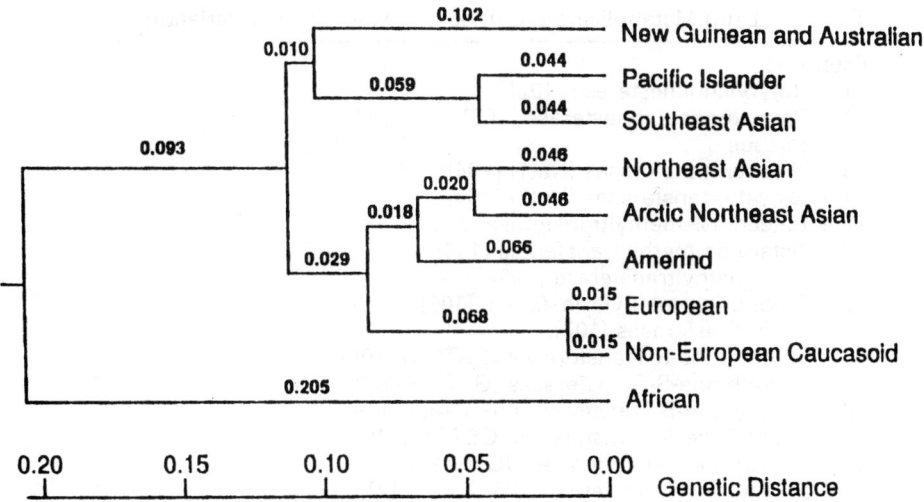

FIGURE 1 Linkage tree. Analysis of nine population clusters, condensed from data obtained by studying 42 populations. The genetic distance 0.2 represents approximately 150,000 years. (From Ref. 10.)

2.2 Individual and Ethnic Differences in Drug Metabolism

As time went on, it became more and more clear that many genetic variations of drug metabolising enzymes that determine inter-individual differences of drug clearance, also show differences between populations. There are two possible kinds of difference: First, it is an almost universal observation that the frequency of a polymorphism is found to differ between populations. Of the numerous drug-metabolising enzymes that show pharmacogenetic variation between individuals, at least 77% show an interethnic difference of variant frequency (Table 1). In many or most cases for which no inter-ethnic difference is on record, such difference has not yet been searched for; the class 2 glucuronosyl transferases are clear-cut examples because their genetic variants are relatively new observations [11]. In any case, one can say with assurance that interindividual differences of drug-metabolizing enzymes are usually paralleled by interethnic differences in allele frequencies.

Second, there are often different variants in different populations; some phenotypic consequences of CYP2D6 variations are shown as an example in Figure 2 [1]. There is a lower average enzyme activity in both Chinese and Africans than in Europeans. These differences in activity represent structural changes of the CYP2D6 protein that affect enzyme function. However, the enzyme struc-

TABLE 1   Drug Metabolising Enzymes Showing Genetic Variation*

Esterases
  1 + Butyrylcholinesterase [102]
  2 + Paraoxonase/arylesterase [103]
Transferases
  3 + N-acetyltransferases (Nat1) [104]
  4 + N-acetyltransferases (Nat2) [104]
  5 + Catechol-0-methyltransferase [105]
  6 0 Histamine methyltransferase [106]
  7 0 Thiol methyltransferase [106]
  8 + Thiopurine methyltransferase [106]
  9 + Sulfotransferases [107]
10 + Glutathione-S-Transferases (GSTM1) [108]
11 + Glutathione-S-Transferases (GSTT1) [108]
12 0 Glutathione-S-Transferases (GSTM3) [109]
13 0 Glutathione-S-Transferases (GSTP1) [110]
14 + Glucuronosyltransferase (UGT1A1) [111]
15 0 Glucuronosyltransferase (UGT2B4) [112]
16 0 Glucuronosyltransferase (UGT2B7) [113]
17 0 Glucuronosyltransferase (UGT2B15) [114]
18 + Amobarbital-glucosyltransferase [115]
Reductases
19 + NAD (P) H:quinone oxidoreductase [116]
20 + Glucose-6-phosphate dehydrogenase [117]
21 0 Epoxide hydrolase, microsomal [118]
Oxidases
22 + Alcohol dehydrogenase, class 1, *ADH2* (β) [119]
23 + Alcohol dehydrogenase, class 1, *ADH3* (Γ) [119]
24 + Aldehyde dehydrogenase, mitochondrial [120]
25 0 Monoamine oxidase A [121]
26 0 Monoamine oxidase B [121]
27 + Catalase [122]
28 + Superoxide dismutase [123]
29 + Trimethylamine N-oxidase [124]
30 + Dihydropyrimidine dehydrogenase [125]
Cytochromes P450
31 + CYP1A1 [126]
32 + CYP1A2 [127]
33 + CYP2A6 [128]
34 0 CYP2B6 [129]
35 0 CYP2C8 [130]
36 0 CYP2C9 [131]
37 + CYP2C18 [132]
38 + CYP2C19 [133]
39 + CYP2D6 [134]
40 0 CYP2E1 [135]
41 + CYP3A4 [136]
42 + CYP3A5 [137]

---

* A pharmacogenetic list of variable enzymes, marked + if the occurrence of interethnic differences in variant frequency is known. ("0" usually means absence of interethnic comparisons.)

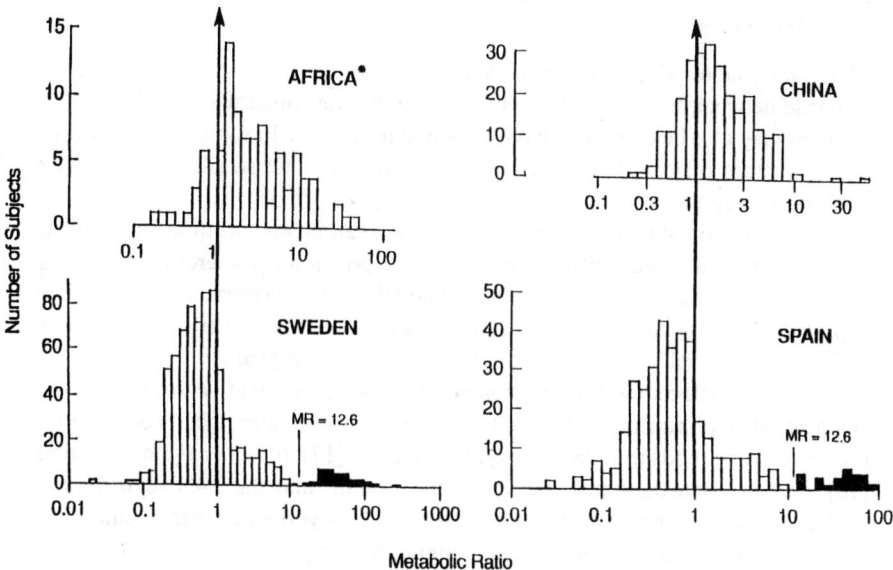

FIGURE 2 Frequency distributions of debrisoquine metabolic ratios (MR) in four populations. An alignment of data from four separate studies. The abscissa indicates on a logarithmic scale the metabolic ratio debrisoquine/4-OH-debrisoquine in urine after administration of a test dose of debrisoquine; these are conventional plots in which the increasing ratios reflect decreasing metabolism. The black bars indicate subjects classified as genetically poor metabolizers, usually defined as subjects with a metabolic ratio >12.6. Each of the four inserts represents an adaptation of a published illustration so that their abscissas are comparable and aligned for metabolic ratios of unity. The insert marked China represents a study of 269 Han [98]; Africa, a study of 92 Venda [99]; Sweden, a study of 752 Swedes [100]; and Spain, a study of 377 Spaniards [101]. The entry for Africa is marked with an asterisk because it represents tribal data of unknown generality. The measurements from China and Sweden were comparable, as assured by controls. (From Ref. 1.)

tures that cause the lower activities are different in the Chinese [12] and in the African populations [13]. It is an independent fact that enzyme absence is more rare in Asians and Africans than in Europeans [5].

2.3 Not All Interethnic Differences in Drug Response Are Genetic

While this chapter aims to describe genetic factors that cause differences in drug response between human populations, one should not forget that population differences may also be caused by environmental influences. In some cases, environmental factors may be increased by genetic variants that should not be called pharmacogenetic.

As pointed out by Anderson et al. [14], starvation, malnutrition, and protein deficiency may all cause differences in drug disposition and thereby differences of drug action. Even relatively minor food deficiencies as observed in Berlin after World War II [15] caused some unusual reactions, e.g., death from injection of the old and generally safe local anesthetic drug procain [16].

Climate affects food production and is thus a factor that determines ethnic characteristics of nutrition. Different food intakes may cause differences in drug response: some foods may cause enzyme induction [17], others enzyme inhibition [18]. In this context, it may be worth mentioning that the P450 cytochrome CYP2A6, which metabolizes nicotine [19] and which varies between populations, does cause interethnic differences in smoking habits [20]; since cigarette smoking causes enzyme induction, there must be population differences of drug-metabolizing capacity on that basis.

In some African and Polynesian populations, cardiovascular diseases often have other biochemical causes than in Caucasians. Different drug responses to these diseases may therefore have pathological rather than pharmacogenetic causes [21,22].

Also, cultural differences exist. There are population differences in attitude toward disease and cure [23]. These could affect compliance and perception of therapeutic benefits, and thereby psychologically influence the responsiveness to drug therapy. In Western medicine, the occurrence of placebo effects are well documented; this is the name for imagined effects occurring when people are fooled into thinking that they had a drug while they were given only a little sugar or other fake.

Thus, while most interethnic differences in drug response are now known to have a genetic basis, it would be wrong to assume automatically that there must be a genetic cause.

3 SOME SPECIFIC EXAMPLES

A good understanding of the pharmacogenetic features of interethnic differences in drug-metabolizing enzymes should be obtainable by careful consideration of data obtained with some widely studied enzymes. We will therefore present some pertinent data of two P450 cytochromes in human liver, of the N-acetyltransferases, of G-6-PD deficiency enzymes, and of the ethanol-metabolizing enzymes. These should serve to illustrate principles and difficulties encountered by the student of interethnic pharmacogenetics, but there will be no attempt to provide a comprehensive overview over the many existing examples.

3.1 The P450 Cytochromes

As indicated in Table 1, differences between human populations are known for at least eight P450 cytochromes. Particularly well documented are the data for CYP2D6 and for CYP2C19. These will be briefly reviewed in the following paragraphs; they show instructive differences and similarities. In pharmacogenetics, the last named of these two enzymes is the most investigated of all; the Medline quotes 1477 publications on this topic.

3.1.1 CYP2D6

Mutations in CYP2D6 may lead to three kinds of functional changes: absence, decrease, or increase of enzyme activity. Lack of enzyme activity indicates in most cases a frameshift mutation or a splicing defect, but there is also a case of totally missing enzyme formation. Decreases of enzyme activity indicate a change of enzyme structure; these can be clinically treacherous since the decrease may differ in severity for different sustrates. Enhanced enzyme activity usually indicates gene duplication, sometimes multiplication; a case of 13-fold multiplication has been observed. Every one of these enzyme changes may differ among human populations.

Marez et al. [24] described 48 different DNA variants in human CYP2D6, leading to 53 different alleles, which means that some alleles contain several DNA changes. Daly et al. [25] developed a rational nomenclature for CYP2D6 variants, and they also indicated the biochemical changes characterizing each variant. Lack of enzyme activity occurs with a high frequency of ~7% in all Caucasian populations, and a frequency usually <1% in all Asian populations. In ~75% of the Caucasian cases, the enzyme lack represents the frameshift mutations of CYP2D6*4. This mutation is absent in Asians, accounting for the low incidence of enzyme lack. On the other hand, the splicing mutant CYP2D6*5 occurs with low but similar frequency in all major population groups and accounts for the fact that poor metabolizers are occurring everywhere, even when rarely so.

Table 2 gives a list of different CYP2D6 mutations and indicates their occurrences in some major human populations. Note that the gene may carry as many as seven mutations in Europe and up to four mutations in China, while only three were seen in Japan. Only one nucleotide change (G4268C) occurs in all populations. One must assume the this is a very old mutation which occurred

TABLE 2 Mutations in Cytochrome CYP2D6 Nucleotide Changes and Their Locations

CYP2D6 allele	C>T	C>A	A>G	C>G	C>T	G>C	G>C	G>A	C>T	G>C	People from
*2							1749		2938	4268	Europe
*4A	188	1062	1072	1085			1749	1934		4268	Europe
*4B	188	1062	1072	1085			1749	1934		4268	Europe
*10A	188						1749			4268	Japan
*10B	188				1127		1749			4268	China
*10C	188				1127		1749			4268+	China
*17					1111	1726			2938	4268	Africa

The variants *4A and *4B represent enzymes without activity, all others have reduced activity compared to the wildtype. The + sign at CYP2D6*10C indicates exon 9 conversion into that of pseudogene CYP2D7.

before *Homo sapiens* left Africa, and therefore is seen everywhere. Mutations specific for any given population are probably relatively recent events. Thus, the time of mutation seems to explain at least some population differences.

The deficiency of CYP2D6 was discovered in England by testing debrisoquine as a substrate [26], in Germany by testing sparteine [27]. That the deficiency of a single enzyme was responsible for both deficiencies was demonstrated later [28]; the correlation coefficient of the rates of metabolism of the two substrates was found to be $r = .91$ in Europe. The presence or absence of enzyme activity is a straightforward phenomenon, but problems may be encountered if structural variants occur. Woolhouse et al. [29] observed in a Ghanaian population that many poor metabolizers of debrisoquine could readily metabolize sparteine. Masimirembwa et al. [13] made a similar observation comparing the metabolisms of debrisoquine and metropolol (another CYP2D6 substrate) in Zimbabwe. It is a general truth that structural enzyme variants do not always have the same binding affinities for all substrates.

Many African data were due to the variant CYP2D6*17 which has reduced activity. This variant occurred with an allele frequency of 37% in Zimbabwe, 17% in Tanzania, and 9% in Ethiopia. The reduced enzyme activity in Asia is due to a different variant, CYP2D6*10 characterized by C188T, which has in China a frequency of 51%. Besides their generally reduced activity, the Asian and African variants have no similarity. The activities of these variants toward different substrates requires much additional investigation.

Gene duplication (or multiplication) representing abnormally high enzyme activity occurred in about 1–2% of the Swedish population, was 3.7% in Germany, 7–10% in Spain, 20% in Saudi Arabia, and 29% in Ethopia (B&K 2000). Europeans with gene duplication are ultrarapid metabolizers of debrisoquine. The enzyme activity in Ethiopia is not as high as one might expect from the number of duplicants; the reason is not entirely clear. Perhaps a CYP2D6 variant with reduced activity is duplicated. The relatively high duplication frequency in Spain is almost certainly a remnant of the historical invasion of Spain by Arabs.

3.1.2 CYP2C19

The drug that led to the discovery of the polymorphic variation of CYP2C19 was mephenytoin [30,31], an anticonvulsant agent that is no longer in regular therapeutic use. It is a racemic drug of which the R-enantiomer is generally demethylated at a slow rate, while the S-enantiomer is hydroxylated at a very fast rate in some people and slowly in others [for review see 32]. Wrighton et al. [33] and Goldstein et al. [34] identified the P450 cytochrome CYP2C19 as the variable enzyme that caused this metabolic difference between people.

Some observations which carried this topic to prominence may be summarized by the statement that slow metabolizers of S-mephenytoin were found with a frequency of 2.8% in several Caucasian populations [35], but with considerable higher frequencies (20–30%) in Asians [8]. Measurements of mephenytoin metabolism in Africa indicate generally low frequencies of the slow-metabolizer genotypes [35].

Besides the wild-type CYP2C19*1, there are two major low-activity alleles, CYP2C19*2 and *3 (formerly called CYP2C19m$_1$ and m$_2$). Both alleles cause a lack of enzyme formation, and any person homozygous for these two alleles or with their combination will register as having the metabolic deficiency; wild-type heterozygotes are as a rule not phenotypically distinguished from wild-type homozygotes. The higher frequency of the deficiency in Asians is mostly due to CYP2C19*3. On Vanuatu and other Pacific islands this latter allele occurred in 70% of the populations [36].

Substrates other than mephenytoin that have caused clinical disturbances in people with deficient CYP2C19 alleles include omeprazol [37], proguanil [38], and citalopram [39]. Additional substrates listed [8] include clomipramine, imipramine, diazepam, and propanolol.

3.1.3   Comparison of CYP2D6 and CYP2C19

It is possible that further genetic variants of CYP2C19 will be discovered. Nevertheless, the large number of nucleotide changes in CYP2D6 deserves attention. Perhaps this fact points to a relative lack of any physiological importance of CYP2D6, allowing the enzyme to be eliminated without danger in a drug-free environment. On the other hand, this enzyme occurs in human brain, and its absence seems to cause a difference of mental attitudes [40].

Another major difference lies in the fact that the genetic variation of CYP2C19 seems to always cause enzyme absence, while CYP2D6 shows many structural changes which affect different substrates differently. This seems to have a peculiar consequence.

Observations cited above from Ghana indicated a lack of correlation of the metabolic rates of debrisoquine and sparteine, and from Zimbabwe a similar lack of correlation for debrisoquine and metropolol. We took this to indicate structural variation of CYP2D6. A recent review [8] quoted data of different investigators indicating interethnic differences in the kinetics of diazepam, omeprazol, and clomipramine, all CYP2C19 substrates; their fate must be affected by that enzyme's activity. The pharmacokinetic differences affecting these substrates could not be fully explained by the absence of CYP2C19. While CYP2C19 may be present or absent, the kind of structural changes and consequent race-dependent substrate selectivities known for CYP2D6 are not known for CYP2C19. Hence, the interethnic variations in the metabolism of these CYP2C19 substrates must mean that other enzymes which marginally participate in their metabolism show interethnic variability. This marginal participation becomes visible in the absence but is not noted in the presence of CYP2C19 activity.

3.2 N-Acetyltransferases

The introduction of isoniazid into medicine was an exciting advance because of its revolutionary capability to cure tuberculosis, a kind of cure never seen before [41]. When it was found that the drug caused tingling in the hands or feet and other neurological disturbances in some but not all subjects, the cause was intensely investigated. It turned out that people with this side effect did not properly metabolize isoniazid [42,43]. The faulty drug-metabolizing enzyme was identified as a form of N-acetyltransferase. This was a major discovery in support of the then young science of pharmacogenetics.

Not very long after the discovery of the deficiency of isoniazid acetylation, it turned out that the frequency of this phenotypic fault also differed much between the world's populations [44]. Today, the reason for this particular interethnic variability is still unknown; an influence of geographical latitude and climate is suspected. Such scientific uncertainty is common in this field of research, and it contrasts with the clear-cut findings relating malaria resistance and G6PD deficiency (see below).

Later it was found that there are two N-acetyltransferases, designated NAT1 and NAT2 [45,46]. Isoniazid is metabolized only by NAT2, so its variability was thus early recognized. Vatsis and Weber [47] reported evidence of genetic variation of NAT1.

Grant et al. [48] described seven nucleotide changes in the *NAT2* gene which gave rise to 15 variant alleles; of these, four resulted in rapid and nine in slow acetylator phenotypes, and the remaining two are undetermined. In vitro tests indicated that most slow acetylations were due to instability of the enzyme; only one case showed decreased V_{max}. They listed the frequency of three selected slow acetylator alleles in 16 populations together with >4000 subjects.

Their set of data may be summarized by the statements that the $T^{341}C$ allele was the cause of slow acetylation in most Caucasians and Africans (with frequencies of 0.450 and 0.350, respectively), but was much rarer in all other populations. The slow acetylator allele $G^{590}A$ occurred in all populations except in Amerindians with the relatively high average frequency of 0.275 ± .073, and thus was most often responsible for slow acetylation in Asians.

Grant et al. [48] also reported 10 nucleotide changes in the *NAT1* gene which formed eight allelic variants. The functional activities of most of these are still unknown, but NAT1*14 with the amino acid change $Arg^{187}Gln$ has reduced substrate affinity, and NAT1*15 ($Arg^{187} \rightarrow Stop$) has a stop codon that prevents enzyme formation. Both have been found with low but significant frequencies (0.01 and 0.03, respectively) in Caucasian populations. However, Dhaini and Levy [49] reported a frequency of 0.238 for NAT1*14 in a Lebanese population. Other interethnic comparisons do not yet seem to exist.

Commonly used drugs (other than isoniazid) affected by NAT2 polymorphism were procainamide, hydralazine, dapsone, and sulfonamides with an increase of side effects in all cases. A selective substrate of NAT1 is p-aminosalicylic acid (PAS), but its genetic variation was never clinically important [50]. Because of such lack of importance, more attention is often paid to the fact that various industrial chemicals with carcinogenic potential, and mutagenic heterocyclic amines are substrates of both N-acetyltransferases. The presence or absence of these transferases will determine some incidences of cancer [51]. Attempts have been made to ascribe cancer incidences in different populations to acetyltransferase differences [52].

3.3 Glucose-6-Phosphate Dehydrogenase (G-6-PD)

In the historical introduction to this book (Chap. 1, Sect. 2.1), I mentioned primaquine hemolysis and G6PD deficiency during World War II in American soldiers. I did not indicate the remarkable fact that virtually only black soldiers developed this disease. The explanation for the interethnic difference was found later [53,54]. The hemolysis-associated variant of the G6PD enzyme protected its carriers from malaria infection with *Plasmodium falciparum*; it therefore occurred mainly in populations that came from countries in which malaria was prominent [55].

Glucose-6-phosphate dehydrogenase is a large structure with many genetic variants–perhaps more than any other human protein [56–59]. It is an almost ubiquitous cytosolic enzyme which catalyzes the first step in the hexose monophosphate pathway [59]. Its most essential function is to produce the NADPH required to maintain the concentration of reduced glutathione (GSH) in the face of oxidative stress. GSH and catalase and glutathione peroxidase represent the defense against hydrogen peroxide; this is particularly true in red blood cells.

There are different kinds of genetic variants of G6PD. Some of these generate serious disease in the form of chronic hemolytic anemia and therefore tend to be rare. This is not the pharmacogenetic problem; this results from the fact that hydrogen peroxide is often a byproduct arising during drug oxidation, and thus some drugs tend to produce destruction of the red cells—that is, hemolysis. These deficiencies are the ones which are frequent in some populations because they protect against malaria. They tend to be symptomless unless a drug or an infection overwhelms the protective function of the enzyme; persons with these variants may go through life without ever realizing that they have G6PD deficiency. On the other hand, there may be pathological consequences for infants (see below). In addition to the life-threatening and the pharmacogenetic variants, there are neutral variants; Caucasians usually have a G6PD form called B+, while A+ is frequent in Africa. Approximately one-tenth of the world population has one or other of the 300-odd functionally different variants of G6PD.

The gene *Gd* producing G6PD is located on the X chromosome at Xq28 [60]. It means that the deficiency is sex linked, and it is mostly the males who show the deficiency. Males either do or do not have the deficiency, but females with their two X chromosomes may be heterozygous. In females during early embryogenesis, each cell eliminates at random one of the two X chromosomes so that in heterozygotes, approximately half the cells are normal and the other half are G6PD deficient. The protective effect of G6PD deficiency against malaria operates mostly via the heterozygous females.

However, the mechanism of the malaria protection is complex [55,61]. It probably involves a sufficient survival time of the malaria-infected heterozygous infant girls to allow them to develop immunological defenses against malaria. This could mean that after puberty, their better state of health might render them more fertile than their less protected sisters. Since G6PD deficiency, sickle cell anemia, and thalassemia all seem to be related to the incidence of malaria, combinations of these traits are not uncommon.

About 20% of the X chromosomes in American blacks contain A+. It has about the same enzymatic activity as B+ but has higher electrophoretic mobility because aspartate replaces asparagine due to a A→G mutation at nucleotide (nt) 376 [62]. The G6PD deficiency typical of blacks is A−; this has always one amino acid substitution in addition to the mutation which characterizes A+. The most common second mutation in A− is G→A at nt 202. However, there may be mutations at nt 680 or nt 968 instead. Thus, at the molecular level, there are three A− variants instead of one. On the other hand, a few separately recorded variants were at first erroneously thought to be distinct from A−. In any case, all African deficiency variants are descendants of A+ [63].

One of the more common variants in the Orient is G6PD Canton, which has a mutation at nt 1376 [58]; the same mutation turned out to be present in three other variants which had been thought to be independent. An equivalent situation occurred in Europe. G6PD Mediterranean is characterized by a C→T substitution at nt 563. The four variants formerly distinguished as G6PD Cagliari, Dallas, Birmingham, and Sassari turned out to be identical with G6PD Mediterranean.

However, there is a peculiar observation in that virtually all persons from southern Europe and the Near East who have G6PD Mediterranean also have the noncoding mutation at nt 1311. In addition, this noncoding mutation is common in the area and present in 20% of the Mediterranean population. Since subjects from India with G6PD Mediterranean did not have the 1311 mutation, Beutler [64] suggested that G6PD Mediterranean arose as independent mutations in Europe and in India.

Some pathological effects of G6PD deficiency are neonatal jaundice and hemolysis. Neonatal jaundice can be due to overproduction or undersecretion of bilirubin and thus can have many causes, but the likelihood of its occurrence is much enhanced in the presence of G6PD deficiency. Neonatal jaundice on the basis of G6PD deficiency is a relatively prominent problem in China and in Greece. The prevalence of G6PD deficiency in the Chinese and Malayan population of Singapore is on the order of 1.4%, but about 25% of newborns with jaundice have the deficiency. The relative magnitude of these figures varies: in Greece, with an adult deficiency rate of slightly less than 5%, the rate is ~15% of cases with neonatal jaundice. Such population differences are compatible with the recently provided evidence by Kaplan et al. [65] that it is the combination of deficiencies of G6PD and glucuronyltransferase UDPGT1 (Gilbert syndrome) that causes neonatal jaundice.

A much investigated but not yet fully understood happening is the cause of favism, the hemolytic episode occurring in some Mediterranean people after eating fava beans; favism occurs only in persons with G6PD deficiency but not in all persons with this deficiency [66]. It seems that the fate of the glycoside divicine, a component of the fava been, varies metabolically or immunologically among persons.

3.4 Ethanol-Metabolizing Enzymes

In the current context, we will use the term "alcohol" not in its chemical sense in which there are many different alcohols with various (often poorly investigated) metabolic fates. This overview will be confined to the variable elements of ethanol metabolism.

Ethanol is mainly metabolized by alcohol dehydrogenase (ADH) to acetaldehyde which in turn is oxidized by aldehyde dehydrogenase (ALDH) to acetic acid. Genetic variation of alcohol dehydrogenase was discovered in 1964 by Von Wartburg et al. [67]; that of aldehyde dehydrogenase, in 1978 by Harada et al. [68]. In the years since these discoveries, both variations have become targets of many investigations, and topics of specialized books [69–71]. Alcohol dependence is influenced by many factors other than the dehydrogenases [72,73]. Hence, the clinical significance of alcohol dehydrogenase variants is still unraveling. On the other hand, aldehyde dehydrogenase genotypes have been known for many years to influence drinking behavior in populations and alcohol-induced liver damage.

4 ALCOHOL DEHYDROGENASE

There are seven different ADH classes (gene families) which are expessed in different but overlapping sets of tissues [74]. Here we will be concerned only with Class I ADH, consisting of three genes—*ADH1*, *ADH2*, and *ADH3*—located on chromosome 4 between 4q21 and 4q24. Their products are referred to as alpha, beta, and gamma ADH, respectively [75]. All these dehydrogenases are expressed in adult liver; beta and gamma also in kidney.

The ADH Class I molecules are dimers, composed of two subunits. They may be homodimers composed of alpha/alpha, beta/beta, gamma/gamma units or they are the heterodimers alpha/beta, alpha/gamma, and beta/gamma. There is genetic variation of the beta and gamma subunits. There are three beta variants—$beta_1$, $beta_2$, and $beta_3$. If for instance somebody is heterozygous having $beta_1$ and $beta_2$, the ADH is expected to consist of 10 dimers formed by random association. If this person were also heterozygous at the ADH_3 locus to produce $gamma_1$ and $gamma_2$ subunits, his or her alcohol dehydrogenase should consist of 18 different dimers. In vitro, the "atypical" ($beta_2$) variant is the better catalyst than is $beta_1$ [76], while $beta_3$ may be less efficient than $beta_1$.

The three subunits alpha or ADH1, beta or ADH2, and gamma or ADH3, are structurally similar. Each consists of 374 amino acids [77]. In the context of ethnic comparisons, the most important difference is between the "typical" subunit $beta_1$ which is predominant in Caucasians and the "atypical" $beta_2$ subunit which is prominent in Orientals. The occurrence of $beta_3$ in American blacks is a comparatively new observation.

If the reoxidation of NADH to cofactor NAD is the rate-limiting step of ethanol oxidation in vivo [78], the different capabilities of alcohol dehydrogenase may not be fully reflected in the elimination rate of ethanol. There are also the possibilities that the effect of the variants depends on ethanol concentration, or that $beta_2$ causes an initial spurt of ethanol oxidation in Orientals which is not seen in Caucasians who have the $beta_1$ allele or in blacks who have the $beta_3$ allele.

Some functional clarification of these problems has been provided by recent comparative genotyping of alcoholics and nonalcoholics. Studies in Chinese [79–81] and in Japanese [82,83], supported by meta-analysis [84], indicated significantly reduced frequencies of $beta_2$ and $gamma_1$ in alcoholics, besides the usually present aldehyde dehydrogenase deficiency (see below). It means that the high rate of ethanol conversion to the toxic and unpleasant acetaldehyde tends to reduce ethanol consumption, particularly if acetaldehyde is slowly metabolized.

In short, the interethnic differences in the structure of alcohol dehydrogenase appear to have sufficient effects upon the fate of ethanol to be one of the determinants of alcoholism. Furthermore, one should not exclude the possibility that variation of alcohol dehydrogenase matters for the fate of endogenous [85,86] or exogenous substrates [87,88]. Ethanol is also metabolized by CYP2E1, but this enzyme is quantitatively less important than are the alcohol dehydrogenases [89].

5 ALDEHYDE DEHYDROGENASE

The clinical importance of ALDH2 deficiency for alcohol ingestion rests on the chemical reactivity and therefore toxicity of the ethanol-derived substrate acetaldehyde. If the enzymatic removal of acetaldehyde is not fast enough, ethanol intake tends to cause facial flushing and a drop in blood pressure with tachycardia [90], effects which are perceived as unpleasant. The unpleasantness, or even an embarassed reaction to the visual flushing, have been deterrents of excessive ethanol consumption and thereby of alcoholism. In Japan, however, the deterrent effect of these sensations has been claimed to be gradually diminishing [91].

Traditionally established as being of clinical significance is variation of the mitochondrial aldehyde dehydrogenase referred to as ALDH2 [92]. There are additional and different aldehyde dehydrogenases which are cytosolic enzymes and which seem to be also relevant in the present context [93], but this review will be confined to ALDH2, the best-investigated enzyme of this group. Virtually all recent studies of alcoholism in Asians include data on ALDH2. The gene for this enzyme is located on chromosome 12 [94]. ALDH2 occurs mostly in liver and kidney and takes the form of a tetramer which consists normally of four identical subunits.

This tetrameric composition is important: there is an inactive genetic variant of ALDH2 which represents a point mutation. Glutamic acid at position 14 from the C-terminus is substituted in the deficient enzyme by lysine [95]. Even if the tetramer contains only one genetically inactive subunit, the whole tetramer is inactive. This means that there is enzyme deficiency even in the heterozygote; in other words, ALDH2 deficiency is inherited as a dominant trait [96]! Most published population comparisons therefore simply list the percentages of deficiency subjects.

Goedde and Agarwal [92] list test results from 29 different populations and a total of 3248 subjects. The data can be summarized by the statements that Central Asian, East Asian, and Southeast Asian populations showed deficiencies in the order of 30–50%. The deficiency was absent in European, Middle Eastern, and African populations. North American Indians showed deficiency rates of 2–5%; South American Indians of 40–45%. O'Dowd et al. [97] have shown that the functional enzyme deficiency in South American Indians must be due to a different mutation from the deficiency in Asians. This observation raises interesting questions regarding the biological significance of the mitochondrial aldehyde dehydrogenase.

6 CONCLUSIONS

More than interindividual comparisons, interethnic studies require the use of genotyping rather than phenotyping methodology. DNA analysis has shown that many, perhaps most, differences in drug response between populations have a genetic basis. At the same time, there are many nonpharmacogenetic or environ- mental factors capable of producing such differences, so a genetic cause of inter- ethnic differences requires specific demonstrations.

Whenever interindividual pharmacogenetic differences are observed, a proper search showed the existence of equivalent interethnic differences. It is not entirely clear whether this rule applies specifically to pharmacogenetics, or whether it affects all genetic variations to the same extent.

The number of mutant forms of an enzyme in a population varies widely from enzyme to enzyme. In most cases of pharmacogenetics, the reason for such enzyme differences is not clear. This is particularly striking since the variability of drug-metabolizing enzymes often seems to have nonfunctional consequences in the absence of drugs.

In some cases, biological reasons for ethnic differences in drug-metaboliz- ing capacity have been established, but usually they are not understood.

Genetic variation of a drug-metabolizing enzyme can have divergent func- tional consequences. The easiest to deal with are usually cases of absence of enzyme activity, even if it may occur as a dominant or recessive feature. The most complicated tend to be structural enzyme variants which may affect differ- ent ligands differently. Hence, functional predictions for a new population can often not be made on the basis of established experiences.

The same experiences as obtained with drugs in different populations apply principally to environmental chemicals. This opens new prospects for the investi- gation of environmentally caused intoxications, including cancer.

REFERENCES

1. W Kalow. Interethnic variation of drug metabolism. Trends Pharmacol Sci 12:102– 107, 1991.
2. AJ Wood, HH Zhou. Ethnic differences in drug disposition and responsiveness. Clin Pharmacokinet 20:350–373, 1991.
3. EC Kudzma. Drug response: all bodies are not created equal. Am J Nurs 92:48– 50, 1992.
4. KM Lin, RE Poland, G Nakasaki, eds. Psychopharmacology and Psychobiology of Ethnicity. Washington: American Psychiatric Press, 1993.
5. W Kalow, L Bertilsson. Interethnic factors affecting drug response. Adv Drug Res 25:1–59, 1994.
6. MW Smith, RP Mendoza. Ethnicity and pharmacogenetics. Mt Sinai J Med 63: 285–290, 1996.
7. WW Weber. Pharmacogenetics. Oxford: Oxford University Press, 1997.
8. L Bertilsson, W Kalow. Interindividual variability in drug metabolism in humans. In: GM Pacifici, O Pelkonen, eds. Interethnic Differences in Drug Disposition and Effects. London: Taylor & Francis, in press.

9. M Nei. Molecular Evolutionary Genetics. New York: Columbia University Press, 1987.

10. LL Cavalli-Sforza, P Manozzi, A Piazza. The History and Geography of Human Genes. Princeton, NJ: Princeton University Press, 1994.

11. B Burchell, M Soars, G Monaghan, A Cassidy, D Smith, B Ethell. Drug-mediated toxicity caused by genetic deficiency of UDP-glucuronosyltransferases. Toxicol Lett 112:333–340, 2000.

12. I Johansson, M Oscarsson, Q-Y Yue, L Bertilsson, F Sjoqvist, M Ingelman-Sundberg. Genetic analysis of the Chinese CYP2D locus. Characterization of variant CYP2D6 genes present in subjects with diminished capacity for debrisoquine hydroxylation. Mol Pharmacol 46:452–459, 1994.

13. CM Masimirembwa, JA Hasler, L Bertilsson, I Johansson, O Ekberg, M Ingelman-Sundberg. Phenotype and genotype analysis of debrisoquine hydroxylase (CYP2D6) in a black Zimbabwean population. Reduced enzyme activity and evaluation of metabolic correlation of CYP2D6 probe drugs. Eur J Clin Pharmacol 51: 117–122, 1996.

14. KE Anderson, AH Conney, A Kappas. Nutrition as an environmental influence on chemical metabolism in man. In: W Kalow, HW Goedde, DP Agarwal, eds. Ethnic Differences in Reactions to Drugs and Xenobiotics. New York: Alan R. Liss, 1986, pp 39–54.

15. H Herken. Untersuchungen an Serumproteinen bei Eiweißmamgelernährung. Arztl Wochenschr 4:297–302, 1949.

16. H Herken, W Kalow. Photometometrische Bestimmung der Enzymatischen Novocain-Hydrolyse. Klin Wochenschr 29:90–91, 1951.

17. AB Okey. Enzyme induction in the cytochrome P-450 system. In: W Kalow, ed. Pharmacogenetics of Drug Metabolism. New York: Pergamon Press, 1992, pp 549–608.

18. U Fuhr, G Strobl, F Manaut, EM Anders, F Sorgel, E Lopez-de-Brinas, DT Chu, AG Pernet, G Mahr, F Sanz. Quinolone antibacterial agents: relationship between structure and in vitro inhibition of the human cytochrome P450 isoform CYP1A2. Mol Pharmacol 43:191–199, 1993.

19. ES Messina, RF Tyndale, EM Sellers. A major role for CYP2A6 in nicotine C-oxidation by human liver microsomes. J Pharmacol Exp Ther 282:1608–1614, 1997.

20. EM Sellers. Pharmacogenetics and ethnoracial differences in smoking. JAMA 280: 179–180, 1998.

21. AD Richardson, RW Piepho. Effect of race on hypertension and antihypertensive therapy. Int J Clin Pharmacol Ther 38:75–79, 2000.

22. WC Cushman, DJ Reda, HM Perry, D Williams, M Abdellatif, BJ Materson. Regional and racial differences in response to antihypertensive medication use in a randomized controlled trial of men with hypertension in the United States. Department of Veterans Affairs Cooperative Study Group on Antihypertensive Agents. Arch Intern Med 160:825–831, 2000.

23. HP Lefley. Culture and chronic mental illness. Hosp Commun Psychiatry 41:277–286, 1990.

24. D Marez, M Legrand, N Sabbagh, JM Lo Guidice, C Spire, JJ Lafitte, UA Meyer, F Broly. Polymorphism of the cytochrome P450 CYP2D6 gene in a European population: Characterization of 48 mutations and 53 alleles, their frequencies and evolution. Pharmacogenetics 7:193–202, 1997.

25. AK Daly, J Brockmoller, F Broly, M Eichelbaum, WE Evans, FJ Gonzalez, JD Huang, JR Idle, M Ingelman-Sundberg, T Ishizaki, E Jacqz-Aigrain, UA Meyer, DW Nebert, VM Steen, CR Wolf, UM Zanger. Nomenclature for human CYP2D6 alleles. Pharmacogenetics 6:193–201, 1996.

26. A Mahgoub, LG Dring, JR Idle, R Lancaster, RL Smith. Polymorphic hydroxylation of debrisoquine in man. Lancet 2:584–586, 1977.

27. M Eichelbaum, N Spannbrucker, B Steincke, HJ Dengler. Defective N-oxidation of sparteine in man: a new pharmacogenetic defect. Eur J Clin Pharmacol 16:183–187, 1979.

28. M Eichelbaum, L Bertilsson, BJ Sawe, C Zekorn. Polymorphic oxidation of sparteine and debrisoquine: related pharmacogenetic entities. Clin Pharmacol Ther 31:184–186, 1982.

29. NM Woolhouse, M Eichelbaum, NS Oates, JR Idle, RL Smith. Dissociation of coregulatory control of debrisoquin/phenformin and sparteine oxidation in Ghanaians. Clin Pharmacol Ther 37:512–521, 1985.

30. A Kupfer, R Preisig. Pharmacogenetics of mephenytoin: a new drug hydroxylation polymorphism in man. Eur J Clin Pharmacol 26:753–759, 1984.

31. PJ Wedlund, WS Aslanian, CB McAllister. Mephenytoin hydroxylation deficiency in Caucasians: frequency of a new oxidative drug metabolism polymorphism. Clin Pharmacol Ther 36:773–780, 1984.

32. GR Wilkinson, FP Guengerich, RA Branch. Genetic polymorphism and S-mephenytoin hydroxylation. In: W Kalow, ed. Pharmacogenetics of Drug Metabolism. New York: Pergamon Press, 1992, pp 657–685.

33. SA Wrighton, JC Stevens, GW Becker. Isolation and characterization of human liver cytochrome P4502C19: correlation between 2C19 and S-mephenytoin 4′-hydroxylation. Arch Biochem Biophys 306:240–245, 1993.

34. J Goldstein, S de Morais. Biochemistry and molecular biology of the human CYP2C subfamily. Pharmacogenetics 4:285–299, 1994.

35. HG Xie, RB Kim, CM Stein, GR Wilkinson, AJ Wood. Genetic polymorphism of (S)-mephenytoin 4′-hydroxylation in populations of African descent. Br J Clin Pharmacol 48:402–408, 1999.

36. A Kaneko, JK Lum, L Yaviong, N Takahashi, T Ishizaki, L Bertilsson, T Kobayakawa, A Bjorkman. High and variable frequencies of CYP2C19 mutations: medical consequences of poor drug metabolism in Vanuatu and other Pacific islands. Pharmacogenetics 5:581–590, 1999.

37. T Andersson, CG Regardh, YC Lou, Y Zhang, ML Dahl, L Bertilsson. Polymorphic hydroxylation of S-mephenytoin and omeprazole metabolism in Caucasian and Chinese subjects. Pharmacogenetics 2:25–31, 1992.

38. SA Ward, NA Helby, E Skjelbo. The activation of the biguanide antimalarial proguanil co-segregates with the mephenytoin oxidation polymorphism—a panel study. Br J Clin Pharmacol 31:689–692, 1991.

39. SH Sindrup, K Brosen, MG Hansen, T Aaes-Jorgensen, KF Overo, LF Gram. Pharmacokinetics of citalopram in relation to the spartcine and the mephenytoin oxidation polymorphisms. Ther Drug Monit 15:11–17, 1993.

40. L Bertilsson, C Alm, C de las Carreras, J Widen, G Edman, D Schalling. Debrisoquine hydroxylation polymorphism and personality. Lancet 1:555, 1989.

41. EH Robitzek, IJ Selikoff, GG Ornstein. Chemotherapy of human tuberculosis with hydrazine derivatives of isonicontinic acid. Q Bull Sea View Hosp 13:27–51, 1952.

42. R Bonicke, W Reif. Enzymatische inaktivierung von Isonicotinsaure-hydrazid im menschlichen und tierischen Organismus. Arch Exp Pathol Pharmakol 220:321–333, 1953.

43. HB Hughes, JP Biehl, AP Jones, LH Schmidt. Metabolism of isoniazid in man as related to the occurrence of peripheral neuritis. Am Rev Tuberculosis 70:266–273, 1954.

44. S Sunahara, M Urano, M Ogawa. Genetical and geographical studies on isoniazid inactivation. Science 134:1530–1531, 1961.

45. M Blum, DM Grant, OW McBride, M Heim, UA Meyer. Human arylamine N-acetyltransferase genes: isolation, chromosomal localization and functional expression. DNA Cell Biol 9:193–203, 1990.

46. DM Grant, M Blum, M Beer, UA Meyer. Monomorphic and polymorphic human arylamine N-acetyltransferases: a comparison of liver isozymes and expressed products of two cloned genes. Mol Pharm 39:184–191, 1991.

47. KP Vatsis, WW Weber. Structural heterogeneity of Caucasian N-acetyltransferase at the NAT1 gene locus. Arch Biochem Biophys 301:71–76, 1993.

48. DM Grant, NC Hughes, SA Janezic, GII Goodfellow, IIJ Chen, A Gaedigk, VL Yu, R Grewal. Human acetyltransferase polymorphisms. Mutat Res 376:61–70, 1997.

49. HR Dhaini, GN Levy. Arylamine N-acetyltransferase 1 (NAT1) genotypes in a Lebanese population. Pharmacogenetics 10:79–83, 2000.

50. NC Hughes, SA Janezic, KL McQueen, MA Jewett, T Castranio, DA Bell, DM Grant. Identification and characterization of variant alleles of human acetyltransferase NAT1 with defective function using p-aminosalicylate as an in-vivo and in-vitro probe. Pharmacogenetics 8:55–66, 1998.

51. A Hirvonen. Chapter 20. Polymorphic NATs and cancer predisposition. IARC Sci Publ 148:251–270, 1999.

52. N Brockton, J Little, L Sharp, SC Cotton. N-acetyltransferase polymorphisms and colorectal cancer: a HuGE review. Am J Epidemiol 151:846–861, 2000.

53. AG Motulsky. Metabolic polymorphisms and the role of infectious diseases in human evoluation. Hum Biol 32:28, 1960.

54. AC Allison. Glucose 6-phosphate dehydrogenase deficiency in red blood cells of East Africans. Nature 186:531, 1960.

55. T Vulliamy, P Mason, L Luzzatto. The molecular basis of glucose-6-phosphate dehydrogenase deficiency. Trends Genet 8:138–143, 1992.

56. A Yoshida, E Beutler. Glucose-6-Phosphate Dehydrogenase. Orlando, FL: Academic Press, 1986.

57. L Luzzatto. Glucose-6-phosphate dehydrogenase and other genetic factors inter-

acting with drugs. In: W Kalow, HW Goedde, D Agarwal, eds. Ethnic Differences in Reactions to Drugs and Xenobiotics. New York: Alan R. Liss, 1986, pp 385–399.

58. E Beutler. Study of glucose-6-phosphate dehydrogenase: history and molecular biology. Am J Hematol 42:53–58, 1993.

59. L Luzzatto, A Mehta. Glucose 6-phosphate dehydrogenase deficiency. In: CR Scriver, AL Beaudet, WS Sly, D Valle, eds. The Metabolic and Molecular Bases of Inherited Disease, Vol. 111. New York: McGraw-Hill, 1995, pp 3367–3398.

60. E Beutler. The genetics of glucose-6-phosphate dehydrogenase deficiency. Semin Hematol 27:137–164, 1990.

61. EA Usanga, L Luzzatto. Adaptation of plasmodium falciparum to glucose 6-phosphate dehydrogenase-deficient host red cells by production of parasite-encoded enzyme. Nature 313:793–795, 1985.

62. A Hirono, E Beutler. Molecular cloning and nuicleotide sequence of cDNA for human glucose-6-phosphate dehydrogenase variant A(−). Proc Natl Acad Sci USA 85:3951–3954, 1988.

63. AC Kay, W Kuhl, J Prchal, E Beutler. The origin of glucose-6-phosphate-dehydrogenase (G6PD) polymorphisms in African-Americans. Am J Hum Genet 50:394–398, 1992.

64. E Beutler. The molecular biology of G6PD variants and other red cell enzyme defects. Annu Rev Med 43:47–59, 1992.

65. R Kaplan, M Becker, L Broadman. Isolated masseter muscle spasm versus generalized rigidity? Anesth Analg 141:156, 1992.

66. C Kattamis. Favism: epidemiological and clinical aspects. In: A Yoshida, E Beutler, eds. Glucose-6-Phosphate Dehydrogenase. Orlando: Academic Press, 1986, pp 25–43.

67. JP von Wartburg, JL Bethune, BL Vallee. Human liver alcohol dehydrogenase. Kinetic and physicochemical properties. Biochemistry 3:1775–1782, 1964.

68. S Harada, DP Agarwal, HW Goedde. Isozyme variations in acetaldehyde dehydrogenase (EC1.2.1.3.) in human tissues. Hum Genet 44:181–185, 1978.

69. HW Goedde, DP Agarwal. Aldehyde dehydrogenase polymorphism: molecular basis and phenotypic relationship to alcohol sensitivity. Alcohol Alcoholism Suppl 1:47–54, 1987.

70. JC Crabbe, RA Harris, eds. The Genetic Basis of Alcohol and Drug Actions. New York: Plenum Press, 1991.

71. H Weiner, R Lindahl, DW Crabb, TG Flynn. Enzymology and Molecular Biology of Carbonyl Metabolism 6. New York: Plenum Press, 1997.

72. RA Ferguson, DM Goldberg. Genetic markers of alcohol abuse. Clin Chim Acta 257:199–250, 1997.

73. T Reich, HJ Edenberg, A Goate, JT Williams, JP Rice, P van Eerdewegh, T Foroud, V Hesselbrock, MA Schuckit, K Bucholz, B Porjesz, TK Li, PM Conneally, JI Nurnberger Jr, JA Tischfield, RR Crowe, CR Cloninger, W Wu, S Shears, K Carr, C Crose, C Willig, H Begleiter. Genome-wide search for genes affecting the risk for alcohol dependence. Am J Med Genet 81:207–215, 1998.

74. HJ Edenberg, CJ Brown, MW Hur, S Kotagiri, M Li, L Zhang, X Zhi. Regulation

of the seven human alcohol dehydrogenase genes. In: H Weiner, R Lindahl, DW Crabb, TG Flynn, eds. Enzymology and Molecular Biology of Carbonyl Metabolism 6. New York: Plenum Press, 1996, pp 339–345.

75. H Jornvall, JO Hoog. Nomenclature of alcohol dehydrogenases. Alcohol Alcoholism 30:153–161, 1995.

76. TD Hurley, T Ehrig, HJ Edenberg, WF Bosron. Characterization of human alcohol dehydrogenases containing substitutions at amino acids 47 and 51. In: H Weiner, B Wermuth, DW Crabb, eds. Enzymology and Molecular Biology of Carbonyl Metabolism 3. New York: Plenum Press, 1990, pp 271–275.

77. WF Bosron, TK Li. Genetic polymorphism of human liver alcohol and aldehyde dehydrogenases, and their relationship to alcohol metabolism and alcoholism. Hepatology 6:502–510, 1986.

78. RF Suddendorf. Research on alcohol metabolism among Asians and its implications for understanding causes of alcoholism. Public Health Reports 104:615–620, 1989.

79. HR Thomasson, HJ Edenberg, DW Crabb, XL Mai, RE Jerome, TK Li, SP Wang, YT Lin, RB Lu, SJ Yin. Alcohol and aldehyde dehydrogenase genotypes and alcoholism in Chinese men. Am J Hum Genet 48:677–681, 1991.

80. YC Chao, SR Liou, YY Chung, HS Tang, CT Hsu, TK Li, SJ Yin. Polymorphism of alcohol and aldehyde dehydrogenase genes and alcoholic cirrhosis in Chinese patients. Hepatology 19:360–366, 1994.

81. YC Shen, JH Fan, HJ Edenberg, TK Li, YH Cui, YF Wang, CH Tian, CF Zhou, RL Wang, J Zhou, ZL Zhao, GY Xia. Polymorphism of ADH and ALDH genes among four ethnic groups in China and effects upon the risk for alcoholism. Alcohol Clin Exp Res 21:1272–1277, 1997.

82. S Higuchi. Polymorphisms of ethanol metabolizing enzyme genes and alcoholism. Alcohol Alcoholism Suppl 2:29–34, 1994.

83. F Shiratori, Y Tanaka, O Yokosuka, F Imazeki, Y Tsukada, M Omata. High incidence of ADH2*1/ALDH2*1 genes among Japanese alcohol dependants and patients with alcoholic liver disease. Hepatology 23:234–239, 1996.

84. JB Whitfield. Meta-analysis of the effects of alcohol dehydrogenase genotype on alcohol dependence and alcoholic liver disease. Alcohol Alcoholism 32:613–619, 1997.

85. F Strasser, MN Huyng, BV Plapp. Activity of liver alcohol dehydrogenases of steroids. In: H Weiner, R Lindahl, DW Crabb, TG Flynn, eds. Enzymology and Molecular Biology of Carbonyl Metabolism 6. New York: Plenum Press, 1996, pp 313–320.

86. NY Kedishvili, CL Stone, KM Popov, EAG Chernoff. Role of alcohol dehydrogenases in steroid and retinoid metabolism. In: H Weiner, R Lindahl, DW Crabb, TG Flynn, eds. Enzymology and Molecular Biology of Carbonyl Metabolism 6. New York: Plenum Press, 1996, pp 321–329.

87. JP Kassam, BK Tang, D Kadar, W Kalow. In vitro studies of human liver alcohol dehydrogenase variants using a variety of substrates. Drug Metab Dispos 17:567–572, 1989.

88. JC Burnell, WF Bosron. Genetic polymorphism of human liver alcohol dehydrogenase and kinetic properties of the isoenzymes. In: KE Crow, RD Batt, eds. Human Metabolism of Alcohol, Vol. 2. Boca Raton, FL: CRC Press, 1989, pp 65–75.

89. Y Maezawa, M Yamauchi, G Toda, H Suzuki, S Sakurai. Alcohol-metabolizing enzyme polymorphisms and alcoholism in Japan. Alcohol Clin Exp Res 19:951–954, 1995.

90. S Higuchi, KM Parrish, MC Dufour, LH Towle, TC Harford. The relationship between three subtypes of the flushing response and DSM-III alcohol abuse in Japanese. J Stud Alcohol 53:553–560, 1992.

91. Y Hasumura, J Takeuchi. Alcoholic liver disease in Japanese patients: a comparison with Caucasians. J Gastroenterol Hepat 6:520–527, 1991.

92. HW Goedde, DP Agarwal. Pharmacogenetics of aldehydo dehydrogenase. In: W Kalow, ed. Pharmacogenetics of Drug Metabolism. New York: Pergamon Press, 1992, pp 281–311.

93. W Ambroziak, R Pietruszko. Metabolic role of aldehyde dehydrogenase. In: H Weiner, R Lindahl, DW Crabb, TG Flynn, eds. Enzymology and Molecular Biology of Carbonyl Metabolism 4. New York: Plenum Press, 1993, pp 5–15.

94. V Vasiliou. Appendix B, Aldehyde dehydrogenase genes. In: H Weiner, R Lindahl, DW Crabb, TG Flynn, eds. Enzymology and Molecular Biology of Carbonyl Metabolism 6. New York: Plenum Press, 1997, pp 595–600.

95. J Hempel, R Kaiser, H Jörnvall. Mitochondrial aldehyde dehydrogenase from human liver: primary structure, differences in relation to the cytosolic enzyme and functional correlations. Eur J Biochem 153:13–28, 1985.

96. S Singh, G Fritze, B Fang, S Harada, YK Paik, R Eckey, DP Agarwal, HW Goedde. Inheritance of mitochondrial aldehyde dehydrogenase: genotyping in Chinese, Japanese and South Korean families reveals dominance of the mutant allele. Hum Genet 83:119–121, 1989.

97. BF O'Dowd, F Rothhammer, Y Israel. Genotyping of mitochondrial aldehyde dehydrogenase locus of native American Indians. Alcoholism Clin Exp Res 14:531–533, 1990.

98. YC Lou, L Ying, L Bertilsson, F Sjoqvist. Low frequency of slow debrisoquine hydroxylation in a native Chinese population. Lancet 2:852–853, 1987.

99. DK Sommers, J Moncrieff, J Avenant. Non-correlations between debrisoquine and metoprolol polymorphism in the Venda. Hum Toxicol 8:365–368, 1989.

100. E Steiner, L Bertilsson, J Sawe, I Bertling, F Sjoqvist. Polymorphic debrisoquine hydroxylation in 757 Swedish subjects. Clin Pharmacol Ther 44:431–435, 1988.

101. J Benitez, A Llerena, J Cobaleda. Debrisoquin oxidation polymorphism in a Spanish population. Clin Pharmacol Ther 44:74–77, 1988.

102. SL Primo-Parmo, CF Bartels, B Wiersema, AF van der Spek, JW Innis, BN LaDu. Characterization of 12 silent alleles of the human butyrylcholinesterase (BCHE) gene. Am J Hum Genet 58:52–64, 1996.

103. DN Nevin, A Zambon, CE Furlong, RJ Richter, R Humbert, JE Hokanson, JD Brunzell. Paraoxonase genotypes, lipoprotein lipase activity, and HDL. Arterioscler Thromb Vasc Biol 16:1243–1249, 1996.

104. DM Grant, NC Hughes, SA Janezic, GH Goodfellow, HJ Chen, A Gaedigk, VL Yu, R Grewal. Human acetyltransferase polymorphisms. Mutat Res 376:61–70, 1997.

105. HM Lachman, J Kelsoe, L Moreno, S Katz, DF Papolos. Lack of association of catechgol-O-methyltransferase (COMT) functional polymorphism in bipolar affective disorder. Psychiatr Genet 7:13–17, 1997.

106. RM Weinshilboum, DM Otterness, CL Szumlanski. Methylation pharmacogenetics: catechol O-methyltransferase, thriopurine methyltransferase, and histamine N-methyltransferase. Annu Rev Pharmacol Toxicol 39:19–52, 1999.

107. RM Weinshilboum, DM Otterness, IA Aksoy, TC Wood, C Her, RB Raftogianis. Sulfation and sulfotransferases 1: sulfotransferase molecular biology: cDNAs and genes. FASEB J 11:3–14, 1997.

108. JG Hengstler, A Kett, M Arand, B Oesch-Barthlomowicz, F Oesch, H Pilch, B Tanner. Glutathione S-transferase T1 and M1 gene defects in ovarian carcinoma. Cancer Lett 14:43–48, 1998.

109. N Jourenkova-Mironova, A Voho, C Bouchardy, H Wikman, P Dayer, S Benhamou, A Hirvonen. Glutathione S-transferase GSTM1, GSTM3, GSTP1 and GSTT1 genotypes and the risk of smoking-related oral and pharyngeal cancers. Int J Cancer 31:44–48, 1999.

110. MJ Harris, M Coggan, L Langton, SR Wilson, PG Board. Polymorphism of the Pi class glutathione S-transferase in normal populations and cancer patients. Pharmacogenetics 8:27–31, 1998.

111. B Burchell, CH Brierley, G Monaghan, DJ Clarke. The structure and function of the UDP-glucuronosyltransferase gene family. Adv Pharmacol 42:335–338, 1998.

112. E Levesque, M Beaulieu, DW Hum, A Belanger. UGT2B4 (E458): a UDP-glucuronosyltransferase encoded by a polymorphic gene with differential substrate specificity. Pharmacogenetics 9:207–216, 1999.

113. M Patel, BK Tang, W Kalow. (S) Oxazepam glucuronidation is inhibited by ketoprofen and other substrates of UGT2B7. Pharmacogenetics 5:43–49, 1995.

114. E Levesque, M Beaulieu, MD Green, TR Tephly, A Belanger, DW Hum. Isolation and characertization of UGT2B15 (Y85): a UDP-glucuronosyltransferase encoded by a polymorphic gene. Pharmacogenetics 7:317–325, 1997.

115. W Kalow, BK Tang, D Kadar, T Inaba. Distinctive patterns of amobarbital metabolites in man. Clin Pharmacol Ther 24:576–582a, 1978.

116. WA Schulz, A Krummeck, I Rosinger, P Eickelmann, C Neuhaus, T Ebert, BJ Schmitz-Drager, H Sies. Increased frequency of a null-allele for NAD(P)H: quinone oxidoreductase in patients with urological malignancies. Pharmacogenetics 7:235–239, 1997.

117. T Vulliamy, E Beutler, L Luzzatto. Variants of glucose-6-phosphate dehydrogenase are due to missense mutations spread throughout the coding region of the gene. Hum Mutat 2:159–167, 1993.

118. EM Laurenzana, C Hassett, CJ Omiecinski. Post-transcriptional regulation of human microsomal epoxide hydrolase. Pharmacogenetics 8:157–167, 1998.

119. DW Crabb, KM Dipple, HR Thomasson. Alcohol sensitivity, alcohol metabolism, risk of alcoholism, and the role of alcohol and aldehyde dehdrogenase genotypes. J Lab Clin Med 122:234–240, 1993.

120. A Novoradovsky, SJ Tsai, L Goldfarb, R Peterson, JC Long, D Goldman. Mitochondrial aldehyde dehydrogenase polymorphism in Asian and American Indian populations: detection of new ALDH2 alleles. Alcohol Clin Exp Res 19:1105–1110, 1999.

121. M Nakatome, Z Tun, S Shimada, K Honda. Detection and analysis of four polymorphic markers at the human monoamine oxidase (MAO) gene in Japanese controls

and patients with Parkinson's disease. Biochem Biophys Res Commun 247:452–456, 1998.

122. EJ Calabrese, AT Canada. Catalase: its role in xenobiotic detoxification. In: W Kalow, ed. Pharmacogenetics of Drug Metabolism. New York: Pergamon Press, 1992, pp 397–410.

123. AT Canada, EJ Calabrese. Superoxide dismutase: its role in xenobiotic detoxication. In: W Kalow, ed. Pharmacogenetics of Drug Metabolism. New York: Pergamon Press, 1992, pp 383–396.

124. SC Mitchell, AQ Zhang, T Barrett, R Ayesh, RL Smith. Studies on the discontinuous N-oxidation of trimethylamine among Jordanian, Ecuadorian and New Guinean populations. Pharmacogenetics 7:45–50, 1997.

125. PM Fernandez-Salguero, A Sapone, X Wei, JR Holt, S Jones, JR Idle, FJ Gonzalez. Lack of correlation between phenotype and genotype for the polymorphically expressed dihydropyrimidine dehydrogenase in a family of Pakistani origin. Pharmacogenetics 7:161–163, 1997.

126. S Munoz, V Vollrath, MP Vallejos, JF Miquel, C Covarrubias, A Raddatz, J Chianale. Genetic polymorphisms of CYP2D6, CYP1A1 and CYP2E1 in the South-Amerindian population in Chile. Pharmacogenetics 8:343–351, 1998.

127. M Nakajima, T Yokoi, M Mizutani, M Kinoshita, M Funayama, T Kamataki. Genetic polymorphism in the 5′-flanking region of human CYP1A2 gene: effect on the CYP1A2 inducibility in humans. Nature Biotechnol 125:803–808, 1999.

128. P Fernandez-Salguero, SMG Hoffman, S Cholerton, H Mohrenweiser, H Raunio, A Rautio, O Pelkonen, J Huang, WE Evans, JR Idle, FJ Gonzalez. A genetic polymorphism in coumarin 7-hydroxylation: sequence of the human CYP2A genes and identification of variant CYP2A6 alleles. Am J Hum Genet 57:651–660, 1995.

129. RJ Edwards, DA Adams, PS Watts, DS Davies, AR Boobis. Development of a comprehensive panel of antibodies against the major xenobiotic metabolising forms of cytochrome P450 in humans. Biochem Pharmacol 1:377–387, 1998.

130. RJ Riley, G Smith, CR Wolf, VA Cook, JS Leeder. Human anti-endoplasmic reticulum autoantibodies produced in aromatic anticonvulsant hypersensitivity reactions recognise rodent CYP3A proteins and a similarly regulated human P450 enzyme. Biochem Biophys Res Commun 191:32–40, 1993.

131. SJ London, AK Daly, JBS Leathart, WC Navidi, JR Idle. Lung cancer risk in relation to the CYP2C9*1/CYP2C9*2 genetic polymorphism among African-Americans and Caucasians in Los Angeles County, California. Pharmacogenetics 6:527–533, 1996.

132. K Komai, K Sumida, H Kaneko, I Nakatsuka. Identification of a new non-functional CYP2C18 allele in Japanese: substitution of T204 to A in exon 2 generates a premature stop codon. Pharmacogenetics 6:117–119, 1996.

133. HI Daniel, TI Edeki. Genetic polymorphism of S-mephenytoin 4′-hydroxylation. Psychopharmacol Bull 32:219–230, 1996.

134. UA Meyer, UM Zanger. Molecular mechanisms of genetic polymorphisms of drug metabolism. Annu Rev Pharmacol Toxicol 37:269–296, 1997.

135. KS Fairbrother, J Grove, I de Waziers, DT Steimel, CP Day, CL Crespi, AK Daly. Detection and characterization of novel polymorphisms in the CYP2E1 gene. Pharmacogenetics 8:543–552, 1998.

136. F Sata, A Sapone, G Elizondo, P Stocker, VP Miller, W Zheng, H Raunio, CL Crespi, FJ Gonzalez. CyP3A4 allelic variants with amino acid substitutions in exon 7 and 12: evidence for an allelic variant with altered catalytic activity. Clin Pharmacol Ther 67:48–56, 2000.

137. SK Janardan, KS Lown, P Schmiedlin-Ren, KE Thummel, PB Watkins. Selective expression of CYP3A5 and not CYP3A4 in human blood. Pharmacogenetics 379: 385, 1996.

7

Pharmacogenetics
Clinical Viewpoints

Urs A. Meyer
Biocenter of the University of Basel, Basel, Switzerland

1 INTRODUCTION

Individual variation in drug response is a major problem in clinical practice and in drug development. Variation can range from therapeutic failure to adverse or even fatal effects of drugs in some patients. The incidence of serious or fatal adverse drug reactions (ADRs) has been extensively analyzed in hospital patients. A recent meta-analysis of 39 prospective studies from U.S. hospitals suggests that 6.7% of patients have serious and 0.32% have fatal ADRs, the latter causing ~100,000 deaths per year in the United States. This would make ADRs between the fourth and sixth leading cause of death [1].

Pharmacogenetics and pharmacogenomics have contributed to understand the inherited risk of an individual patient to develop an ADR or to have no beneficial drug effect. This chapter will discuss how one important part of pharmacological variability can be predicted by pharmacogenetic testing and how this knowledge can be applied in clinical practice and in drug development.

The risk for drug inefficacy or toxicity is a product of the interaction of genes and the environment. Risk factors include drug-drug interactions, the patient's age, renal and liver function, or other disease factors or clinical variables

TABLE 1 Clinically Important Genetic Polymorphisms of Drug Metabolism Influencing Drug Response

Gene	Incidence of individuals at risk	Drug	Drug effect or ADR linked to polymorphism	References
CYP2C9	14–28% (heterozygotes)	Warfarin	Hemorrhage	14
	0.2–1% (homozygotes)	Tolbutamide	Hypoglycemia	Rev. by 15
		Phenytoin	Phenytoin toxicity	Rev. by 16
		Glipicide	Hypoglycemia	Rev. by 16
		Losartan	Decreased antihypertensive effect	Rev. by 15
CYP2D6	5–10% (poor metabolizers)	Antiarrhythmics	Proarrhythmic and other toxic effects	Rev. by 11
		Antidepressants	Toxicity in poor metabolizer, inefficacy in ultrarapid metabolizers	Rev. by 11
		Antipsychotics	Tardive dyskinesia	Rev. by 11
		Opioids	Inefficacy of codeine as analgesic, narcotic side effects and dependence	Rev. by 11
		β-Adrenoceptor antagonists	Increased β-blockade	Rev. by 11

Enzyme	Frequency	Drug	Clinical effect	Ref.
CYP2C19	3–6% (Caucasians) 8–23% (Asians)	Omeprazol	Higher cure rates when given together with clarithromycin	28
Dihydropyrimidine dehydrogenase (DPD)	0.1%	Diazepam Fluorouracil	Prolonged sedation Neurotoxicity, myelotoxicity	Rev. by 11 Rev. by 17
Plasma pseudocholinesterase	1.5%	Succinylcholine	Prolonged apnea	Rev. by 11
N-Acetyltransferase (NAT2)	40–70% (Caucasians)	Sulfonamides Amonafide	Hypersensitivity Myelotoxicity (rapid acetylators)	Rev. by 11 Rev. by 17
	10–20% (Asians)	Procainamide, hydralazine, isoniazid	Drug-induced lupus erythematosus	Rev. by 11
Thiopurinemethyltransferase (TPMT)	0.3%	Mercaptopurine, thioguanine, azathioprine	Myelotoxicity	Rev. by 17
UDP-glucuronosyltransferase (UGT1A1)	10–15%	Irinotecan	Diarrhea, myelosuppression	Rev. by 17

such as smoking and alcohol consumption. As described in the previous chapters of this book a major part of individuality of drug response is inherited. Genetic variation in genes for drug-metabolizing enzymes, drug receptors, and drug transporters has been associated with individual variability in the efficacy and toxicity of drugs (reviewed in Sect. 2.6). It is of course difficult to disentangle the contribution of environmental and genetic factors in an individual patient. A major difference between genetic and environmental variation is that an inherited mutation or trait is present throughout life and has to be tested for only once in a lifetime whereas environmental effects are continually changing. Genetic polymorphisms of genes that influence the kinetics or dynamics of drug action explain why a fraction of the population may be at higher risk for drug inefficacy or toxicity and have given rise to the field of pharmacogenetics.

The initial clinical events that uncovered genetic variants of drug-metabolizing enzymes or drug targets, a selection of which are listed in Table 1, were ADRs. Thus, genetic polymorphisms were discovered by incidental observations that some patients or volunteers experienced unpleasant and disturbing ADRs on standard recommended doses of drugs.

2 GENOTYPES AND PHENOTYPES OF INDIVIDUAL VARIATION

Molecular genetics and genomics have profoundly transformed pharmacogenetics in the last decade. The two alleles (or alternate genes) carried by an individual at a given gene locus, e.g., at the CYP2D6 locus on chromosome 22q13, referred to as the *genotype*, can now be characterized with accuracy and high sensitivity at the DNA level, and their influence on the disposition of the drug or a receptor function, the *phenotype*, can be determined by advanced analytical methods for detection of the drug itself or its metabolites or by sophisticated clinical investigations, e.g., receptor density studies by positron emission tomography (PET). Molecular studies in pharmacogenetics started with the initial cloning and characterization of the drug-metabolizing enzyme CYP2D6 [2,3] and now have been extended to numerous human genes, including more than 20 drug-metabolizing enzymes and drug receptors and several drug transport systems as summarized in this book. For instance, >70 variant alleles of the CYP2D6 locus have been described (regular update on www.imm.ki.se/CYPalleles/cyp2d6.htm), of which at least 15 encode nonfunctional gene products. These alleles are different from the normal or "wild-type" gene by one or multiple mutations, but also include gene deletions and gene duplications or multiduplications. The mutations may have no effect on enzyme activity, or lead to enzymes with decreased or absent activity, duplications lead to increased enzyme activity. The consequent categories of phenotypes are called *extensive metabolizers* (EM) for individuals homozygous or heterozygous for the wild-type or normal activity enzymes (75–85%

of population), *intermediate metabolizers* (IM) (10–15%, [4]) or *poor metabolizers* (PM) (5–10%) for carriers of two decreased-activity or loss-of-function alleles, and *ultrarapid metabolizers* (UM) (2–7%) for carriers of duplicated or multiduplicated active genes [reviewed in 3,5]. Although the number and complexity of the mutations may be large overall, only a small number of mutant genes, usually three to five alleles, are common and account for most (usually >95%) of mutant alleles. These alleles can easily be detected by modern DNA methods (see Chap. 9) including DNA chip microarrays and mass spectrometry, and can assign most patients to a particular phenotype group.

CYP2D6 remains one of the best-studied polymorphic genes of clinical interest; numerous other genes have been or are being studied by identical approaches. The PM phenotype for most of the polymorphic genes is inherited as an autosomal-recessive trait, requiring the presence of two mutant alleles; the UM phenotype of CYP2D6 is inherited as a dominant trait. These considerations apply to monogenic traits, where one gene locus has a major effect on the phenotype and divides the population into two or three distinct groups. However, it has to be realized that the responses to most medications are not monogenic but involve the interaction of multiple genes involved in drug disposition and drug action. Polygenic inheritance is more difficult to detect and to distinguish from environmental factors. The analysis of these conditions is similar to the analysis of complex diseases (e.g., cancer, mental diseases, arthritis, asthma, etc.), where primary genes, modifier genes, and environmental factors interact, as discussed in other chapters and in [6,7].

A strikingly simple method to distinguish between hereditary and environmental components of variability is the comparison of series of mono- and dizygotic twins or the repeated drug administration and comparison of the variability of the responses within and between individuals as recently proposed by Kalow et al. [8]. These techniques have demonstrated important genetic factors in the pharmacokinetics of numerous drugs—e.g., dicoumarol, halothane, phenytoin, tolbutamide, and midazolam.

3 WHAT MAKES A PHARMACOGENETIC TRAIT CLINICALLY RELEVANT?

In principle, three genetic mechanisms can influence pharmacotherapy. First and best studied to date are genetic polymorphisms of genes which are associated with altered metabolism of drugs (e.g., metabolism of tricyclic antidepressants). Increased or decreased metabolism of a drug may change its concentration and of that of active, inactive, or toxic metabolites. Second, genetic variants may produce an unexpected drug effect outside of its therapeutic indication (e.g., hemolysis in glucose-6-phosphate dehydrogenase deficiency). Third, genetic variation in a drug target may alter the clinical response and frequency of side effects

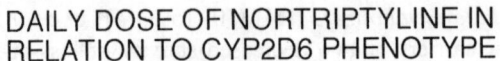

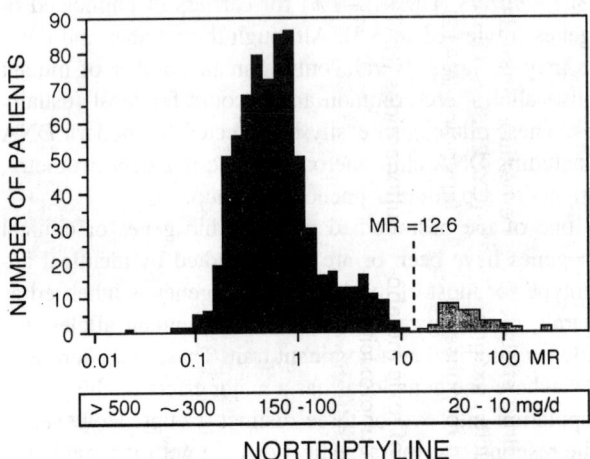

FIGURE 1   Different dose requirement for nortriptyline (mg/d) in patients with depression with different CYP2D6 phenotypes, determined by the debriso-quine urinary metabolic ratio (MR). Poor metabolizers are defined as individuals with a MR >12.6. (From Refs. 12 and 27.)

(e.g., variants of the β-adrenergic receptor alter response to β-agonists in asthma patients).

Whether a genetic polymorphism has relevance for drug therapy mainly depends on the characteristics of the drug in question. The quantiative role of a drug-metabolizing enzyme (e.g., CYP2D6) or a drug uptake mechanism (e.g., by the multidrug-resistance protein MDR1) in the overall kinetics of a drug and the agent's therapeutic range will determine how much the dose has to be adjusted in a PM or UM individual. The example of the CYP2D6 polymorphism again

TABLE 2   Clinical Issues Raised by Polymorphically Metabolized Drugs

Difficulties in dose setting
Ethnic variation in the frequency of occurrence
Failure to achieve therapeutic effect in poor metabolizers treated with prodrugs or in ultrarapid metabolizers
Administration of drugs that inhibit/compete for polymorphic enzyme may create phenocopy—poor metabolizers

TABLE 3 Pharmakokinetic and Clinical Consequences of Polymorphic Drug Metabolism in Poor (PM), Extensive (EM), and Ultrarapid Metabolizers of Debrisoquine/Sparteine

Kinetic consequences			
PM individuals	EM individuals	Clinical consequences	Examples
1. Reduced first-pass metabolism, increased oral bioavailability, and elevated plasma levels		Exaggerated drug response, potential drug toxicity	Metoprolol, encainide (CYP2D6)
2. Reduced overall metabolic clearance, prolonged half-life, drug accumulation		Prolonged drug effect, drug toxicity, exaggerated drug response	Perhexiline, thioridazine (CYP2D6), isoniazid, sulfapyridine (NAT2)
3. Alternative pathway of metabolism		Formation of toxic metabolites, immunotoxicity	Sulfonamides (NAT2)
4. Failure to generate active metabolite		Altered concentration/effect relationship between EM and PM	Encainide, propafenone, codeine (analgesic effect) (CYP2D6)
	1. Multiple substrates and inhibitors competing at active site of enzyme	Drug interactions with substrates of polymorphic enzyme	Quinidine, propafenone, flecainide, metoprolol, etc. (CYP2D6)
	2. Ultrarapid metabolism of compound	Therapeutic failure	Tricyclic antidepressants (CYP2D6)

PM: poor metabolizer (genotype or phenotype); EM: extensive or "normal" metabolizer.

provides incontroversible clinical data for these concepts. The majority of patients (~90%) require 75–150 mg/d of nortriptyline to reach a "therapeutic" plasma steady-state concentration of 200–600 nmol/L (50–150 µg/L), but PM individuals need only 10–20 mg/d, to reach the same levels. Ultrarapid metabolizers, on the other extreme, may require 300–500 mg or even >500 mg/d to reach the same plasma concentration (Fig. 1). Obviously, without knowing about the genotype or phenotype of the patient, PMs will be overdosed and be at high risk of drug toxicity, whereas UMs will be underdosed. Clinical observations have repeatedly confirmed these predictions.

Another situation is presented if the therapeutic effect depends on the formation of an active metabolite (e.g., morphine from codeine). Poor metabolizers will have no drug effect and ultrarapid metabolizers may have exaggerated drug responses [9]. These concepts are summarized in Tables 2 and 3. The drug-related criteria that make a genetic polymorphism clinically relevant are similar to those for drug concentration monitoring, i.e., narrow therapeutic range or large interindividual variation in kinetics or suspicion of overdose. In pharmacogenetics, however, a single DNA test done once in a lifetime can identify the predisposition of patients, at least at the extremes of the phenotypes.

4   WHO SHOULD BE PHENOTYPED OR GENOTYPED?

At present, pharmacogenetic testing is restricted to a limited number of patients or volunteers in academic institutions and clinical drug trials, although the evidence is accumulating that prospective testing could be of major benefit to many patients. The lack of large prospective studies to evaluate the impact of genetic variation on drug therapy is one reason for the slow acceptance of these principles. On the other hand, pharmacogenetic information is increasingly included in product information or drug data sheets alerting the physician to dosing problems. Recent retrospective analysis of psychiatric patients treated with drug substrates of CYP2D6 strongly indicates that genotyping can improve efficacy, prevent ADRs, and lower the costs of therapy with these agents [10].

Phenotyping tests require the administration of a specific marker drug or test drug, and collection of urine, blood, or saliva for analysis of drug and metabolite concentrations. These tests are time-consuming, expensive, and subject to drug-drug interactions or other influences. Genotyping tests have the advantage of having to be done only once in a lifetime and providing unequivocal genetic information. However, gentoyping tests only identify a group or category association (e.g., poor metabolizer, ultrarapid metabolizer) and do not predict the exact individual metabolic capacity or receptor interaction, because there still is considerable variation between individuals of the same genotype.

There are convincing arguments to use genotyping in volunteers or patients in clinical drug trials with known polymorphically metabolized drugs. Thereby patients can be recruited who will best respond to the medication, having the lowest risk of ADRs, resulting in smaller, less costly, and more efficient clinical trials.

The most widely accepted use of genotyping is testing for the five common mutations of CYP2D6 in patients with mental disease for the reasons discussed below.

5 THE FUTURE OF GENOTYPING

In the future, discovery of pharmacogenetic traits will change with the new technologies coming from genomics. Rapid sequencing and socalled single nucleotide polymorphisms (SNPs, or ''snips'') will play a major role in associating sequence variations with heritable clinical phenotypes of drug response. SNPs occur approximately once every 300–1500 bp if one compares the genomes of two unrelated individuals. Any two individuals thus differ by ~3 million bp, i.e., only in ~0.1% of the ~3 billion bp of the haploid genome (23 chromosomes). Common or informative SNPs are those that occur at frequencies of at least 1% or even higher proportions of the population. Once a large number of these SNPs and their frequencies in different populations are known, they can be used to correlate a patient's or volunteer's genetic ''fingerprint'' with the probable individual drug response [6,7]. SNPs in coding regions of genes (cSNPs), estimates are ~30,000–100,000 per genome, can cause amino acid changes and changes in protein function or can be neutral. SNPs inside genes or in regulatory regions (perigenic or pSNPs) can cause differences in protein expression. High-density maps of SNPs in the human genome will allow to use these SNPs as markers of drug responses even if the drug target remains unknown, providing a ''drug response profile'' associated with contributions from multiple genes to a drug response phenotype [6,7] (see also http://snp.cshl.org). The ability to predict interindividual differences in drug efficacy or toxicity based on genetic factors will thus be a realistic scenario for future drug treatments.

6 GENETIC POLYMORPHISMS OF CLINICAL RELEVANCE

6.1 Drug Metabolism

Many or most of the 50–100 drug-metabolizing enzymes expressed in a human organism are subject to common genetic polymorphisms. In Table 1 some are listed in which clinically important differences in drug response have been documented. Drug classes rather than single drugs are given, e.g., for CYP2D6, because ~100 drug substrates are known for this enzyme [11]. Similarly, CYP2C9, CYP2C19, and NAT2 each catalyze the metabolism of more than 15 different drugs.

6.1.1 CYP2D6

There is substantial interindividual variation in plasma concentrations of antidepressants [11,12]. The metabolism of the *tricyclic* antidepressants amitriptyline,
clomipramine, desipramine, imipramine, nortriptyline and of the *tetracyclic compounds* maprotiline and mianserin is influenced by the CYP2D6 polymorphism
to various degrees. For these agents, there are clearly two patient groups that
may pose clinical problems. The PMs (and to a lesser degree the IMs) predictably
have increased plasma concentrations on recommended doses of tricyclic antidepressants. The other group are the UMs, who are prone to therapeutic failures
because the drug concentrations at normal doses are by far too low (Fig. 1).

Five percent to 20% of patients may belong to one of these risk groups,
depending on the population studied. Adverse effects clearly occur more frequently in poor metabolizers and may be one of the causes of poor compliance.
Moreover, toxic reactions may be misinterpreted as symptoms of depression and
lead to erroneous further increases in the dose.

The metabolism of the recently introduced antidepressant drug venlafaxine
is controlled by CYP2D6, and poor metabolizers have a markedly decreased oral
clearance and increased cardiovascular toxicity [13]. This has been documented,
however, in only a few patients so far. Another group of antidepressants are the
selective serotonin reuptake inhibitors (SSRIs) which interact with CYP2D6 in
three different ways. Paroxetine, fluvoxamine, and fluoxetine are in part metabolized by CYP2D6. However, the phenotype differences in clearance or plasma
levels are small in relation to the relatively large therapeutic index of these drugs.
Of considerable importance is the effect of these agents as potent competitive
inhibitors of CYP2D6 (paroxetine, fluoxetine) with the consequence that the
elimination of other CYP2D6 substrates, e.g., of tricyclic antidepressants, is
markedly impaired and that phenotyping with debrisoquine, sparteine, or dextro-
metorphan results in false-positive results or "phenocopies" of poor metabolizers, if SSRIs are coadministered. These interactions are phenotype dependent,
i.e. restricted to extensive metabolizers.

Citalopram, fluvoxamin, and sertraline do not share this inhibitory property
and do not cause CYP2D6-specific interactions. Fluvoxamine is also a substrate
and potent inhibitor of CYP1A2 causing important interactions with drugs in
part metabolized by this cytochrome P450 such as amitriptyline, clomipramin,
imipramine, clozapine, or theophylline. Thus, polymorphic drug metabolism affects a large number of drugs used in psychiatric patients (Table 1), and the
question arises how this information will be used by physicians in the future.
Obviously, prospective trials are needed to prove the value of phenotyping or
genotyping in patients with depression in selecting the proper starting dose to
increase therapeutic efficacy and prevent toxicity.

Marked differences in the effect and ADRs of *opioids* are associated with the CYP2D6 polymorphism. Dextromethorphan, codeine, hydrocodon, oxycodone, ethylmorphine, and dehydrocodeine are dealkylated by polymorphic CYP2D6. The polymorphic O-demethylation of codeine is of clinical importance when this drug is given as an analgesic. Approximately 10% of codeine is O-demethylated to morphine, and it is this pathway that is deficient in poor metabolizers. PMs therefore experience no analgesic effect of codeine, as demonstrated in several studies [reviewed in 9,11]. Similarly, respiratory, psychomotor, and pupillary effects of codeine are decreased in PMs in comparison to EMs. Codeine is frequently recommended as a drug of first choice for treatment of chronic severe pain. The physician must appreciate that no analgesic effect is to be expected in the 5–10% of Caucasians who are of the PM phenotype, or who are EMs and receive concomitant treatment with a potent inhibitor of CYP2D6 such as quinidine. It is controversial if the inability to form active metabolites from opioids may protect PMs against oral opiate dependence.

6.1.2 CYP2C9

Another example of a clinically important genetic polymorphism of drug metabolism is the recent observation that variant alleles of CYP2C9 are associated with lower *warfarin* dose requirements. In a retrospective study of an anticoagulant clinic population, the CYP2C9 alleles (*2, *3) associated with diminished enzyme activity were found to be overrepresented in patients stabilized on low doses of warfarin. These patients had an increased incidence of major and minor hemorrhage [14]. Up to 37% of a British population were carriers of one mutant allele (*2 or *3) and therefore at higher risk for hemorrhage (Table 1). Homozygous carriers of mutant alleles of CYP2C9 are rare (0.2–1% of the population), and this genotype predictably is associated with an even higher risk for warfarin ADRs and with severe impairment of the metabolism of tolbutamide, glipicide, and phenytoin [15,16].

6.1.3 Pharmacogenetics of Cancer Chemotherapy

The severe and potentially fatal bone marrow toxicity (acute leucopenia, anemia, and pancytopenia) in patients with thiopurine methyltransferase (TPMT) deficiency treated with standard doses of mercaptopurine, thioguanine, and azathioprine is a rare (~1 in 300) event in the treatment of acute lymphoblastic leukemia (ALL) in children. TPMT-deficient patients may require up to a 15-fold reduction in the dose of mercaptopurin to prevent fatal hematotoxicity [reviewed in 17–19]. The myelosuppression and neurotoxicity of 5-fluorouracil in patients with (1) deficiency of *dihydropyrimidine dehydrogenase* (DPD), (2) the myelosuppression and diarrhoe after the topoisomerase I inhibitor irinotecan in patients with an inherited deficiency in glucuronidation by a promoter polymorphism of *UGT-*

glucuronosyltransferase UGT1A1, and (3) the greater bone marrow toxicity of the topoisomerase II inhibitor amonafide in *N-acetyltransferase 2* (NAT2) rapid acetylators (30–60% of Caucasians, 80–90% of Asians) are other genetic polymorphisms complicating cancer treatment. These situations have recently been reviewed [17,18].

6.2 Drug Transport (see also Chap. 5)

A number of membrane transporters are involved in the absorption of drugs in the intestinal tract, the uptake into brain and other tissues or in the transport into specific sites of action, e.g., in the synaptic cleft. However, little is known about transporter variants in relation to drug response. A first such variant was recently discovered for the *multidrug resistance gene MDR-1*, an ATP-dependent transmembrane efflux pump (P-glycoprotein, P-gp), whose function is the export of numerous substances including drugs from the inside of cells to the outside, protecting cells from accumulation of toxic substances or metabolites. A mutation in exon 26 of the MDR-1 gene (C3435T) correlated with the expression levels and the function of intestinal P-gp. Thus, the digoxin plasma levels were up to 4 fold higher in individuals homozygous for this mutation after a single oral dose of digoxin, the C_{max} of digoxin was also increased after chronic administration [20]. Homozygozity of this variant was observed in 24% of a German population. Substrates of P-gp include numerous important drugs with narrow therapeutic ranges including chemotherapeutic agents, cyclosporin A, verapamil, terfenadine, fenoxifenadin, and most HIV-1 protease inhibitors. Therefore, this polymorphism could have a major impact on the requirement for individual dose adjustments for carriers of this mutation. Mutations of other transporters, particularly those involved in reuptake of serotonin, dopamine, and GABA, are studied in regard to clinically relevant changes in drug response. Transporter pharmacogenetics is a rapidly developing field.

6.3 Drug Targets (Receptors, Enzymes)

The effects of most drugs is exerted via interaction of the compound with membrane receptors (~50%), enzymes (~30% of drugs) or ion channels (~5%) [21]. Many of the genes encoding these drug targets have been found to exhibit polymorphisms which may alter drug response. Clinically relevant examples are summarized in Table 4. One of the best-studied drug receptors is the β_2 adrenergic receptor (β_2 AR) and some of its mutations (e.g., the common mutation Arg→Gly at amino acid 16) are major determinants of β_2-agonist bronchodilator response [22]. Similarly, mutations in the *angiotensin converting enzyme* (ACE) have been proposed to account for differences in the response to ACE inhibitors, but the data from different studies remain controversial [reviewed in 23]. A combination of two mutations of the gene for a high-affinity *sulfonylurea receptor* (SUR1)

TABLE 4 Clinically Important Genetic Polymorphisms of Drug Targets and Drug Transporters

Gene	Incidence of individuals at risk	Drug	Drug effect or ADR linked to polymorphism	References
Multidrug-resistance gene (MDR1)	24%	Digoxin	Increased plasma levels	21
β_2-Adrenergic receptor (β_2AR)	37%	Albuterol	Decreased response to β_2-adrenergic agonists	23
Sulfonylurea receptor (SUR1)	2–3%	Tolbutamide	Decreased insulin response	25
LQT 1–5 (mutations on five genes coding for cardiac ion channels)	1–2% (?)	Antiarrhythmics, terfenadine, many other drugs	Sudden cardiac death due to long QT syndrome	27

leads to a 40% reduction in the insulin response to tolbutamide [24] and genetic polymorphisms of the *5-hydroxytryptamin (serotonin) receptor HTR2A* may be associated with the response to clozapine in patients with schizophrenia [25].

Mutations in five genes each encoding structural subunits of cardiac ion channels, have been identified to affect the risk of drug-induced long-QT syndrome (LQT), a potential cause of sudden cardiac death in young individuals without structural heart disease. The prevalence of LQT has been estimated ~1/10,000. All five genes code for membrane ion channels affecting sodium or potassium transport and are differentially influenced by antiarrhythmics and other drugs [for review, see 26].

7 CONCLUSIONS

Pharmacogenetics and pharmacogenomics are related fields involving the study of interindividual differences in drug responses. A rapidly expanding knowledge base on genetic variation in drug response could lead within the next few years to prospective genotyping and thereby to more affective and safer drug therapy. The possibility to identify individuals at increased risk for ADRs or ineffective therapy before drug treatment may have a major impact on health care in general and on drug development. However, there also are many legal, regulatory, and ethical issues that have to be addressed.

REFERENCES

1. J Lazarou, BH Pomeranz, PN Corey. Incidence of adverse drug reactions in hospitalized patients: a meta-analysis of prospective studies. JAMA 279:1200–1205, 1998.
2. FJ Gonzalez, RC Skoda, S Kimura, M Umeno, UM Zanger, DW Nebert, HV Gelboin, JP Hardwick, UA Meyer. Characterization of the common genetic defect in humans deficient in debrisoquine metabolism. Nature 331:442–446, 1988.
3. UA Meyer, UM Zanger. Molecular mechanisms of genetic polymorphisms of drug metabolism. Annu Rev Pharmacol Toxicol 37:269–296, 1997.
4. S Raimundo, J Fischer, M Eichelbaum, E-U Griese, M Schwab, UM Zanger. Elucidation of the genetic basis of the common "intermediate metabolizer" phenotype for drug oxidation by CYP2D6. Pharmacogenetics 10:1–5, 2000.
5. M Ingelman-Sundberg, M Oscarson, RA McLellan. Polymorphic human cytochrome P450 enzymes: an opportunity for individualized drug treatment. Trends Pharmacol Sci 20:342–349, 1999.
6. AD Roses. Pharmacogenetics and future drug development and delivery. Lancet 355:1358–1361, 2000.
7. AJ Brookes. The essence of SNPs. Gene 234:177–186, 1999.
8. W Kalow, B-K Tang, L Endrenyi. Hypothesis: comparison of inter- and intra-individual variations can substitute for twin studies in drug research. Pharmacogenetics 8:283–289, 1998.

9. SH Sindrup, K Brosen. The pharmacogenetics of codeine hypoalgesia. Pharmacogenetics 5:335–346, 1995.

10. WH Chou, F-X Yan, J Dc Lcon, J Barnhill, R Rogers, M Cronin, M Pho, V Xiao, T Ryder, WW Liu, C Teiling, PJ Wedlund. Extension of a pilot study: impact from the cytochrome P4502D6 polymorphism on outcome and costs associated with severe mental illness. J Clin Psychopharmacol 20:246–251, 2000.

11. UA Meyer. Drugs in special patient groups: clinical importance of genomics in drug effects In: GS Carruthers, BB Hoffmann, KL Melmon, DW Nierenberg, eds. Melmon and Morelli's Clinical Pharmacology. New York: McGraw-Hill, 2000, pp 1179–1205.

12. L Bertilsson, M-L Dahl, G Tybring. Pharmacogenetics of antidepressants: clinical aspects. Acta Psychiatr Scand 96:14–21, 1997.

13. E Lessard, M-A Yessine, BA Hamelin, G O'Hara, J LeBlanc, J Turgeon. Influence of CYP2D6 activity on the disposition and cardiovascular toxicity of the antidepressant agent venlafaxine in humans. Pharmacogenetics 9:435–443, 1999.

14. GP Aithal, CP Day, PJ Kesteven, AK Daly. Association of polymorphisms in the cytochrome P450 CYP2C9 with warfarin dose requirement and risk of bleeding complications [see comments]. Lancet 353:717–719, 1999.

15. JO Miners, DJ Birkett. Cytochrome P4502C9: an enzyme of major importance in human drug metabolism. Br J Clin Pharmacol 45:525–538, 1998.

16. RS Kidd, AB Straughn, MC Meyer, J Blaisdell, JA Goldstein, JT Dalton. Pharmacokinetics of chlorpheniramine, phenytoin, glipizide and nifedipine in an individual homozygous for the CYP2C9*3 allele. Pharmacogenetics 9:71–80, 1999.

17. L Iyer, MJ Ratain. Pharmacogenetics and cancer chemotherapy. Eur J Cancer 34: 1493–1499, 1998.

18. WE Evans, MV Relling. Pharmacogenomics: translating functional genomics into rational therapeutics. Science 286:487–491, 1999.

19. RM Weinshilboum, DM Otterness, CL Szumlanski. Methylation pharmacogenetics: catechol O-methyltransferase, thiopurine methyltransferase, and histamine N-methyltransferase. Annu Rev Pharmacol Toxicol 39:19–52, 1999.

20. S Hoffmeyer, O Burk, O von Richter, HP Arnold, J Brockmoller, A Johne, I Cascorbi, T Gerloff, I Roots, M Eichelbaum, U Brinkmann. Functional polymorphisms of the human multidrug-resistance gene: multiple sequence variations and correlation of one allele with P-glycoprotein expression and activity in vivo. Proc Natl Acad Sci USA 97:3473–3478, 2000.

21. J Drews, S Ryser. The role of innovation in drug development. Nat Biotechnol 15: 1318–1319, 1997.

22. SB Liggett. The pharmacogenetics of beta$_2$-adrenergic receptors: relevance to asthma. J Allergy Clin Immunol. 105:487–492, 2000.

23. G Navis, FG van der Kleij, D de Zeeuw, PE de Jong. Angiotensin-converting enzyme gene I/D polymorphism and renal disease. J Mol Med 77:781–791, 1999.

24. T Hansen, SM Echwald, L Hansen, AM Moller, K Almind, JO Clausen, SA Urhammer, H Inoue, J Ferrer, J Bryan, L Aguilar-Bryan, MA Permutt, O Pedersen. Decreased tolbutamide-stimulated insulin secretion in healthy subjects with sequence variants in the high-affinity sulfonylurea receptor gene. Diabetes 47:598–605, 1998.

25. MJ Arranz, J Munro, P Sham, G Kirov, RM Murray, DA Collier, RW Kerwin. Meta-

analysis of studies on genetic variation in 5-HT2A receptors and clozapine response. Schizophr Res 32:93–99, 1998.

26. SG Priori, J Barhanin, RN Hauer, W Haverkamp, HJ Jongsma, AG Kleber, WJ McKenna, DM Roden, Y Rudy, K Schwartz, PJ Schwartz, JA Towbin, AM Wilde. Genetic and molecular basis of cardiac arrhythmias: impact on clinical management parts I and II*. Circulation 99:518–528, 1999.

27. P Dalén, M-L Dahl, ML Bernal Ruiz, J Nordin, L Bertilsson. 10-Hydroxylation of nortriptyline in white persons with 0, 1, 2, 3, and 13 functional CYP2D6 genes. Clin Pharmacol Ther 63:444–452, 1998.

28. T Furuta, K Ohashi, K Kobayashi, I Iida, H Yoshida, N Shirai, M Takashima, K Kosuge, H Hanai, K Chiba, T Ishizaki, E Kaneko. Effects of clarithromycin on the metabolism of omeprazole in relation to CYP2C19 genotype status in humans. Clin Pharmacol Ther 66:265–274, 1999.

8

Tools of the Trade
The Technologies and Challenges of Pharmacogenetics

Glenn A. Miller

Genzyme Corporation, Framingham, Massachusetts

1 INTRODUCTION

As the 20th century ends, the field of drug discovery is filled with opportunity and challenge. The ability of the pharmaceutical industry of the 21st century to take advantage of the opportunities and meet the challenges while maintaining a significant growth rate will be determined by the success with which the industry makes use of the rich sources of information at its disposal.

The field of pharmacogenetics is one of the many disciplines that will produce insights and avenues of opportunity for drug discovery. The facility with which the pharmaceutical industry uses this information will have a major impact on the safety, efficacy, and time to market of a wide variety of therapeutic compounds in the future.

The use to which pharmacogenetics is put will be determined by how the information is collected, organized, and disseminated. The technologies brought to bear on the problems that pharmacogenetics presents will be critical to the effective use of pharmacogenetics information in the therapeutic development process. The current state of technological development has permitted investigators to address an array of previously unapproachable genetic questions. This has, in turn, created an ever-growing library of DNA sequence information, cDNA clones, genes, mutations, and polymorphisms available for use in target discovery, lead identification, lead optimization, preclinical testing, and clinical trials. The high per-patient cost of these technologies does not, however, permit the wide-scale use of this information resource. The development of new technologies providing low-cost, high-throughput alternatives to genetic testing will permit the application of pharmacogenomic information across a broad range of therapeutic development. This review will endeavor to provide an overview of the current state of the art in genetic technologies along with those technologies that may facilitate the widespread use of pharmacogenetics information.

2   TECHNOLOGY SELECTION

The selection of an appropriate technology is best based on the requirements of a project or area of investigation. Technologies that are appropriate for gene discovery are not universally applicable to population studies or patient group stratification.

Figure 1 depicts the most common areas of use for genomic and genetic technology in the drug development pathway. As the process moves from initial target identification through development of lead compounds, the impact of genomic technology lessens while that of genetics technology increases. The impact of the limited number of technologies applicable to clinical diagnostic laboratory use is reserved for those compounds well into the development process where

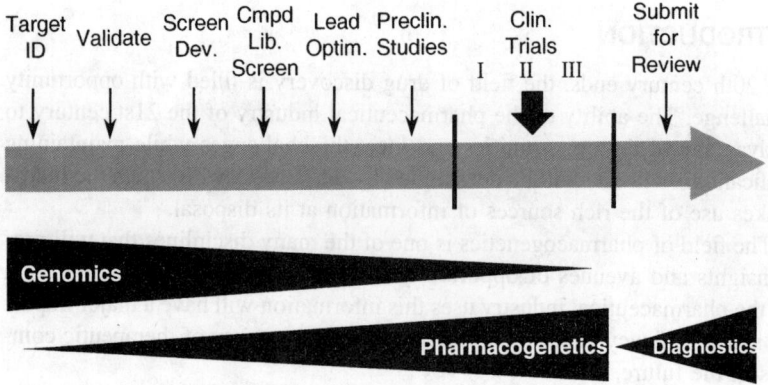

FIGURE 1   The steps involved in drug development and the relative use of genomics, pharmacogenetics, and diagnostics during this process.

a genetic test is being considered as an adjunct or requirement for therapeutic selection.

The selection of an appropriate technology can take two forms depending upon the state of knowledge concerning a gene, locus, or disease. In one form technology selection will be guided by a relative lack of knowledge concerning mutations and polymorphisms. The technologies selected in this manner will rely heavily on gene scanning methods and/or sequencing. In another form technology selection will be guided by a relative abundance of knowledge. The technologies selected in this environment will rely on high-throughput, reliable, robust methods of identifying known mutations or polymorphisms. The driving force behind the selection of technology is the detailed knowledge of gene sequence and variation.

2.1 Identification of Gene Variants

The completion of the final version of the sequence of the human genome in the near future will provide an unparalleled resource for the identification of mutations and polymorphisms. Knowing the location and sequence of genes important to the cause and treatment of disease will permit the rapid collection of sequence variations in a wide variety of potential patient populations. The tools used in that variant discovery fall into two categories—those technologies that are information rich but relatively costly in capital and man-hour terms (i.e., sequencing), and those technologies that are less information rich but relatively less expensive (i.e., gene scanning).

2.2 Brute Force Variant Identification

The use of DNA sequencing to identify population wide variation is, except for the largest commercial and governmental operations, a labor intensive and costly exercise. With the completion of the first draft of the Human Genome Project the task of finding appropriate primer sites for both PCR and sequencing has been simplified. The most practical sequencing based method of variant detection is via one of the various automated DNA sequencers currently on the market. All take advantage of substantially similar sequencing chemistry while using a variety of labeling technologies. The major difference between manufacturers, marketing claims aside, is the number of different labels that can be loaded into one lane of a gel or capillary at one time. By detecting multiple labels one is able to perform all four sequencing reactions in a single tube and/or load more than one sequencing reaction into a sequencing gel lane. The throughput advantage of automated sequencers able to detect multiple labels is a strong point in their favor when variant detection on a large scale is planned.

For most laboratories, however, variant detection via sequencing remains less a completely automated collection of data and more a task composed of visually sifting through quantities of sequence data in search of variants from a "normal." Advances in DNA analysis software have automated a portion of this task but the efficiency of this process varies by sequencing chemistry and automated analyzer. The major difficulty in sequence analysis is the determination of heterozygotes and true SNPs versus sequencing artifact. The SNP Consortium has addressed this difficulty in two ways. The genome centers that are identifying the sequence variants are re-sequencing randomly selected SNPs for verification and, secondly, the consortium has contracted with Orchid Biosciences (Princeton, NJ) to verify and develop assays for 4500 randomly selected SNPs [1]. In this way it is hoped that the accuracy level of SNPs collected by the consortium will reach a 95% standard level.

When one looks back on the SNP discovery process in the future, it is likely that the majority of sequence variants will have been identified using a brute force sequencing approach. This will no doubt be as a direct result of the amount of raw sequencing horsepower being applied to the task. There will, however, be a portion of the SNPs that will have been identified through the use of a variety of gene scanning methods. The use of such methods is appropriate for those laboratories that do not have access to large scale sequencing operations.

2.3   Gene Scanning Technologies

The identification of sequence variants in the absence of a large-scale sequencing capability can be accomplished through the use of gene scanning techniques. This collection of technologies are capable, at varying degrees of precision, of comparing a "normal" DNA (and in some instances RNA) sample to a test sample. The result of this comparison is either complete identity with the standard sequence or the identification of a variant at some point within the sequence under comparison. The common weakness of virtually all such scanning technologies is the requirement for a sequencing step to characterize the variant.

The technologies that purport to identify sequence variants generally fall into two categories: gel shift assays and mismatch identification.

2.3.1   Gel Shift Assays

The mobility of DNA, either single or double stranded, through a gel matrix is determined by a number of factors. By comparing the mobility of a test DNA sample to that of a normal control sample it is possible to determine the presence of a sequence alteration in the test sample. The major factors that affect DNA mobility are listed below:

Sequence length
Base composition
Single-strand secondary structure
Double-strand melting characteristics
Double-strand mobility in the presence of mismatched strands

A variety of techniques are used to take advantage of these factors in order to discover previously unknown mutations and polymorphisms. Two excellent reviews of these technologies have been published, by Cotton [2] and Schaefer et al. [3]. The following list outlines several of these techniques and a selection of their related methods.

Single-strand conformation polymorphism (SSCP)
    Restriction endonuclease fingerprinting (REF)
    Dideoxy fingerprinting (ddF)
Denaturing gradient gel electrophoresis (DGGE)
    Temperature gradient gel electrophoresis (TGGE)
Heteroduplex analysis (HA)

2.3.2 SSCP

This technique is perhaps the easiest of all of the variant detection methods to establish and perform. Developed by Orita et al. [4], PCR amplified fragments are heat denatured and then rapidly cooled to prevent reassociation of the complementary strands. The single-stranded DNA is then electrophoresed through a native acrylamide gel. The rate of transit through the gel is dependent upon sequence length and single-strand secondary structure. Variations in the sequences of single-stranded DNA fragments will, in theory, produce a change in the secondary structure of the DNA thereby affecting its progress through the gel matrix. It is this change in mobility that is resolved by the gel matrix producing additional or displaced bands as compared to a normal control. The resolving power of the gel matrix is affected by temperature and gel additives such as glycerol which enhance variant detection. The detection rates for SSCP can fall into the 60% to 95% range depending upon the sequence context in which the variants occur. By maintaining a relatively small fragment size ($\sim$200 bp) and selecting appropriate gel conditions it is possible to routinely achieve variant detection rates of >85%.

2.3.3 REF

Originally described by Liu and Sommer [5], this technique takes advantage of the capabilities of SSCP and restriction fragment length polymorphism (RFLP) analysis to increase the amount of information available to an investigator in an alteration discovery process. A restriction fragment analysis of a normal control region of interest is completed to select a collection of restriction enzymes capable of generating a series of fragments resolvable on a standard acrylamide gel. A PCR amplified segment of DNA up to 1–2 kb in length is restricted using the preselected enzyme set. The fragments are then radioactively or fluorescently labeled, heat denatured, and run as single-stranded segments on a native acrylamide gel. The electrophoretic step is identical to an SSCP gel with the resulting fragment pattern providing multiple bands whose mobility would be potentially affected by an alteration present in a fragment. In addition, the loss or gain of a restriction site would be identified by the gain or loss of an expected fragment and the increase or decrease in length of another fragment. Thus, REF provides two concurrent methods of alteration analysis, SSCP with the advantage of multiple analyzable bands and an RFLP component. The major advantage of this technique is the increased number of bands that are available for analysis using the SSCP component. While the RFLP analysis component is useful, it is not likely to provide consistently valuable information as the statistical likelihood of an alteration creating or eliminating an enzyme site that is also a member of the REF set is low. The multiple banding pattern, however, creates several opportunities for shifts in mobility to be identified. The increased fragment size available for analysis is also a major advantage of REF over SSCP and favorably impacts throughput for this technique. The detection rate for this technique has been reported to be in the 90–95% range [5]. One of the difficulties in this technique is the selection of the enzyme set. It is often a difficult task of balancing informativeness, exotic enzyme expense and fragment size. A subsequent publication from the Sommer group described a computer program which aided the enzyme selection process [6]. As with SSCP, the detection rate is dependent upon conformation changes and their resolvability on an acrylamide gel. The read-out of the assay provides a great deal of information for analysis which can be difficult to interpret on a routine basis. Precise localization of a variant for subsequent sequence identification is also difficult given the number of fragments which must be analyzed.

2.3.4   ddF

This technique uses a combination of SSCP and Sanger sequencing to create a larger set of bands for analysis in a native acrylamide gel [7]. In this method an amplified fragment is sequenced using a standard Sanger protocol and primers spaced at a SSCP friendly size of approximately 200–250 bp throughout the amplified fragment. One modification to the Sanger protocol is the use of a single dideoxy nucleotide to create the banding pattern. The change in banding pattern as compared to a normal control is then indicative of a sequence alteration in that region. This technique has been adapted to fluorescence as well as using primers running in both directions to increase detection rates. Through the appropriate selection of dideoxy nucleotide, fragment size and gel running conditions a significant improvement in detection rate over SSCP can be achieved. In addition, a degree of alteration localization can be determined by noting the location of the shift in banding patterns. The ability to perform a single PCR amplification followed by multiple Sanger reactions also reduces the overall cost of the assay. The fragment size used for variant detection remains in the SSCP range thus decreasing assay throughput. The original paper [7] suggests that reaching the 90–95% detection rate range may be difficult for some genes and some mutation types. In this event ddF would be useful as an adjunct to SSCP rather than a subsitute.

2.3.5   DGGE

This technique makes use of the reduced double-stranded melting characteristics inherent in heteroduplexed DNA as compared to a normal homoduplex control to identify novel sequence alterations [8]. A key modification to DGGE was made by Myers et al. [9,10] whereby a DNA sequence of interest is amplified using a specialized PCR primer pair consisting of one standard, sequence-specific primer and an opposing primer containing sequence specific information at the primer's 3' end and a GC-enriched sequence at the primer's 5' end. The purpose of the GC-enriched sequence (often called a GC clamp) is to normalize the melting profile of the sequence of interest. The GC clamp acts as a high-melting-temperature region of the resulting amplicon, stabilizing the melting characteristics over the entirety of the sequence. Without this normalization of amplicons containing multiple melting domains, the domains would denature at different temperatures. The lower-melting-temperature domains would denature first, obscuring the decrease in melting temperature contributed by sequence variants present in higher-temperature-melting domains.

In performing DGGE the sample is heat denatured, allowed to slowly reanneal, and then electrophoresed through an acrylamide gel containing a gradient of denaturant (usually formamide). As the double-stranded amplicon progresses through the gel matrix, it encounters an increasing denaturant concentration and the amplicon begins to denature. This denaturation slows the progression of the amplicon through the gel. Any alteration in a heteroduplex DNA sequence will result in decreased mobility, yielding a multiple banding pattern. By comparing the extent of mobility in the gradient matrix to a normal control, it is possible to determine the presence of a sequence change. In theory, any sequence alteration which changes the melting characteristics will result in additional bands being produced on the gel.

The melting profile of any sequence can be predicted using an algorithm created by Lerman and Silverstein [11]. If the sequence under investigation is amplified as a single melting domain using the GC clamp method it is then possible to design denaturing gradient conditions under which all sequence alterations in that single domain would be identified. The commonly accepted detection rates for DGGE are in the 90–95% range given an amplicon containing a single melting domain. The size of the routinely analyzable fragments (up to ~650 bp) is greater than the 200–250 bp for SSCP. The pouring of gradient gels is a technically difficult task requiring considerable experience and patience to achieve consistent results. The cost of the clamped primers is greater than nonclamped primers due to the addition of as many as 40 or more additional bases at the 5' end of the primer to produce the clamp. Alterations closer than 40–50 bp from the 3' end of the clamped primer are unlikely to be identified due to the increase thermal stability of this region. This requires the design of a second set of clamped primers opposing the initial set of primers for each region of interest. In this manner the region nearest one clamp and thus refractory to analysis is accounted for by the 3′ end of the opposing clamped amplicon. This necessarily doubles the cost of the assay from the PCR step onward.

2.3.6 TGGE and dHPLC

These variants of DGGE make use of a carefully controlled temperature gradient as a substitute for chemical denaturation. The simplest form of this method from an equipment standpoint immerses a uniform denaturant gel in a temperature-controlled buffer chamber. The buffer temperature is gradually increased during the running of the gel providing the denaturing gradient range desired.

Another modification of this type of denaturing gradient methodology uses the high-resolution characteristics of high-performance liquid chromatography (HPLC) to physically separate sequences which differ in their denaturing characteristics [12]. The main advantage is the rapid nature of HPLC coupled with the fine temperature control of HPLC, resulting in an ability to resolve small differences in melting characteristics. The semiautomated manner in which the samples can be loaded into the HPLC and the potential for customizing the run characteristics is also a favorable feature for this approach. The use of dHPLC does not provide any inherent improvements over traditional DGGE other than in the area of automation as detection for all variants must still labor under the constraints of DNA melting theory. The major advantage of dHPLC over DGGE is more one of process and throughput for the end user.

2.3.7 HA

This technique makes use of the change in mobility caused by mismatched hetero-duplexed DNA strands as compared to perfectly homoduplexed DNA strands [13]. In this technique a DNA sample is amplified, heat denatured, and then reannealed. This results in a fraction of the single-stranded DNA reannealing with a complementary strand from an opposing allele, thus forming a hetero-duplex. When this mixture is subsequently electrophoresed through a nondenatur-ing acrylamide gel a mobility shift can be resolved indicating the presence of a sequence alteration as compared to a normal control homoduplex. The relative ease of this protocol is the major advantage to this technique. The generally accepted detection rates for a specific PCR run on an appropriate acrylamide gel ranges from the low 80% range to the 90–95% range. Modifications to the assay to generate heteroduplexes may increase the detection rate to a more routine 90–95%. The major difficulty with this technique is the establishment of sufficiently specific PCR amplification conditions to avoid missing important heteroduplexes or the creation of false alterations. The lack of resolution of the acrylamide matrix is another area of false-negative results. In practice, the amplicon size range for routine detection is 250–500 bp, thus limiting the use of this technique for very large genes.

2.4 Mismatch Identification

The discovery of sequence alterations can be accomplished by the creation of mismatched base pairs which occur when a test sample containing a sequence alteration is denatured and reannealed with an otherwise complementary normal control sequence. The routine and specific discovery of these mismatches and their localization to within an easily sequenced region is the goal of several techniques. There are two general methods for identification of mismatched sequences: chemical and enzymatic.

2.4.1 Chemical

The major method involving chemical identification of mismatched sequences is a modification of Maxam-Gilbert sequencing termed chemical cleavage of mismatch (CCM) [14]. Using the C- and T-specific reactivity of hydroxylamine and osmium tetroxide, respectively, to identify mismatched bases followed by piperidine cleavage of the modified products, it is possible to not only scan a genomic segment for mismatched bases but also localized the site of the mismatch. When optimized, this technique is highly efficient in alteration discovery (nearly 100%). The current practical limit of the size of a fragment suitable for analysis is in the 1- to 1.5-kb range. A considerable disadvantage, however, to CCM is the use of highly toxic chemicals in a clinical environment. Hydroxylamine and osmium tetroxide both require chemical-grade fume hoods for use. The relatively large number of manipulations associated with the technique and the toxic nature of the chemicals render this technique a difficult choice for a clinical lab. A recent improvement on the assay has substituted potassium permangenate for osmium tetroxide making the manipulations involving these chemicals less toxic and more attractive for the routine laboratory [15].

2.4.2 Enzymatic

This set of methods makes use of specific enzymes to recognize mismatched base pairs in heteroduplexed DNA strands. In general a test sample is amplified and heat-denatured in the presence of a normal control sample. This combination of test and normal control samples is allowed to slowly reanneal forming a mixture of homo- and heteroduplexes. The mixture is then exposed to any one of a number of enzymes which recognize mismatched base pairs at various efficiencies and the sample is then analyzed for these recognized mismatches. There are several types of enzymes and assays available which purport to recognize mismatched base pairs in a heteroduplex or secondary structures formed by mismatches. A short selection of these enzymes and assays are discussed below.

2.4.2.1 Ribonuclease Cleavage.   This technique, developed by Myers et al. [16], is useful for sequence alteration discovery due to its ability to cleave double stranded RNA, or RNA:DNA hybrid sequence at areas of mismatch. The mismatched areas form single stranded regions in a heteroduplex which are then amenable to cleavage by the RNAses. A significant improvement in the assay was published by Murthy et al. [17] whereby an amplified product is produced following a standard PCR of regions of interest. The test sample DNA is then mixed with a normal control RNA sample to produce a normal/test duplex which creates the potential for mismatched heteroduplexes open to cleavage by RNAse. The cleaved products are then electrophoresed on a standard agarose gels (this is the most recent form of the assay which has been reduced to its simplest practice) and the banding pattern is compared to a normal control. Relative to SSCP and DGGE this technique offers slightly longer analyzable read lengths and the potential for multiple bands for analysis. RNA handling requirements, however, are often a negative factor in a high throughput or clinical environment.

2.4.2.2   T4 Endonuclease VII.   Mashal et al. [18] originally described the use of two bacteriophage resolvases to identify mismatches in heteroduplexed DNA. The current technique depends upon one of those enzymes, T4 endonuclease VII, to recognize and cleave double stranded DNA at the site of the mismatch. This technology is now incorporated into kit form by Amersham Pharmacia Biotech (Piscataway, NJ). The length of fragment amenable to this sort of scanning is approximately 1kb. The assay is essentially the same as a restriction enzyme analysis with respect to ease of use. The size of the generated cleaved fragment is then used to roughly localize the site of the alteration for subsequent sequencing.

2.4.2.3   Cleavase.   This enzyme cleaves secondary structure in single-stranded DNA. The principle used here, as described by Brow et al. [19], is one of secondary folding structure of single stranded DNA being altered when the underlying sequence is changed by polymorphism or mutation. Cleavase acts as a structure-specific endonuclease by cutting at the 3′ end of a loop structure in a single-stranded DNA producing a characteristic banding pattern. When compared to a normal control sample a cleaved test sample containing a different base composition would demonstrate an altered banding pattern. This method has been developed for commercial use by Third Wave Technologies (Madison, WI).

The main advantages of any enzyme based gene scanning system is the relative ease of use and cost effectiveness when compared to full gene sequencing. The ability to scan through large amounts of genetic real estate identifying only those individuals demonstrating variations from a control reduces the overall amount of DNA sequencing required to characterize the panoply of genetic variation in a population. A significant disadvantage, however, is the amount and types of variations that the enzymatic methods have difficulty identifying. Depending upon the sequence context and variant type the enzyme may not recognize the mismatched base pair leading to a false negative result. This may not be a significant difficulty in the context of a large variant discovery effort where missing one polymorphism is not of great import. In a clinical diagnostic effort where each patient sample must be completely and accurately scanned enzymatic based assays must be designed with great care to reduce the false negative rate to an absolute minimum. All of the described methods are now offered commercially so it remains the consumers challenge to sort through the various detection claims and identify the enzyme which works best in their hands and for the sequence to be scanned.

2.5 Variant Identification

The technologies available to the research pharmacogenetics community are varied and numerous. The task confronting the end user in the selection of the appropriate tool set is one of overall throughput, accuracy and thoroughness. How one goes about using the vast quantities of variants which are discovered is the subject of the next section.

2.6 Testing for Previously Identified Gene Variants

The development of large and publicly available SNP and mutation databases provides ample intellectual material for pharmacogenetics. The real value of this information glut will be in using it to design appropriate therapeutics and to select individuals most likely to benefit from these new treatments. The techniques and reagents which were included in the description of variant identification methods are not universally applicable to the task of genotyping individuals on a clinical basis. There are several technologies which are useful to perform this type of known variant detection. Virtually all of these technologies use probes of one sort or another to detect variants. The probes in these cases are highly specific for a particular known variant and are therefore not useful for generalized gene scanning. The universe of variant detection can be broken into two categories: array-based and non-array-based.

2.6.1 Array-Based Systems

The use of a fixed-probe system with a test sample in solution has promised to revolutionize genetic testing for nearly a decade [20,21]. The promise has not entirely become a reality as of yet but the uses of arrays have increased over the decade to accommodate the potential to screen individuals for thousands of discrete polymorphisms in a single hybridization [22]. In fixed array systems the probes are attached to a surface by a number of methods. The method pioneered by Fodor et al. [20] uses a modification of the photolithographic system used to manufacture computer chips. In this method a mask is placed over the surface of the DNA chip covering those regions to be protected from the light activated oligonucleotide synthetic process. The process is completed and the mask realigned to uncover subsequent areas. In this manner a series of chemical reactions can take place in a defined order resulting in the building of an oligonucleotide probe of a specific design at a known location on the array. By carefully controlling the synthetic process it is possible to increase the number of probes on the array to the hundreds of thousands or greater. Other fixed array types attach fully preconstructed probes to a number of different substrates by a variety of chemical means [23–27].

The process of analyzing a sample on fixed arrays generally takes place in several steps. The sample must first be amplified for the specific region of the genome to be probed. The sample must then be fragmented in order for optimal hybridization to a static probe. The hybridization then occurs and analysis of the hybridization pattern takes place. The number of probes able to be queried on a fixed array is not equal to the number of separate elements fixed to the substrate. Due to the detection limits of the fluorescent technology which underlies the majority of fixed array systems multiple probe elements must hybridize to the test sample in order for a sufficient signal to be measured. The hybridization characteristics of oligonucleotide probes are often difficult to normalize when dealing with large numbers of probes. This is exacerbated when a probe must be placed in a sequence context of unfavorable hybridization characteristics due to the presence of an important sequence variant. As a result, there are regions of the genome and types of variants that are not easily amenable to oligonucleotide hybridization. Nanogen (San Diego, CA) has approached the hybridization problem with a methodology involving control of the hybridization and denaturation of disparate oligonucleotides by varying the electric field strength of the hybridization repelling molecules with reduced affinity for the probe [28].

One of the drawbacks of a fixed-array system in an era where not all the relevant information concerning a biologic system may be present is the relatively inflexible nature of a fixed system. In order to add elements to a fixed array one needs to return to the chip manufacture process and redesign the array. Not all array-based systems, however, make use of a fixed solid support. Two types of arrays make use of bead technologies to permit rapid rearrangement and alteration of the components of an array. Luminex (Austin, TX) attaches oligonucleotide probes to polystyrene beads that have been colored with one of a number of colors separately identifiable by a fluorescence activated cell sorter. It is then possible to perform a standard oligonucleotide hybridization to a collection of these probe-bound beads using test sample material that has been labeled with another identifiable fluorescent tag. The beads are then washed and run through the cell sorter, producing a profile of test sample-bound and -unbound beads. The colors of the bound beads are then correlated to the type of oligonucleotide previously attached to them and a positive identification of the probe is made. This process has the advantage of speed and thus throughput as well as flexibility of array composition. In order to change the array one only needs to mix the appropriate combination of beads. A second type of non-fixed array was developed at Tufts University using beads similarly color coded with oligonucleotide probes covalently attached [29]. In this method, however, the beads are deposited onto the ends of fiber optic cable following a process of etching carefully controlled pits into the end of the fiber optic. The amplified test sample is labeled with a fluorescent tag and is hybridized to the beads. The laser excitation of the fluorescent tag and the colored beads provides evidence of a positive hybridization and identification of the probe. This technology is now under further development at Illumina (San Diego, CA).

2.6.2 Non-Array-Based Systems

Hybridization-based array systems are not the only method of analyzing test samples for known genetic variants. One of the most effective methods of analyzing SNPs is a technique known as minisequencing or single-base extension. This technique is described in detail later in this volume and is used by Orchid BioScience (Princeton, NJ) as well as Sequenom (San Diego, CA) to type SNPs. The method takes advantage of DNA sequencing technology and the chain terminating effect of dideoxynucleotides to determine the presence of particular nucleotide at a known position. A primer specific for a region immediately adjacent to the SNP under study is hybridized to a test sample. A dideoxynucleotide corresponding to one of the two bases indicative of the SNP is then added to the reaction. If the SNP corresponding to the particular dideoxynucleotide is present the reaction is terminated. By labeling the dideoxynucleotide with a fluorescent tag (or a mass tag for mass spectrometry-based methods), it is possible to perform these assays in an automated manner increasing throughput and decreasing manpower requirements.

Another SNP detection system that does not rely on fixed arrays is being developed by Third Wave Technologies (Madison, WI). The Invader assay [30–32] makes use of two probe molecules which partially overlap a known SNP site. The probes compete for hybridization to the specified genetic sequence. When one probe binds specifically to the test sample it forces the overlapping probe to leave a portion of the overlapping region non hybridized. The Cleavase endonuclease described earlier in this review then cleaves the overlapping flap releasing a small fragment which is either directly labeled or used as an ''invading'' oligonucleotide itself in a secondary reaction which releases labeled sequence producing a detectable signal. This isothermal reaction is compatible with several assay formats and has been developed for a number of clinical assays, most notably Factor V Leiden [32,33]. The isothermal nature of the assay and the single base discriminatory nature of the probe reactions make this system an attractive choice for those laboratories seeking an alternative to PCR-based systems.

3   REDUCTION TO PRACTICE

The construction of large-scale databases and genotype/phenotype correlations within large population groups is of great value to the future of medical care. This large-scale research effort will create opportunities for the genetic testing community previously seen as mere science fiction. For the testing community to take advantage of these opportunities a shift in technologies must take place on a scale which is not possible at present. The volume of assays that might be expected over the next decade or more will be far closer to that seen in the clinical chemistry laboratories. If one considers the development of clinical chemistry testing on an industrial scale a few similarities to the challenges that pharmacogenetics will face in the future can be seen.

The major development which permitted clinical chemistry to achieve the volumes of testing that laboratories currently handle was the wide scale adoption of automation. The modern clinical chemistry laboratory receives samples for testing, bar codes each sample and places the sample tube into an automated system. This system reads the bar code, consults a database to determine the requested testing, and proceeds to perform the necessary procedures often without any human intervention. There is no currently available system for widespread genetic analysis that approaches this level of automation for even the most straightforward of test protocols. As it is unlikely that a pharmacogenetics test will involve a single SNP as the definitive predictor of therapeutic response a new generation of molecular genetic technologies and automation must be developed that can perform this highly complex testing in a clinical chemistry-like atmosphere. An example of the scale that the testing industry will have to face in the not too distant future is that presented by the volume of testing for a pharmaceutical that has a rather modest market size and a different pharmaceutical with a large market size.

One of the assumptions that is often made in pharmacogenetics is that there will eventually be a pharmaceutical product whose prescription will be linked to a genetic test. This will probably not be a safety related issue but one of selecting those patients who will benefit most from being treated by a drug or to determine an appropriate dosage level. If one creates a hypothetical drug whose market size is ~$200 million, the monthly new prescriptions can be in the range of 18,000. The market size for such a genetic test would be >200,000 tests per year. If one increases the market for the drug to the $1 billion size the monthly new prescription rate can equal the number of prescriptions written in an entire year for the smaller market example. In this scenario the yearly testing market for a $1 billion drug with a genetic test linked to prescription would be over 2 million tests per year. To put this into context, the current market size for cystic fibrosis testing in the United States prior to population screening is ~100,000 tests annually. The molecular genetics technology development community and the genetic testing community do not currently have the ability to perform that level of genetic testing.

The caveat to the argument, however, is that there are unlikely to be $1 billion drugs that have a genetic test linked to them in the near future. The problem becomes essentially identical to the billion dollar drug issue, however, when one envisions multiple smaller drugs on the market that have a linked genetic test for therapeutic efficacy. This is an issue that will only increase in seriousness as more information concerning genetic markers of drug response become an increasing part of routine medical practice.

4 THE FUTURE

The promise of pharmacogenetics to enhance the future of pharmaceutical development and medical care has been discussed in this volume as well as a number of others. The technological task challenging the scientific community is twofold. The first challenge is identifying the relevant genetic markers that will provide significant and medically relevant information to the clinician. This effort will require the establishment of large, well annotated databases linking information concerning disease pathogenesis, functional genomics, proteomics and genetic variation. The most useful data will be those correlating the large databases with subpopulations of individuals particularly susceptible to severe disease or to particular sequelae, or in need of or obtaining a particular benefit from a specific treatment regimen significantly different from a larger population group. As the future of pharmacogenetics unfolds it will hold opportunities for the developers of novel, highly specific and efficient technologies which provide valuable information to the medical community. Those successful in the development effort will have solved the many layered problem of medical relevance, technological possibility, and cost-effectiveness. The technologies and concepts described in this volume go a long way down this path.

REFERENCES

1. A Holden. The SNP consortium: a case study in large pharmaceutical company research and development collaboration. J Comm Biotech 6(4):320–332, 2000.
2. RG Cotton. Mutation detection and mutation databases. Clin Chem Lab Med 36(8): 519–522, 1998.
3. A Schafer, JR Hawkins. DNA variation and the future of human genetics. Nature Biotech 16:33–39, 1998.
4. M Orita, H Iwahana, H Kanazawa, K Hayashi, T Sekiya. Detection of polymorphisms of human DNA by gel electrophoresis as single-strand conformation polymorphisms. Proc Natl Acad Sci USA 86:2766–2770, 1989.
5. Q Liu, SS Sommer. Restriction endonuclease fingerprinting (REF): a sensitive

method for screening mutations in long, contiguous segments of DNA. Biotechniques 18(3):470–477, 1995.

6. WA Scaringe, Q Liu, SS Sommer. REF Select: expert system software for selecting restriction endonucleases for restriction endonuclease fingerprinting. Biotechniques 27(6):1188 passim, 1999.

7. G Sarkar, HS Yoon, SS Sommer. Dideoxy fingerprinting (ddE): a rapid and efficient screen for the presence of mutations. Genomics 13(2):441–443, 1992.

8. S Fischer, LS Lerman. DNA fragments differing by single base pair substitutions are separated in denaturing gradient gels: correspondence with melting theory. Proc Natl Acad Sci USA 80:1579–1583, 1983.

9. RM Myers, SG Fischer, LS Lerman, T Maniatis. Nearly all single base substitutions in DNA fragments joined to a GC-clamp can be detected by denaturing gradient gel electrophoresis. Nucleic Acids Res 13(9):3131–3145, 1985.

10. RM Myers, SG Fischer, T Maniatis, LS Lerman. Modification of the melting properties of duplex DNA by attachment of a GC-rich DNA sequence as determined by denaturing gradient gel electrophoresis. Nucleic Acids Res 13(9):3111–3129, 1985.

11. LS Lerman, K Silverstein. Computational simulation of DNA melting and its application to denaturing gradient gel electrophoresis. Methods Enzymol, 155:482–501, 1987.

12. PA Underhill, AA Lin, SQ Mehdi, T Jenkins, D Vollrath, RW Davis, LL Cavalli-Sforza, PJ Oefner. Detection of numerous Y chromosome biallelic polymorphisms by denaturing high-performance liquid chromatography. Genome Res 7(10):996–1005, 1997.

13. MB White, D Derse, SJ O'Brien, M Dean. Detecting single base substitutions as heteroduplex polymorphisms. Genomics 12:301–306, 1992.

14. R Cotton, NR Rodrigues, RD Campbell. Reactivity of cytosine and thymine in single-base-pair mismatches with hydroxylamine and osmium tetroxide and its application to the study of mutations. Proc Natl Acad Sci USA 85:4397–4401, 1988.

15. E Roberts, VJ Beeble, CG Woods, GR Taylor. Potassium permanganate and tetraethylammonium chloride are a safe and effective substitute for osmium tetroxide in solid-phase fluorescent chemical cleavage of mismatch. NAR 25:3377–3378, 1997.

16. R Myers, Z Larin, T Maniatis. Detection of single base substitutions by ribonuclease cleavage at mismatches in RNA:DNA duplexes. Science 230(4731):1242–1246, 1985.

17. K Murthy, SH Shen, D Banville. A sensitive method for detection of mutations— a PCR-based RNase protection assay. DNA Cell Biol 14(1):87–94, 1995.

18. R Mashal, J Koontz, J Sklar. Detection of mutations by cleavage of DNA heteroduplexes with bacteriophage resolvases. Nat Genet 9(2):177–183, 1995.

19. M Brow, MC Oldenburg, V Lyamichev, LM Heisler, N Lyamicheva, JG Hall, NJ Eagan, DM Olive, LM Smith, L Fors, JE Dahlberg. Differentiation of bacterial 16S rRNA genes and intergenic regions and Mycobacterium tuberculosis katG genes by structure-specific endonuclease cleavage. J Clin Microbiol 34(12):3129–3137, 1996.

20. SP Fodor. Light-directed, spatially addressable parallel chemical synthesis. Science 251(4995):767–773, 1991.

21. H Erlich. HLA-DR, DQ and DP typing using PCR amplification and immobilized probes. Eur J Immunogenet 18(1-2):33–55, 1991.

22. M Chee. Accessing genetic information with high-density DNA arrays. Science 274(5287):610–614, 1996.

23. N Zammatteo. Comparison between different strategies of covalent attachment of DNA to glass surfaces to build DNA microarrays. Anal Biochem 280(1):143–150, 2000.

24. FN Rehman. Immobilization of acrylamide-modified oligonucleotides by copolymerization. Nucleic Acids Res 27(2):649–655, 1999.

25. YH Rogers. Immobilization of oligonucleotides onto a glass support via disulfide bonds: a method for preparation of DNA microarrays. Anal Biochem 266(1):23–30, 1999.

26. M Beier, JD Hoheisel. Versatile derivatisation of solid support media for covalent bonding on DNA-microchips. Nucleic Acids Res 27(9):1970–1977, 1999.

27. T Okamoto, T Suzuki, N Yamamoto. Microarray fabrication with covalent attachment of DNA using bubble jet technology [see comments]. Nat Biotechnol 18(4):438–441, 2000.

28. RG Sosnowski. Rapid determination of single base mismatch mutations in DNA hybrids by direct electric field control. Proc Natl Acad Sci USA 94(4):1119–1123, 1997.

29. BG Healey, RS Matson, DR Walt. Fiberoptic DNA sensor array capable of detecting point mutations. Anal Biochem 251(2):270–279, 1997.

30. RW Kwiatkowski. Clinical, genetic, and pharmacogenetic applications of the invader assay. Mol Diagn 4(4):353–364, 1999.

31. RC Cooksey. Evaluation of the invader assay, a linear signal amplification method, for identification of mutations associated with resistance to rifampin and isoniazid in *Mycobacterium tuberculosis*. Antimicrob Agents Chemother 44(5):1296–1301, 2000.

32. D Ryan, B Nuccie, D Arvan. Non-PCR-dependent detection of the factor V Leiden mutation from genomic DNA using a homogeneous invader microtiter plate assay. Mol Diagn 4(2):135–144, 1999.

33. MJ Hessner, MA Budish, KD Friedman. Genotyping of factor V G1691A (Leiden) without the use of PCR by invasive cleavage of oligonucleotide probes. Clin Chem 46(8 Pt 1):1051–1056, 2000.

9

Molecular Diagnostics and Development of Biotechnology-Based Diagnostics

Tracy L. Stockley and Peter N. Ray
Hospital for Sick Children, Toronto, Ontario, Canada

1 INTRODUCTION

Adverse drug reactions are a leading cause of death in current medical treatment regimes [1]. Some adverse drug reactions may be due in part to individual variability in drug response, as there are to date many known genetic variations that affect pharmacological differences [2]. The use of molecular diagnostic techniques to identify individuals with genetic changes relevant to drug response is an essential component of pharmacogenomics. The detection of these individuals prior to drug administration will result in increased safety and efficacy of pharmacological treatments. This chapter will focus on issues related to molecular diagnosis that are relevant to pharmacogenomic applications, and the molecular diagnostic tests required to identify variants in genetic loci known to affect drug metabolism.

Molecular pharmacogenomic applications are rapidly evolving in response to the new technologies and new genetic information provided by the Human Genome Project (HGP). Traditional methods to determine individual differences in drug responses involve the administration of drugs to subjects and examination of biological markers [3,4]. However, the potential for using molecular diagnostic methods to determine pharmacological variation is becoming more relevant as the genetic basis for variations in drug responses is discovered. This is especially relevant at the present time due to the ongoing discovery of novel genes by the HGP, and the shift in focus from single genes to whole genomes is reflected in the transition from *pharmacogenetics* to *pharmacogenomics* [5].

At present, molecular diagnosis is costly and is restricted to a limited number of individuals at high risk, typically people who are suspected of being affected or carriers of a particular monogenic disorder. Large-scale diagnostic applications such as molecular pharmacogenomic testing will require the development of high-throughput, cost-effective molecular diagnostic tests suitable for screening a large number of individuals. As the technology for molecular diagnosis improves, molecular testing will assume an increasingly significant role in the application of drug administration to patients on a large scale.

Another important issue in applying molecular diagnostics to pharmacogenomics is the difference in testing for mutations in a single gene disorder versus testing for mutations involved in multifactorial disorders. The majority of current molecular diagnostic assays are used to test for mutations causing monogenic disorders. For example, cystic fibrosis is a relatively common single-gene disorder, and is caused by mutations in the cystic fibrosis transmembrane conductance regulator (CFTR) gene. Many diagnostic laboratories routinely test for 10–30 of the most common CFTR mutations, which account for the majority of cystic fibrosis mutations in the Caucasian population. The finding of a mutation is diagnostic in that a prediction of disease can be made on the basis of finding two mutations in the CFTR gene carried by an individual.

In contrast, multifactorial diseases such as hypertension and obesity are more complex as disease onset is likely to be dependent on changes in several genetic regions, each with a different influence on disease progression, plus environmental factors [6]. For example, individuals with a family history of hypertension may carry mutations in genetic regions that lead to an increased susceptibility for hypertension. However, due to environmental differences only a portion of the individuals who carry these mutations will develop hypertension. The application of molecular testing to multifactorial diseases is complex, as it requires testing of several genetic regions and involves unknown gene-environment interactions that are difficult to predict. Many individual drug responses are likely to be multifactorial traits, and these same issues will complicate prediction of drug response outcome based on molecular diagnostic test results.

In order to highlight some of the considerations of molecular diagnostics that will be relevant to pharmacogenomics, we will discuss some common types of genetic variation and current molecular diagnostic methods used to detect these variations. Important recent developments in the biotechnology field that will have an impact on future molecular diagnostic testing will also be discussed.

2 TYPES OF GENETIC MUTATIONS

When considering technical approaches to molecular diagnosis, genetic diseases can be segregated by whether they are caused by relatively few common mutations or by many unique mutations. For example Tay-Sachs disease, a fatal neurodegenerative disorder caused by a deficiency of hexosaminidase A, is common in the Ashkenazi Jewish population. Five hexosaminidase mutations account for ~96% of the mutations in the Ashkenazi Jewish population. In contrast, most patients with Fabry disease, a metabolic disorder caused by deficiency of the enzyme galactosidase A, have unique mutations in the galactosidase A gene. This distinction is significant as the detection of a small number of known mutations in a gene requires quite different technologies from the analysis of a complete gene to search for unknown mutations. Therefore, when designing molecular diagnostic assays, the technical approach taken depends on the nature of the mutations that are to be detected.

A complication in analyzing genes for unique mutations is that it is often difficult or impossible to predict the biological consequences of a mutation. A missense mutation that changes an amino acid in the protein may or may not affect protein function, depending on the nature of the amino acid change. An exchange of a basic amino acid for an acidic amino acid would likely have a more significant effect on protein function than an exchange of a basic amino acid for another basic amino acid, although this is not necessarily true. In other cases the pathological consequences of a mutation will be more obvious, as would be the case with a nonsense mutation producing a deleterious premature translation stop codon. The assessment of the functional effect of an identified mutation is a current obstacle for molecular diagnosis, as will also be true for mutation identification in pharmacogenomics.

Other types of genetic variation include deletions and duplications that can range in size from a single base to large regions encompassing whole exons or entire genes. Deletions and duplications are of particular significance in molecular diagnosis, as they require special assays for detection, such as quantitative polymerase chain reaction (PCR) assays to determine gene copy number [7]. Genetic mutations can also alter function at levels other than the DNA coding sequence, such as mutations at conserved splice site sequences which alter RNA splicing [8].

The methods of detection of these different types of genetic changes vary depending on the type of mutation to be detected. Methods of mutation detection include specific assays designed to identify a certain nucleotide change at a particular base pair in a sequence, or the use of direct sequencing to detect many unique mutations. Direct sequencing may be proceeded by scanning methods to highlight particular exons of a gene that may contain a mutation. If a genetic disease is caused by a few recurrent mutations that account for the majority of disease, it is more appropriate to test for these few mutations by a specific assay rather than by sequencing. In contrast, diseases caused by a large number of mutations in a single gene are more appropriately tested by direct sequencing methods [for review, see 9]. Therefore, it is critical that a molecular diagnostic test be appropriately matched to the types of mutations to be detected for a particular gene. The usual methods to test known mutations and the advantages and disadvantages are discussed below, as well as more recent developments to these methods.

3   METHODS TO DETECT KNOWN MUTATIONS

3.1   PCR Restriction Enzyme Assays

Certain genetic changes may alter a restriction enzyme recognition site, either by creating a new site or destroying an existing site. In these cases, a molecular diagnostic assay can be designed in which a region containing the potential mutation site is amplified via PCR and the product is digested with the appropriate restriction enzyme to determine if the restriction digest pattern is altered due to the presence of the mutation. In some cases, designing a PCR primer containing a mismatch that anneals near a mutation site can artificially produce a restriction enzyme site. When combined with the mutant genetic sequence, the mismatched PCR primer sequence and the mutation alters a restriction enzyme site and so produces altered restriction enzyme patterns. Quality control for this type of assay requires that appropriate positive and negative control samples be present in each assay in order to confirm that the enzyme is properly active.

An example of a PCR restriction enzyme assay to detect variation for a pharmacogenomic application is the detection of mutations in the gene for the cytochrome isozyme P250D6 (CYP2D6) which cause the "poor metabolizer" of debrisoquine phenotype [10]. The detection of mutant alleles in the P250D6 gene is an interesting example of the use of molecular diagnostic methods for pharmacogenomics, since several assays using different methods have been designed to detect genetic variation in this gene. This highlights the difficulty in choosing the best method for molecular analysis of mutations in a particular gene.

The main advantage of a PCR restriction enzyme assay is that it is simple to develop and use. The major disadvantage is that the assay is time consuming, as each mutation must be individually analyzed. Although this assay is effective for testing a small number of samples in specific cases, it is not ideal for testing samples for multiple mutations or for screening large numbers of samples.

3.2   Allele-Specific Oligonucleotide Assay

The basis of the allele-specific oligonucleotide (ASO) assay is that DNA duplexes which contain a mismatch are destabilised and have a lower melting temperature than correctly paired duplexes. To test for mutations using this principle two probes, one containing the normal sequence and one containing the mutant sequence, are produced and hybridised sequentially to the patient's DNA. For each normal and mutant probe, conditions can be found where the probe will hybridize to only its perfectly matched duplex. If the patient sample contains only normal sequence, only the normal probe will hybridize. In a heterozygous sample, both the mutant and normal probes will hybridize, and in a homozygous mutant sample only the mutant probe will hybridize.

An advantage of the ASO method is that it can be used to simultaneously test samples for several different mutations by the use of multiple probes bound to a solid matrix. In practice, the success of this method relies on precisely establishing conditions for optimal oligonucleotide hybridization in order to ensure specific probe hybridization, and so multiplex ASO assays can be difficult to develop.

There have been recent improvements to the ASO assay, specifically by development of a multiplex allele-specific diagnostic assay (MASDA) in which the ASO technique is adapted to a solid support and multiple regions are probed simultaneously. This has been achieved by altering probe hybridization conditions, so that hybridization of multiple probes at a single temperature is feasible. Using these improvements it has been possible to analyse >500 samples simultaneously for >100 known mutations in multiple genes [11].

3.3 Allele-Specific Amplification Assay

The allele-specific amplification (ASA) assay is based on the finding that Taq polymerase will not initiate amplification from a primer that has a mismatch at the 3′ end. Two primers are designed so that the 3′ base of the primer corresponds to the site of the genetic mutation to be tested, with either the normal or the mutant sequence at the 3′ base position. An unknown sample can then be tested for the presence of the mutation by using both the normal and the mutant primers in PCR. If the sample contains only normal sequence, a PCR product will only be produced when the normal primer is used, and similarly, when the sample contains mutant sequence, a product will only result from use of the mutant primer. Like the PCR restriction enzyme method discussed, the ASA approach has also been applied to the detection of mutations in the CYP2D6 gene, as described by Heim and Meyer [12].

In the original ASA protocols, the mutant and normal PCR primers were separated into two reactions, so that lack of amplification could occur in one PCR reaction depending on the sequence present in a test sample. This is not ideal for a diagnostic test due to the possible misinterpretation of a false-negative result, and the ASA protocol is usually modified to be a multiplex reaction that includes a positive internal control in each PCR reaction. For example, an ASA assay has been developed which detects 12 common CFTR mutations simultaneously [13]. However, in this assay, two reactions must still be run in parallel for every sample to be analyzed, since the mutant and normal products produced are the same size and so must be physically separated in order to be distinguished.

The ASA can be improved by the use of fluorescent-dye-labeled primers, which avoids the need for two separate reactions by using flourochromes to distinguish normal and mutant sequences. We have developed molecular diagnostic ASA assays to detect mutations causing Tay-Sachs disease using fluorescent-dye-labeled PCR primers. The mutant and normal primers are labelled with different colour dyes, so that the PCR products resulting from either the normal or the mutant allele-specific primer will be a different dye colour, allowing discrimination of normal and mutant sequence. The use of fluorescent dyes thus simplifies the assay, and allows one sample to be tested for multiple mutations in a single reaction.

The advantage of the ASA method is that multiplex reactions to detect several mutations simultaneously can be developed. Multiplex reactions reduce the labour and costs associated with molecular diagnostics and so are ideal for detection of a large number of mutations. The main disadvantage of the ASA method is that achieving specific product amplification can be problematic.

3.4   Oligonucleotide Ligation Assay

The oligonucleotide ligation assay (OLA) is similar to allele-specific amplification in that specific interrogation of a mutation site is achieved by two oligonucleotides that contain the normal or mutant base at the 3' end of the primer. However, in the OLA assay, the normal or mutant primer anneals directly downstream and adjacent to a common primer. The two primers are therefore directly adjacent to one another, and thermostable ligase is able to join the annealed primers. In the case of a normal DNA sequence, only the normal and common primers will anneal and so be ligated, while a mutant DNA sequence will produce ligation of only the mutant and common primers. This method has also been applied to the detection of CYP2D6 alleles as described by Hansen et al. [14].

A recent improvement in the OLA assay is the use of sequence-coded separation (SCS), in which nonnucleic mobility-altering compounds are attached to the specific primers. The mobility-altering compounds are designed so that the products from each primer are a different size, and so will allow discrimination between primer pairs for different mutations. This technology is used in a diagnostic assay for cystic fibrosis in which 32 mutations in the CFTR gene can be detected simultaneously [15]. This novel method of size separation may expand the utility of the OLA assay, as it theoretically will allow multiplex assays for a large number of mutations to be developed.

3.5 Primer Extension Assay

The primer extension assay has similarities to the dideoxy method commonly used in sequence analysis. In the primer extension assay, a region containing the mutation to be assayed is amplified in a first PCR reaction. A specific primer, which is designed to anneal directly upstream of the base that is the site of a known mutation, is then used in a second reaction. Radioactively labeled dideoxy nucleotides corresponding to either the normal or the mutant base at the potential mutation site are added in separate tubes. During the reaction, the labeled nucleotide added to the 3′ end of the primer will depend on the sequence at the potential mutation site. If the normal sequence is present at the potential mutation site, only the reaction containing the normal labeled dideoxy nucleotide will produce a labeled primer. Conversely, if the mutant sequence is present at the mutation site, only the reaction containing the mutant nucleotide will produce a labeled primer. Individuals who are heterozygous for the mutation will produce labeled primers in both dideoxy tubes, due to the presence of both sequences at the potential mutation site.

Primer extension assays are reported to be very sensitive for mutation detection and may be advantageous for large-scale testing with some modifications to the basic protocol. Primer extension assays have been designed to use fluorescent-dye-labeled nucleotides to eliminate the need for radioactivity and may also be adaptable to use on solid supports [16]. The primer extension assay is discussed in further detail in Chapter 11.

4 ROLE OF BIOTECHNOLOGY IN DEVELOPMENT OF DIAGNOSTIC TESTS FOR PHARMACOGENOMICS

In recent years, there have been major technical advances in genetic analysis methods due primarily to ongoing genome research. The completion of the Human Genome Project will lead to identification of more disease genes and eventually information on the deleterious mutations or functionally neutral single nucleotide polymorphisms (SNP) within and surrounding these genes [17]. Databases of SNPs and mutations are rapidly growing [18] and will become more important as our knowledge of the functional significance of the genetic alterations is clarified [19]. In conjunction with this increased knowledge, there will be increasing emphasis on faster, more efficient methods of detecting the identified genetic changes facilitated by the use of novel methods and equipment, with increased automation to reduce labor-intensive steps in genetic analysis.

Major technological advances will be essential for routine diagnosis of genetic changes in large-scale population testing, such as will be required for pharmacogenomic applications. Current molecular diagnostics assays are not highly automated, and are generally labor-intensive and expensive. For large-scale molecular diagnostic testing, more automation with reduced personnel involvement is essential in order to reduce the cost of testing. The use of gel electrophoresis is a common element in most current molecular diagnostic methods, and is labor-intensive as the pouring and loading of gels is time-consuming and cannot be easily automated. The development of methods that do not require traditional gel electrophoresis will allow for reduced diagnostic costs and so will be suitable for large-scale testing. Other requirements of large-scale testing will be improved software programs capable of dealing with large amount of data. We will outline some of the current major advances in biotechnology related to molecular diagnostics in the following section.

4.1 DNA Chip Technology

DNA chips refer to high-density oligonucleotide arrays, in which many short nucleic acid sequences are anchored on glass supports similar in size to microscope slides. DNA chips can be designed in certain formats depending on the application of the chip. The current applications of DNA chip technology include use in determining gene expression profiles from various genes [20], in determining a sequence of an unknown fragment by hybridisation [21], or in detection of SNPs [22]. The major benefit of the use of DNA chips for these applications is that information on thousands of genetic regions can be obtained from a single chip experiment. For example, chips that are used to determine expression profiles from various genes can analyse thousands of RNA fragments on a single chip. This currently has had the most relevance to cancer research, in which gene expression profiles from tumour tissues are compared to normal tissues to determine which genes are differentially regulated in the cancer tissues [23].

The possible applications of DNA chips to molecular diagnostics are in their use for detection of a large number of single-nucleotide polymorphisms [22,24]. DNA chips can be designed to detect sequence variations that have relevance to disease status or altered enzyme activity. Due to the large capacity of the DNA chip, it will be possible to conduct large-scale screening of the genome to detect SNPs that have clinical relevance. The feasibility of this approach to large-scale SNP identification has been demonstrated by a study using DNA chips for detection of >3000 SNPs in a 2.3-megabase genetic region, and the development of "genotyping chips" which could detect hundreds of SNPs simultaneously [25].

Currently, DNA chips for use in gene expression studies work well. However, sequencing and SNP chips are still not accurate enough for routine use in identifying genetic changes in a clinical laboratory. Another disadvantage to widespread use of DNA chip technology at this time is cost. However, as the cost decreases the potential applications will likely escalate, since DNA chips can greatly reduce labour time and have the potential to be fully automated. A more detailed discussion of DNA chips is found in the chapter by Grant and Liggett of this book.

4.2 High-Pressure Liquid Chromatography (HPLC) Analysis

New applications for familiar methods such as HPLC may also have important future applications for testing for genetic variation. HPLC has been adapted to DNA fragment analysis for separation of fragments under partially denaturing conditions. Fragments to be analyzed for the presence of a mutation are amplified by PCR and then run on a denaturing HPLC column. DNA heteroduplexes containing a mismatched base due to the presence of a mutation have a different mobility through the HPLC column from normal matched homoduplexes, due to the altered melting temperature of the heteroduplex. The mobility difference between the normal and the mutant sample allows for screening of fragments for genetic changes [26].

The main application of HPLC technology for diagnostics is likely to be its use as a screening tool for genetic variation prior to sequencing, which is similar in principle to traditional methods of scanning such as single-strand conformational polymorphism (SSCP) and denaturing gradient gel electrophoresis (DGGE) assays. However, the new semiautomated HPLC device is a vast improvement on previous methods due the simplicity of preparing fragments for analysis, having a run time of only minutes to analyze fragments, and direct collection of fragments after analysis on HPLC for use in sequencing. This technique is also applicable to high-throughput applications due to its automated nature, and so is appropriate for large-scale screening of genetic variation.

4.3 Mass Spectrometry

Mass spectrometry is also being applied to genetic analysis by the use of matrix-assisted laser desorption ionization time-of-flight (MALDI-TOF) mass spectrometry. The principle of this application is that sequence differences can be determined by analysing the inherent mass differences of the four nucleotide bases— A, C, G, and T. For molecular diagnostic applications, MALDI-TOF may be applicable to detection of SNPs by the use of modified primer extension assays. In this application, a primer adjacent to a mutation site is extended by one dideoxynucleotide base, and the base added at the mutation site is then identified by the mass added to the primer, which will correspond to one of the four bases [27,28]. This application is promising for high-throughput applications, as more than one primer can be simultaneously extended and then analyzed, and the products for analysis do not require any additional purification after PCR amplification. The reader is referred to the chapter by Ross in this book for a detailed discussion of MALDI-TOF applications.

4.4 Real-Time PCR

New developments have also been made in PCR equipment that may have an impact on molecular diagnostics. One of the most important has been the development of PCR machines that have the capability of detecting product formation during the PCR reaction, known as real-time PCR. Assays can be designed in which the binding of a sequence-specific probe to its homologous PCR product results in an increase in fluorescence during the PCR reaction, allowing for real-time detection of the PCR product. This has been achieved using various probe designs that maintain a fluorescent reporter dye in close proximity to a quencher dye. Upon hybridization to its specific sequence, the quencher is separated from the reporter, thus generating a fluorescent signal from the reporter dye [29,30].

The advantage of real-time PCR techniques is that they do not require any post-PCR analysis such as gel electrophoresis, since the amplification and detection of the specific product are completed within the PCR reaction. However, the design of the probes is complex and is crucial to the success of this application.

4.5 Capillary Electrophoresis

The intensive sequencing programs for the Human Genome Project have lead to major improvements in direct sequencing procedures. Traditional sequencing using slab gels is laborious and time-consuming. A significant advance in sequencing is capillary electrophoresis, in which traditional slab electrophoresis gels are replaced by capillaries. The electrophoresis of samples is carried out in a thin capillary tube filled with a matrix, and the movement of DNA molecules through the tube is detected and recorded. The capillary electrophoresis machine is amenable to automation as samples can be automatically loaded from reaction tubes. Capillary electrophoresis is versatile and can be applied to many genetic tests that traditionally would be analyzed on a slab gel, including fragment analysis and direct sequencing. New capillary electrophoresis models are designed to allow simultaneous analysis of 96–384 samples, and will allow much more rapid analysis of DNA fragments than current slab-sequencing gels. This equipment has only recently been introduced into routine diagnostic laboratories.

For molecular diagnostic applications, capillary electrophoresis will simplify direct sequencing for mutation detection. Traditional sequencing methods are too labor-intensive and expensive for routine diagnostic use. By using capillary electrophoresis to rapidly perform sequencing reactions, the applications of direct sequencing for diagnostics will become more feasible.

4.6 Robotics

A common objective of all of the technical approaches discussed above is the need to reduce the labor and expense required for large-scale testing. High-throughput machines such as capillary electrophoresis require high input rates, which are not feasible without the use of robotics. Robotics will be required to automate the isolation of DNA, to prepare reactions for PCR, and to load detection machines after PCR [31]. For example, the labor associated with manually preparing DNA samples for analysis on a 384-sample capillary electrophoresis machine would negate the benefit of the high-throughput sequencer. Robotics instruments are now available that can perform various functions, including nucleic acid extraction and preparation of PCR reactions. Robotics are likely to become more flexible in future, with robots specifically designed to interact with specialized equipment for specific applications. An important aspect of increased robotic use will be the development of software programs able to perform data analysis on the high volume of data generated. The increasing use of robotics will allow genetic diagnostic laboratories to increase the number of tests it is able to perform, without continually increasing laboratory staff, due to the ability to perform more tasks in less time.

The methods listed above are some of the major areas of interest in the development of biotechnology-based molecular diagnostic procedures. Some private companies are currently offering genetic testing based on new biotechnology-based large-scale molecular diagnostic methods. An overview of some companies involved in developing diagnostic strategies for large-scale genetic testing for pharmacogenomics is provided in Persidis [32].

5 ISSUES OF DIAGNOSTICS SPECIFIC TO PHARMACOGENOMICS

The need to develop high-throughput, sensitive, and cost-effective molecular diagnosis for genetic variation is a significant challenge for the large-scale implementation of pharmacogenomic applications. Several new biotechnology-based methods for molecular diagnosis are discussed above, and these methods or others will have significant impact on the pharmacogenetic field. However, there are still challenges ahead.

The application of molecular diagnostic testing to pharmacogenomics still requires a more thorough understanding of the genetic causes underlying drug response variations. The genetic variations may be simple changes, or they may be complex alterations that are also influenced by environmental factors. Significant research on the effect of genetic variation on enzyme activity and the resultant effect on drug response will be required before molecular diagnosis can be fully implemented for pharmacogenomic purposes.

In parallel with the development of this knowledge, there needs to be a major emphasis on the development of high-throughput, accurate tests for large-scale testing of genetic variation. Since many individuals will require testing, and many genetic changes may need to be tested, the diagnostic methods will need to be robust, cost-effective, and specific. Current methods in molecular diagnostics are not adequate for this volume of testing. However, new technologies for DNA analysis and mutation detection, and the use of robotics to improve the throughput of testing, will make it possible to meet the demands of pharmacogenomic applications.

REFERENCES

1. J Lazarou, BH Pomeranz, PN Corey. Incidence of adverse drug reactions in hospitalized patients: a meta-analysis of prospective studies. JAMA 279:1200–1205, 1998.
2. WW Weber. Pharmacogenetics. Oxford: Oxford University Press, 1997.
3. FJ Gonzalez, RC Skoda, S Dimura, M Umeno, UM Zanger, DW Nebert, HV Gelbion, JP Hardwick, UA Meyer. Characterization of the common genetic defect in humans deficient in debrisoquin metabolism. Nature 331:442–446, 1988.
4. H Madsen, K Kramer Nielsen, K Bronsen. Imipramine metabolism in relation to the sparteine and mephenytoin oxidation polymorphisms—a population study. Br J Clin Pharmacol 39:433–439, 1995.
5. DS Bailey, A Bondar, LM Furness. Pharmacogenomics—it's not just pharmacogenetics. Curr Opin Biotechnol 9:595–601, 1998.
6. J Bell. Medical implications of understanding complex disease traits. Curr Opin Biotechnol 9:573–577, 1998.
7. DJ Allingham-Hawkins, LK McGlynn-Steele, CA Brown, J Sutherland, PN Ray. Impact of carrier status determination for Duchenne/Becker muscular dystrophy by computer-assisted laser densitometry. Am J Med Genet 75:171–175, 1998.
8. DN Cooper. Human gene mutations affecting RNA processing and translation. Ann Med 25:11–17, 1993.
9. RGH Cotton. Mutation Detection. Oxford: Oxford University Press, 1997.
10. AM Douglas, BA Atchison, AA Somogyi, OH Drunmer. Interpretation of a simple PCR analysis of the CYP2D6(A) and CYP2D6(B) null alleles associated with the debrisoquine/sparteine genetic polymorphism. Pharmacogenetics 4:154–158, 1994.
11. AP Shuber, LA Michalowsky, GS Nass, J Skoletsky, LM Hire, SK Kotsopoulos, MF Phipps, DM Barberio, KW Klinger. High throughput parallel analysis of hundreds of patient samples for more than 100 mutations in multiple disease genes. Hum Mol Genet 6:337–347, 1997.
12. M Heim, U Meyer. Genotyping of poor metabolisers of debrisoquine by allele-specific PCR. Lancet 336:529–532, 1990.
13. NH Robertson, SL Weston, SJ Kelly, NJ Duxbury, SR Pearce, P Elsmore, MBT Webb, CR Newton, S Little. Development and validation of a screening test for 12 common mutations of the cystic fibrosis CFTR gene. Eur Respir J 12:477–482, 1998.
14. TS Hansen, NE Petersen, A Iitia, O Blaabjerg, PH Peterson. Robust non-radioactive oligonucleotide ligation assay to detect a common point mutation in the CYP2D6 gene causing abnormal drug metabolism. Clin Chem 41:413–418, 1995.
15. EC Brinson, T Adriano, W Bloch, CL Brown, CC Chang, J Chen, FA Eggerding, PD Grossman, DA Iovannisci, AM Madonik, DG Sherman, RW Tam, ES Winn-

Deen, SL Woo, S Fung. Introduction to PCR/OLA/SCS, a multiplex DNA test, and its application to cystic fibrosis. Gene Test 1:61–68, 1997.

16. T Pastinen, A Kurg, A Metspalu, L Peltonen, AC Syvanen. Mini-sequencing: a specific tool for DNA analysis and diagnostics on oligonucleotide arrays. Genet Res 7: 606–614, 1997.

17. K Uddhav, S Ketan. Advances in the human genome project. Mol Biol Rep 25:27–43, 1998.

18. http://snp.cshl.org; http://www.ncbi.nlm.nih.gov/SNP

19. Dawson E. New collaborations make pharmacogenomics a SNP. Mol Med Today 5:280, 1999.

20. DJ Duggan, M Bittner, Y Chen, P Meltzer, JM Trent. Expression profiling using cDNA microarrays. Nat Genet Suppl 21:10–14.

21. G Yershov, V Barsky, A Belgovskiy, E Kirillov, E Kreindlin, I Ivanov, S Parinov, D Guschin, A Drobishev, S Dubiley, A Mirzabekov. DNA analysis and diagnostics on oligonucleotide microchips. Proc Natl Acad Sci USA 93:4913–4918, 1996.

22. JG Hacia. Resequencing and mutational analysis using oligonucleotide microarrays. Nat Genet Suppl 21:42–47.

23. J DeRisi, L Penland, PO Brown, ML Bittner, PS Meltzer, M Ray, Y Chen, YA Su, JM Trent. Use of a cDNA microarray to analyse gene expression patterns in human cancer. Nat Genet 14:457–460, 1996.

24. JG Hacia, FS Collins. Mutational analysis using oligonucleotide microarrays. J Med Genet 36:730–736, 1999.

25. DG Wang, JB Fan, CJ Siao, A Berno, P Young, R Sapolsky, G Ghandour, N Perkins, E Winchester, J Spencer, L Kruglyak, L Stein, L Hsie, T Topaloglou, E Hubbell, E Robinson, M Mittmann, MS Morris, N Shen, D Kilburn, J Rioux, C Nusbaum, S Rozen, TJ Hudson, R Lipshutz, M Chee, ES Lander. Large-scale identification, mapping, and genotyping of single-nucleotide polymorphisms in the human genome. Science 280:1077–1082, 1998.

26. A Kuklin, K Munson, D Gjerde, R Haefele, P Taylor. Detection of single-nucleotide polymorphisms with the WAVE DNA fragment analysis system. Genet Test 1:201–206, 1997.

27. MT Roskey, P Juhasz, IP Smirnov, EJ Takach, SA Martin, LA Haff. DNA sequencing by delayed extraction-matrix-assisted laser desorption/ionization time of flight mass spectrometry. Proc Natl Acad Sci USA 93:4724–4729, 1996.

28. LA Haff, IP Smirnov. Single-nucleotide polymorphism identification assays using a thermostable DNA polymerase and delayed extraction MALDI-TOF mass spectrometry. Genome Res 7:378–388, 1997.

29. CA Heid, J Stevens, KJ Livak, PM Williams. Real time quantitative PCR. Gen Res 6:986–994, 1996.

30. S Tyagi, FR Kramer. Molecular beacons: probes that fluoresce upon hybridization. Nat Biotechnol 14:303–308, 1996.

31. DS Wilkinson. The role of technology in the clinical laboratory of the future. Clin Lab Manage Rev 11:322–330, 1997.

32. A Persidis. Pharmacogenomics and diagnostics. Nat Biotechnol 16:791–792, 1998.

10

Technologies for the Analysis of Single-Nucleotide Polymorphisms

An Overview

Denis M. Grant and Michael S. Phillips

Orchid BioSciences Inc., Princeton, New Jersey

1 INTRODUCTION

The recent explosion of interest in the use of pharmacogenomics for new-drug development and individualized drug prescribing [1–5] has been accompanied by a flood of new or improved technologies for the analysis of single-nucleotide polymorphisms (SNPs), the commonest form of genetic variant in the human genome [6,7]. Although this review will attempt to mention many of the most important methods currently available and being developed for SNP genotyping, an exhaustive review of available configurations and experimental details is beyond the scope of this chapter. Rather, the primary intention is to briefly highlight some of the issues related to the underlying components of these technologies and how they may influence the choice of an appropriate genotyping methodology for research and clinical settings.

2   SNP ANALYSIS TECHNOLOGIES: BIOCHEMISTRIES, READOUTS, AND PLATFORMS

In comparing currently available and newly emerging technologies for suitability in SNP genotyping assays, it is most important to consider the needs of the variety of potential end users. For academic investigators, assay cost may be a more important driver for adoption of a method, whereas in the clinical diagnostic setting assay accuracy may be paramount. Pharmaceutical industry researchers may value both high throughput (speed and volume of sample processing) and low cost for disease gene discovery studies involving the analysis of large numbers of SNPs in large numbers of clinical DNA specimens. With this in mind, it is likely that a dominant genotyping technology is likely to be one that is flexible enough to adapt to a variety of different throughputs, readouts, and instrumentation platforms to cover the spectrum of cost, throughput, and convenience requirements in a robust and optimally accurate fashion.

An important distinction should also be made between the analytical biochemistries that underlie different SNP genotyping assays and the variety of novel platforms and modes of detection, or readout, of the genotyping results. Such a distinction has sometimes been lacking, leading to confusion on the part of the end user when trying to decide among the various choices. For instance, it is sometimes suggested that mass spectrometry per se is a powerful new method for genotyping, when in reality it is no more than a sophisticated means of detecting a prior genotyping assay result, be it an enzymatic extension followed by mass detection (i.e., Sequenom's MassARRAY; www.sequenom.com) or an allele-selective oligonucleotide hybridization followed by cleavage of mass spectrometry tags (Rapigene/Qiagen's Masscode; www.rapigene.com). DNA microarrays, such as those manufactured by commercial suppliers (i.e., Affymetrix; www.affymetrix.com) or custom made by the end user with arraying equipment, simply represent a means of spatially organizing biochemical reactions—whether hybridization alone or hybridization linked to an enzymatic reaction—so that the end result of the reaction can be efficiently quantified or scored. Such arrays have found utility in a variety of areas ranging from the analysis of differential gene expression to the sorting of genotyping assay products. In a similar fashion, other platforms that allow for sample multiplexing, such as Luminex's fluorescent bead-based flow cytometry (www.luminexcorp.com) or Illumina's parallel fiber optic systems (www.illumina.com), are useful for increasing sample throughput and conserving on the usage of DNA starting material, but still require some form of prior genotyping biochemistry before they can be applied. Microfluidic devices such as those developed by Nanogen (www.nanogen.com) and Orchid BioSciences (www.orchid.com) are designed to transport and deliver small volumes of DNA and reagents for biochemical reactions to occur in defined microreaction chambers. Thus although genotyping readout and platform will influence the throughput and cost components of a given technology, it is important to focus on the fundamental nature of the underlying biochemistry when considering the potential accuracy and robustness of a given genotyping technology. With this in mind, the sections below will focus on a discussion of the different assay biochemistries, the features of which will determine the degree to which they may be ported to various detection or automation platforms.

3 ASSAY BIOCHEMISTRIES

As mentioned above, the central core component of a genotyping technology is contained within the assay biochemistry. A distinction may be made between those methods that rely primarily upon differential hybridization stringency for their specificity, and those that derive specificity primarily from the product of an enzymatic reaction. A number of methods also use combinations of hybridization and enzyme reactions, with varying degrees of contribution to specificity from each of the two components.

3.1 Hybridization-Based Approaches

The specificity of hybridization-based approaches in SNP genotyping relies upon the fact that the melting temperatures of DNA-DNA or DNA-RNA hybrids that perfectly match are different than those that do not. Thus experimental conditions may be found where differential rates or extents of hybridization may be detected even for single-base mismatches such as would occur in the presence of a SNP. Allele-specific oligonucleotide hybridization forms the basis for many of the solid-phase DNA microarray genotyping systems. Drawbacks to this technology in its basic form include the difficulty in achieving the appropriate stringency of hybridization wash conditions so that only perfectly matched oligonucleotides will be retained and provide a positive signal, and the inflexibility of chip design coupled with the expense of chip manufacture. A number of proprietary buffer additives have been developed for increasing the difference in melting temperature between perfectly matched and imperfectly matched DNA hybrids, in an attempt to improve the specificity and overall robustness of hybridization-based assays. Electronically-based control of DNA localization on microarrays and of hybridization conditions [8] can also improve chip flexibility and rate of hybrid formation. In addition, many chip-based hybridization methods are now using universal sequence tags attached to SNP-specific genotyping oligonucleotides [9], which improves the flexibility of chip systems by making the chip a generic signal-sorting device for the products of either solution-phase hybridization reactions or of other biochemical genotyping reactions.

3.2 Enzyme-Based Approaches

Because of the inherent catalytic specificity of enzymes for their substrates, enzyme-based approaches to SNP genotyping generally possess a higher degree of assay fidelity than those primarily dependent upon hybridization for their specificity. The historical standard for genotyping of both SNPs and of other forms of genetic variation, restriction fragment length polymorphism (RFLP) analysis, is an example of an enzymatic approach that relies upon the exquisite selectivity of restriction endonucleases for short.stretches of DNA sequence that act as recognition sites for DNA strand cleavage. Thus, in those instances where a SNP changes a restriction enzyme recognition sequence, differential digestion of normal and variant sequences may be observed. First iterations of this genotyping approach required the endonuclease digestion of large quantities of genomic DNA, electrophoretic size separation of digested fragments, and detection of fragment size differences by hybridization with a labeled probe DNA fragment on Southern blots. Advancements in the method, such as prior PCR amplification of defined DNA segments containing RFLPs and PCR-mediated introduction of novel restriction sites, have improved the conservation of starting DNA material, the ability to detect fragments without subsequent probe hybridization, and the applicability of the method to a wider range of allelic variant sites in the genome. However, the major drawback to such methods is still the requirement for electrophoretic separation of digested products, which severely limits the throughput and automatability of the method and increases reagent and labor costs.

Dideoxy DNA sequencing represents another example of an enzymatic approach to genotyping, which uses the specificity of DNA polymerase to incorporate appropriate nucleotide bases opposite a primed single-stranded DNA template, followed by size separation of terminated polymerase-extended reactions by gel electrophoresis to detect the identity of nucleotide variants at defined sites. DNA sequencing remains the gold standard to which other genotyping methods are generally compared, and is also the method of choice for discovering new SNPs in multiple DNA samples or for confirming those discovered using methods such as single-strand conformation polymorphism (SSCP) analysis or denaturing HPLC. With respect to the analysis of preexisting SNPs, major disadvantages of DNA sequencing are the requirement for electrophoretic separation of extended DNA fragments, which restricts the platform and hampers throughput, potential technical difficulties in detecting heterozygosity at a particular SNP locus when sequencing from uncloned PCR products, and the higher cost of reagents associated with the requirement to extend reactions by many more nucleotide bases than the polymorphic site under investigation. A variant of DNA sequencing (Pyrosequencing; www.pyrosequencing.com) that uses a series of enzymatic steps to enable the continuous readout of short stretches of DNA sequence may be useful for low-throughput research genotyping applications, but the high cost associated with the complex biochemistry may be an issue, especially when there is a need for genotype analysis on a large scale.

Another simple yet very powerful variation of DNA sequencing for SNP scoring is single-base primer extension [10], which in certain embodiments has also been termed "minisequencing" [11] (see Chap. 11). Single-base primer extension in its purest form involves the annealing of an oligonucleotide primer to a single-stranded PCR amplicon (analogous to the primer annealing step in DNA-sequencing reactions) at a location which lies immediately adjacent to, but not including, the polymorphic SNP site, followed by the addition of a DNA polymerase and subsequent enzymatic extension of the primer in the presence only of chain-terminating dideoxynucleotides, which may be labeled in a variety of ways to facilitate subsequent detection of the identity of the single incorporated nucleotide. An important distinguishing feature of primer extension is that assay specificity arises not from the hybridization of the primer, but rather from the catalytic specificity of the polymerase itself. Among the many advantages of the single-base primer extension biochemistry, which is termed SNP-IT™ (single-nucleotide polymorphism identification technology) in its proprietary embodiment from Orchid BioSciences, are its accuracy, robustness, quantal yes/no result, flexibility with respect to detection platform, scalability from benchtop manual assays to high-throughput industrial applications via robotic automation and sample multiplexing, and reagent cost savings. The biochemistry may be employed either in solution followed by solid-phase capture for subsequent detection, or directly on solid supports such as microplate wells, glass slide microarrays, and color-coded microspheres. For many of these reasons, single-base primer extension is being selected as the genotyping biochemistry of choice, and is being licensed and adapted for use on a variety of different platforms, including ELISA-style microtiter plate formats with colorimetric detection (Orchid BioSciences' SNPstream Systems and SNPware Kits), DNA microarray product capture detection systems (SNPcode Kits for use with Affymetrix chips; Asper's APEX [www.asper. ee]), fluorescent bead-based reaction sorting devices (Luminex), solution-phase fluorescence polarization detection systems [12], mass spectrometry [13], and automated capillary DNA sequencing platforms (ABI's SnaPshot [www. appliedbiosystems.com], APB's MegaBase). It is also being adapted for use on standard 96-well plate readers and a number of other readout platforms.

3.3 Combined Hybridization/Enzymatic Approaches

Until recently, one of the most commonly used methods for genotyping in small-scale applications has been allele-specific PCR amplification, which combines selective PCR primer hybridization with a subsequent PCR reaction [14]. Conditions are optimized so that hybridization and subsequent amplification occur only when the PCR priming oligonucleotide is perfectly matched with the target site (usually with the polymorphic site at the 3′ end of the oligonucleotide). The result of the test is therefore determined electrophoretically as either the presence or absence of a PCR product. Again, the major drawback of this method for high-throughput applications is the requirement for gel electrophoresis and visualization of product, a process that is not amenable to automation. Also, it is important to note that in this assay, accuracy is still dependent solely upon differential hybridization, which must be carefully optimized for each polymorphic site to be tested.

Newer assays have been designed to introduce an enzymatic step in an attempt to improve the specificity, and therefore the overall accuracy, of hybridization-based assays. Oligonucleotide ligation assays (OLA) are an example of this approach, where addition of a DNA ligase to a hybridization reaction results in the attachment of an oligonucleotide to an immobilized capture DNA only when the fragments are perfectly matched (for example, ABI's HyChip assay from HySeq). Other combined hybridization/enzymatic methods involve the use of sequence-selective cleavage enzymes, such as Third Wave's Cleavase-based Invader assay (www.twt.com), ABI's TaqMan, the resolvase system from Variagenics (www.variagenics.com), and methods based on rolling circle amplification. Among the stated advantages of the Invader assay is the lack of requirement for a prior PCR amplification step. However, because of the requirement for large quantities of input genomic DNA and the replacement of one expensive enzyme approach (Taq DNA polymerase) for another (Cleavase), it remains to be seen whether this assay will be practical for use on human genomic DNA, which is often available in limited quantities.

4 CONCLUDING REMARKS

From the above brief discussion, it is evident that there are a great number and variety of methodologies now available for the analysis of SNPs in pharmacogenetic studies. It is generally agreed both in academic and industry circles that no single assay/platform combination is likely to meet the needs of all genotyping "customers." The potential user of genotyping assays must therefore carefully assess the needs of his/her own genotyping laboratory, and determine the relative importance of accuracy, cost-efficiency, speed of analysis, laboratory throughput, existing equipment capability, and platform flexibility in making a choice of the appropriate system to meet these needs.

REFERENCES

1. A Marshall. Getting the right drug into the right patient. Nat Biotechnol 15:1249–1252, 1997.

2. JB Lichter, JH Kurth. The impact of pharmacogenetics on the future of healthcare. Curr Opin Biotechnol 8:692–695, 1997.

3. DM Grant. Pharmacogenomics and the changing face of clinical pharmacology. Can J Clin Pharmacol 6:131–132, 1999.

4. WE Evans, MV Relling. Pharmacogenomics: translating functional genomics into rational therapeutics. Science 286:487–491, 1999.

5. DR Pfost, MT Boyce-Jacino, DM Grant. A SNPshot: pharmacogenetics and the future of drug therapy. Trends Biotechnol 18:334–338, 2000.

6. MM Shi, MR Bleavins, FA de la Iglesia. Technologies for detecting genetic polymorphisms in pharmacogenomics. Mol Diagn 4:343–351, 1999.

7. N Spurr, A Darvasi, J Terrett, L Jazwinska. New technologies and DNA resources for high throughput biology. Br Med Bull 55:309–324, 1999.

8. PN Gilles, DJ Wu, CB Foster, PJ Dillon, SJ Chanock. Single nucleotide polymorphic discrimination by an electronic dot blot assay on semiconductor microchips. Nature Biotechnol 17:365–370, 1999.

9. JB Fan, X Chen, MK Halushka, A Berno, X Huang, T Ryder, RJ Lipshutz, DJ Lockhart, A Chakravarti. Parallel genotyping of human SNPs using generic high-density oligonucleotide tag arrays. Genome Res 10:853–860, 2000.

10. TT Nikiforov, RB Rendle, P Goelet, YH Rogers, ML Kotewicz, S Anderson, GL Trainor, MR Knapp. Genetic bit analysis: a solid phase method for typing single nucleotide polymorphisms. Nucleic Acids Res 22:4167–4175, 1994.

11. AC Syvanen. From gels to chips: "minisequencing" primer extension for analysis of point mutations and single nucleotide polymorphisms. Hum Mutat 13:1–10, 1999.

12. X Chen, L Levine, PY Kwok. Fluorescence polarization in homogeneous nucleic acid analysis. Genome Res 9:492–498, 1999.

13. Z Fei, LM Smith. Analysis of single nucleotide polymorphisms by primer extension and matrix-assisted laser desorption/ionization time-of-flight mass spectrometry. Rapid Commun Mass Spectrom 14:950–959, 2000.

14. D See, V Kanazin, H Talbert, T Blake. Electrophoretic detection of single-nucleotide polymorphisms. Biotechniques 28:710–714, 716, 2000.

11

Multiplex Fluorescent Minisequencing Applied to the Typing of Genes Encoding Drug-Metabolizing Enzymes

Gisela Sitbon
PGL Professional Genetics Laboratory AB, Uppsala, Sweden
Ann-Christine Syvänen
Uppsala University, Uppsala, Sweden

1 INTRODUCTION

The sequence variation (SNPs; single-nucleotide polymorphisms) of the human genome ranges from mutations directly causing monogenic inherited diseases or predisposing to multifactorial disorders to neutral polymorphisms that have no influence on the phenotype of the individuals. Moreover, the genome contains sequence variations that can be considered as normal and cause functional differences between individuals in various metabolic pathways. The genes encoding drug-metabolizing enzymes (DMEs), such as the cytochrome P450 enzymes and the N-acetyltransferases, are well-known examples of this type of genetic variation.

One of the most important polymorphic cytochrome P450 enzymes is debrisoquine hydroxylase, denoted CYP2D6. Many commonly used drugs, such as certain antidepressants, neuroleptics, selective serotonin reuptake inhibitors, and cardiovascular drugs, are substrates for this enzyme. The CYP2D locus consists of the intact CYP2D6 gene and two pseudogenes. More than 35 different CYP2D6 alleles have been identified, and their different distributions within populations divide individuals into the phenotypes poor and extensive metabolizers (PM and EM). The terms "intermediate" (IM) and "ultrarapid" metabolizers (UM) have been used to describe phenotypic subgroups. Individuals who are PMs will metabolize CYP2D6 substrates at reduced rate or not at all, which result in too high plasma concentrations of the drugs, and increased risk of adverse effects at normal dosage [1]. The most rational and practical route to information regarding an individual's metabolic status is via genotyping, and it is anticipated that genotyping of the CYP2D6 gene may become a routine part of designing individually optimized drug treatment.

A second example of a DME polymorphism is the "isoniazid acetylation" polymorphism that affects the metabolism of a variety of arylamine and hydrazine drugs, such as sulfonamides, aminoglutethimide, hydralazine, and prizidilol. Individuals are either "rapid acetylators" (RA) or "slow acetylators" (SA) with regard to their metabolic capacity for this type of drugs. Two functional N-acetyltransferase genes (NAT1 and NAT2) and one pseudogene have been identified. The RA and SA phenotype involve principally the NAT2 gene, encoding the NAT2 enzyme. The SA phenotype is conferred by homozygosity or compound heterozygosity for seven mutations in the coding region of the NAT2 gene. Five of the mutations cause amino acid shifts whereas two are silent [1].

Most of the currently used methods for analyzing genetic variation rely on PCR amplification to obtain sufficient sensitivity and specificity for detecting SNPs in the complexity of the human genome. The SNPs can then be analyzed in the amplified target DNA fragments by a variety of methods, of which hybridization with sequence-specific oligonucleotide probes is frequently used, or with the aid of nucleic acid–modifying enzymes, such as DNA ligases or DNA polymerases. The DNA synthesis reaction catalyzed by the DNA polymerases is utilized in the "minisequencing" single-nucleotide primer extension method to distinguish between sequence variants [2]. Many formats of the minisequencing method, including solid-phase assays performed in microtiter plates with colorimetric detection [3], homogeneous fluorescence-based assays [4], and multiplex assays on microarrays [5], have been devised, and are known under a variety of names and acronyms [reviewed in 6].

In a minisequencing reaction the discrimination between the polymorphic nucleotides is based on the high accuracy of the nucleotide incorporation reaction catalyzed by a DNA polymerase. Detection primers that anneal immediately adjacent to the polymorphic nucleotide are extended with single-labeled nucleotide(s) complementary to the nucleotide(s) at the analyzed site. Thus the minisequencing method allows unequivocal discrimination between homozygous and heterozygous genotypes. Because the primer annealing reaction is performed at nonstringent hybridization conditions, the method is robust and insensitive to small variations in the reaction conditions, and the same reaction conditions can be employed for analyzing any SNP, irrespectively of the flanking nucleotide sequence. These features of the method are important advantages when designing multiplex assays for simultaneous detection of many genetic variants per sample. This chapter describes a multiplex fluorescent minisequencing method and its application to the simultaneous detection of multiple polymorphisms in the CYP2D6 and NAT2 genes. The method is flexible in its design, and additional alleles may easily be included or deleted from the analyzed panel of polymorphic nucleotides.

2 PRINCIPLE OF MULTIPLEX FLUORESCENT MINISEQUENCING

DNA fragments spanning the polymorphic sites are first amplified by PCR using one biotinylated and one nonbiotinylated primer followed immobilization of the PCR products on a solid support by mediation of the biotin-streptavidin interaction. The use of a streptavidin-coated manifold support [7] for capturing the amplified templates and for transferring them to the minisequencing reaction mixtures allows practical processing of a large numbers of samples simultaneously. Other solid supports, such as streptavidin-coated microparticles, can also be used

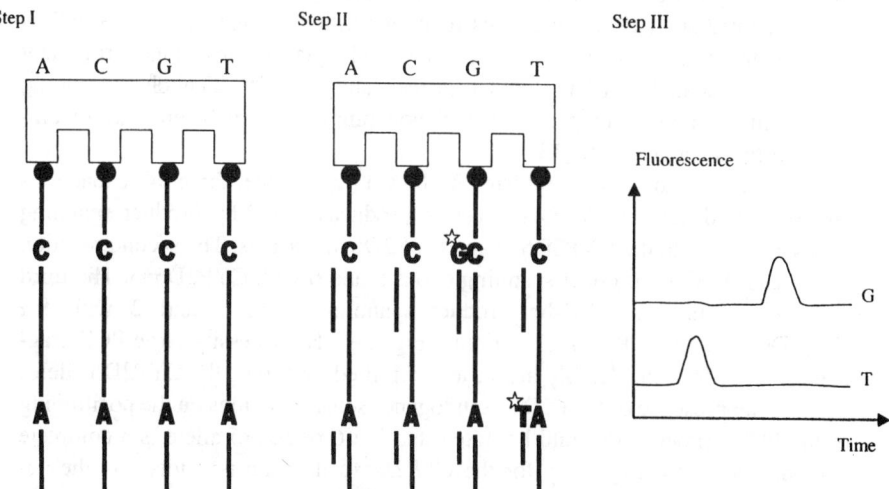

FIGURE 1 Principle and steps of the multiplex fluorescent minisequencing method exemplified by two polymorphic sites. Step I: Capture of biotinylated PCR products on streptavidin-coated manifold support. B. Step II: Multiplex minisequencing reactions. Primers of different length are extended by fluorescent ddNTPs using a DNA polymerase. Step III: The primers are separated by size and detected in an automatic sequencing instrument.

[8]. In the multiplex fluorescent minisequencing, reaction detection primers that differ in size and that anneal immediately adjacent to the variable sites in the captured DNA fragments are extended with fluorescent ddNTPs by a DNA polymerase, followed by detection of the extended primers after electrophoretic separation on a DNA sequencing instrument. The size of the extended primer defines the position of the analyzed polymorphism, and the identity of the incorporated fluorescent ddNTP gives the identity of the nucleotide at each site. Figure 1 illustrates the principle and steps of the multiplex minisequencing method. When a DNA-sequencing instrument that is based on a single label is used for analyzing the extended primers, separate reactions are performed for each of the four fluorescent ddNTPs [9,10]. When a DNA-sequencing instrument equipped with four-color detection is used, four ddNTPS labeled with different fluorophores can be included in a single reaction [11,12].

3 GENOTYPING OF CYP2D6 AND NAT2 POLYMORPHISMS

3.1 Assay Design

One biotinylated and one nonbiotinylated PCR primer per DNA fragment to be analyzed, and one minisequencing detection primer per variable nucleotide position are designed based on the genomic nucleotide sequence information of the genes of interest. It is advantageous if the amplified fragments are as small as possible and of equal size to ensure efficient and equal binding of each fragment to the avidin-coated support. The PCR primers should be 20–23 nucleotides long, have similar melting temperatures and noncomplementary 3′ ends as recommended for standard PCR [13].

For typing the polymorphisms in the CYP2D6 gene, three PCR reactions are performed per sample. One reaction produces a 490-bp product spanning exons 3 and 4 with the CYP2D6*4 and CYP2D6*6 variants. The second reaction produces a 1132-bp product spanning exons 5 and 6 with CYP2D6*3. The third reaction produces a 1363-bp product spanning exons 1 and 2 with the CYP2D6*10 and CYP2D6*17 variants (Fig. 2A). By necessity large PCR fragments that differ considerably in size are amplified for typing the CYP2D6 alleles because the presence of CYP2D6 pseudogenes sets restrictions on the positioning of the PCR primers. It should be noted that the *CYP2D6*5* allele is a complete gene deletion. Homozygosity for the *CYP2D6*5* deletion is evident by the absence of a PCR product, but the deletion should preferably be confirmed by long range PCR or Southern blot analysis [14]. The coding region of the NAT2 gene constitutes a single exon, and hence the seven polymorphic sites defining the mutant NAT2*5B, NAT2*6A, NAT2*5A, NAT2*5C, NAT2*7B, NAT2*13, and NAT2*14A alleles can be amplified within a single PCR fragment of 790 bp in size (Fig. 2B).

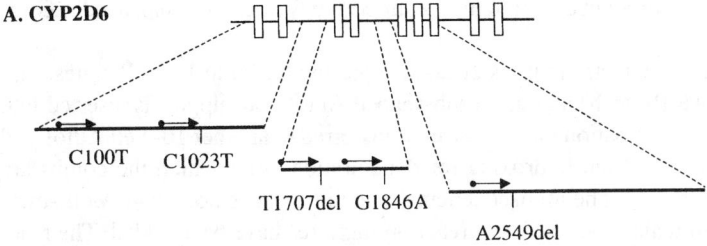

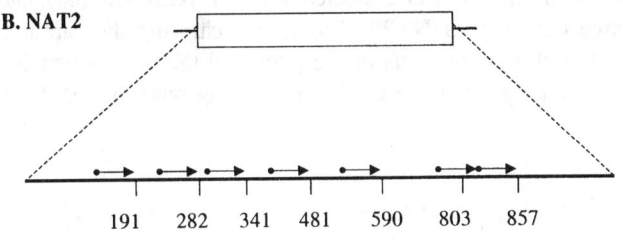

FIGURE 2 Strategy for amplification and genotyping of the CYP2D6 (A) and the NAT2 (B) genes. The polymorphic nucleotides in the CYP2D6 gene are C100T, C1023T, T1707del, G1846A, and A2549del. The polymorphic nucleotides in the NAT2 gene are G191A, C282T, T341C, C481T, G590A, A803G, and G857A.

The multiplex minisequencing primers are designed to be complementary to the biotinylated strand of the PCR products immediately 3′ of the variable nucleotide position. The primers differ in size by three nucleotides, and range from 18 to 36 nucleotides. The primers contain 18 or 21 bases of the gene specific sequence, and the size differences of the longer primers are created by adding a random nucleotide sequence to the 5′ end of the primers.

3.2 Practical Performance

All reagents and equipment required for the fluorescent multiplex minisequencing method are available from common suppliers. DNA is extracted from blood by standard methods, for example using the QIAamp Blood Kit (Qiagen, Germany). Separate PCR reactions are performed, and the three PCR products spanning the CYP2D6 polymorphisms are combined before capturing to the streptavidin-coated support. Particularly when using the manifold supports (AutoLoad Kit, AP Biotech), the size of the PCR products affects the efficiency of the capturing reaction. If the PCR products differ in size, as the CYP2D6 fragments, or the efficiency of PCR differs significantly between the fragments, the relative amounts of PCR product captured on the support may need to be balanced accordingly [10].

The PCR products are transferred in capturing buffer to 10-well plates (AutoLoad Kit, AP Biotech) and the comb-shaped AutoLoad support is inserted into the wells. After incubation the combs are transferred to another 10-well AutoLoad plate containing sodium hydroxide for denaturation, after which the combs are washed in TE buffer. The minisequencing reaction is carried out in 40-well AutoLoad plates to which four different reaction mixtures have been added. The reaction mixtures contain the minisequencing primers, ThermoSequenase DNA polymerase (AP Biotech), one of the four FITC-labeled ddNTPs (NEN/DuPont), and the corresponding three unlabeled ddNTPS. The combs carrying the captured PCR product(s) are inserted into the wells of the plate and the minisequencing reactions are allowed to take place at 55°C. Before loading onto the DNA se-

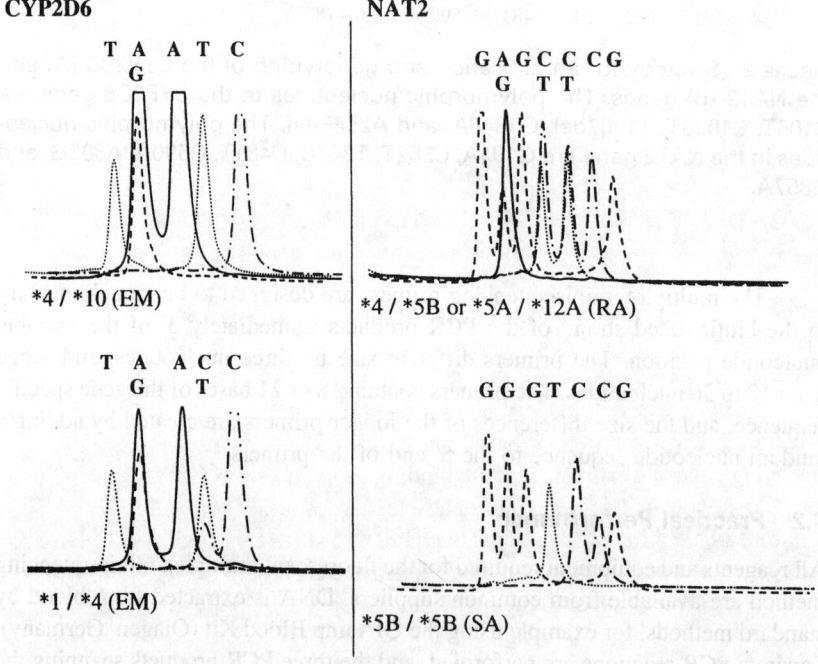

FIGURE 3 Results from typing four samples of different genotype by the multiplex minisequencing method in the CYP2D6 and NAT2 genes, respectively. The alleles identified in the samples and the corresponding phenotypes are given in the figure. Left: CYP2D6*4/*10, EM (top) and CYP2D6*1/*4, EM (bottom). Right: NAT2*4/*5B or *5A/*12A, RA (top) and NAT2*5B/*5B, SA (bottom). EM, extensive metabolizer; RA, rapid acetylator; SA, slow acetylator.

quencer, the combs are washed in TE buffer. The AutoLoad manifolds have been designed to fit the slots of the gel of the ALF DNA-sequencing instrument (AP Biotech), and thus the complete procedure, including loading of the gel, can be carried out without pipetting steps. The extended primers are separated by electrophoresis and detected on an ALF DNA autosequencer. It is of importance to use running conditions at which the separation time between the primer peaks is sufficient to allow for unambiguous peak identification. For more technical details on the performance of the genotyping procedure, see [9,10].

3.2 Interpretation of the Results

The results of the electrophoretic run saved in the computer of the sequencing instrument can be interpreted by direct visual inspection of the electropherograms or using suitable software, such as the AlleleLinks package of the ALF sequencers. In samples from individuals homozygous for the analyzed polymorphism, only one peak is detected at the time point corresponding to the size of a primer, whereas in heterozygous samples there are two peaks at the corresponding time point. Figure 3 shows examples from typing the CYP2D6 and NAT2 genes in samples from individuals of different genotypes.

4 GENOTYPING CAPACITY

Here we describe multiplex typing of polymorphisms in the CYP2D6 and NAT2 genes at four and seven polymorphic sites, respectively. The number of polymorphic sites that can be typed per multiplex minisequencing reaction can be increased significantly, without increasing the amount of work required to carry out the assay, by adding more primers to each reaction. In the application described above we used primers that differed in size by 3 bases, and these were clearly resolved by rapid electrophoresis on short 15-cm gels. Primers differing in size by 2 bases, or even 1 base, can easily be resolved by standard DNA-sequencing gels. We estimate that the binding capacity of the streptavidin-coated manifold support or magnetic microparticles allows capture of 20–30 different biotinylated PCR products, and thus the number of PCR amplified templates that can be analyzed per reaction can also be increased.

The multiplex minisequencing method is generally applicable for detecting variations in any gene employing the same reaction conditions. We have previously used the same protocol based on the ALF DNA-sequencing instrument for multiplex genotyping of nine polymorphic sites in the HLA-DQA1 and DRB1 genes [9]. The number of fluorescent minisequencing reactions per sample is reduced from four to one when the primers are extended with ddNTPs labeled with four different fluorophores followed by multicolor detection in one lane using a PE Biosystems DNA sequencer. This variant of the method has been set up for typing eight mutations in exon 3 of the HPRT gene [11], and validated for a panel of 12 polymorphisms in the control region of the mitochondrial DNA for routine use in forensic analyses [12,15].

The number of genotypes that can be produced in parallel in multiplex genotyping systems is limited by the necessity of amplifying the DNA regions spanning the mutations or SNPs by the PCR. Multiplex PCR amplification is hampered by problems of cross-reactivity arising from the inclusion of multiple sets of primers per amplification reaction [16]. The number of fragments that have been reported to be successfully and reproducibly amplified by multiplex PCR followed by accurate genotyping, irrespective of the genotyping method employed, varies between 2 and 12 fragments per PCR reaction [17–19]. Thus, the multiplexing capacity of PCR is of the same order of magnitude as the multiplexing capacity of the present minisequencing method based on primers of different size. The general availability of all equipment and reagents required renders the multiplex minisequencing method in the format described in the present chapter a powerful method for routine genotyping of SNPs in practice today.

5 ALTERNATIVE SEPARATION METHODS

In an analogous multiplex method that can potentially be fully automated more easily than the methods based on slab gel electrophoresis, separation by capillary electrophoresis and detection by laser-induced fluorescence (CE-LIF) is used for analyzing the extended minisequencing primers [20]. A related semiautomated procedure, in which the products of multiplex primer extension reactions are resolved by high-performance liquid chromatography (HPLC) has the additional advantage that unlabeled nucleotides can be used for distinguishing the polymorphic nucleotides [21]. The separation of the products of primer extension reactions performed with four unlabeled ddNTPs by their differences in molecular weight by mass spectrometry (MALDI-TOF) has been suggested [22,23] and shown to be feasible for multiplex genotyping of PCR-amplified fragments as templates [24].

6 FUTURE PROSPECTS

The large international SNP Consortium will identify hundreds of thousands of human DNA sequence variations among individuals (SNPs) within the next 2 years. SNPs in multiple candidate genes will be analyzed to elucidate the individual variation in drug response caused by variants of multiple genes. The genotyping of pharmacologically relevant genes, such as the CYP2D and NAT2 genes, will extend to variants of genes encoding other drug-metabolizing enzymes as well as drug transporters and receptors affecting an individual's response to drugs, and will allow rational and individualized drug design [25]. Consequently, techniques with higher throughput than the currently available methods for analyzing these functional variants at the DNA level will be required. Given the power of highly specific discrimination of sequence variants by the DNA-polymerase catalyzed minisequencing reaction in various assay formats [6] and the recent advances in technology for miniaturized capillary electrophoresis [26] or other size- or mass-dependent separation systems for DNA molecules [27,28], the concept of multiplex minisequencing with size-tagged primers described in this chapter may well form the basis for future high-throughput genotyping at low reagent costs in pharmacogenetic and other large-scale applications.

ACKNOWLEDGMENTS

We thank Drs. Jörgen Lönngren and Tomi Pastinen for helpful discussions.

REFERENCES

1. UA Meyer, UM Zanger. Molecular mechanisms of genetic polymorphisms of drug metabolism. Annu Rev Pharmacol Toxicol 37:269–296, 1997.
2. A-C Syvänen, K Aalto-Setälä, L Harju, K Kontula, H Söderlund. A primer-guided nucleotide incorporation assay in the genotyping of apolipoprotein E. Genomics 8: 684–692, 1990.
3. G Sitbon, M Hurtig, A Palotie, J Lönngren, A-C Syvänen. A colorimetric mini-sequencing assay for the mutation in codon 506 of the coagulation factor V gene. Thromb Haemost 77:701–703, 1997.
4. X Chen, L Levine, P-Y Kwok. Fluorescence polarization in homogeneous nucleic acid analysis. Genome Res 9:492–498, 1999.
5. T Pastinen, A Kurg, A Metspalu, L Peltonen, A-C Syvänen A-C. Minisequencing: a specific tool for DNA analysis and diagnostics on oligonucleotide arrays. Genome Res 7:606–614, 1997.
6. A-C Syvänen. From gels to chips: ''minisequencing'' primer extension for analysis of point mutations and single nucleotide polymorphims. Hum Mutat 13:1–10, 1999.
7. A Lagerkvist, J Stewart, M Lagerström-Fermer, U Landegren. Manifold sequencing: efficient processing of large sets of sequencing reaction. Proc Natl Acad Sci USA 91:2245–2249, 1994.
8. A-C Syvänen, H Söderlund. Quantification of polymerase chain reaction products by affinity-based collection. In: R Wu, ed. Methods in Enzymology, Vol. 218. Recombinant DNA. Part I. Orlando, FL: Academic Press, 1993, pp 474–490.
9. T Pastinen, J Partanen, A-C Syvänen. Multiplex, fluorescent solid-phase mini-sequencing for efficient screening of DNA sequence variation. Clin Chem 42:1391–1397, 1996.
10. T Pastinen T, A-C Syvänen, C Moberg, G Sitbon, J Lönngren. A fluorescent multi-plex solid-phase minisequencing method for genotyping cytochrome P450 genes. In: M Innis, D Gelfand, J Sninsky, eds. PCR Applications: Protocols for Functional Genomics. Orlando, FL: Academic Press, 1999, pp 521–535.
11. JM Shumaker, A Metspalu, CT Caskey. Mutation detection by solid-phase primer extension. Hum Mutat 7:346–354, 1996.
12. G Tully, KM Sullivan, P Nixon, RE Stones, P Gill. Rapid detection of mitochondrial

sequence polymorphisms using multiplex solid-phase fluorescent minisequencing. Genomics 34:107–113, 1996.

13. CW Dieffenbach, TMJ Lowe, GS Dveksler. General concepts for PCR primer design. PCR Methods Appl 3:S30–S37, 1993.

14. A Wennerholm, I Johansson, AY Massele, M Jande, C Alm, Y Aden-Abdi, M-L Dahl, M Ingelman-Sundberg, L Bertilsson, LL Gustavsson. Decreased capacity for debrisoquine metabolism among black Tanzanians: analyses of the CYP2D6 genotype and phenotype. Pharmacogenetics 9:707–714, 1999.

15. JM Moreley, JE Bark, CE Evans, JG Perry, CA Hewitt, G Tully. Validation of mitochondrial DNA minisequencing for forensic casework. Int J Legal Med 112:241–248, 1999.

16. Q Chou, M Russell, DE Birch, J Raymond, W Bloch. Prevention of pre-pCR mispriming and primer-dimerization improves low-copy number amplifications. Nucleic Acids Res 20:1717–1723, 1992.

17. JS Chamberlain, RA Gibbs, JE Ranier, PN Nguyen, TC Caskey. Deletion screening of Duchenne muscular dystrophy locus via multiplex DNA amplification. Nucleic Acids Res 16:11141–11156, 1988.

18. J Hacia, B Sun, N Hunt, K Edgemon, D Mosbrook, C Robbins, SPA Fodor, DA Tagle, FS Collins. Strategies for mutational analysis of the large multiexon ATM gene using high density oligonucleotide arrays. Genome Res 8:1245–1258, 1998.

19. T Pastinen, M Perola, P Niini, J Terwilliger, V Salomaa, E Vartiainen, L Peltonen, A-C Syvänen. Array-based multiplex analysis of candidate genes reveals two independent and additive risk factors for myocardial infarction in the Finnish population. Hum Mol Genet 7:1453–1462, 1998.

20. CA Piggee, J Muth, E Carrilho, BL Karger. Capillary electrophoresis for the detection of known point mutations by single-nucleotide primer extension and laser induced fluorescence detection. J Chromatogr A781:367–375, 1997.

21. B Hoogendoon, MJ Owen, PJ Oefner, N Williams, J Austin, MC O'Donovan. Genotyping single nucleotide polymorphisms by primer extension and high performance liquid chromatography. Hum Genet 104:89–93, 1999.

22. A Braun, DP Littl, H Köster. Detecting CFTR gene mutations by using primer oligo base extension and mass spectrometry. Clin Chem 43:1151–1158, 1997.

23. LA Haff, IP Smirnov. Single-nucleotide polymorphism identification assays using a thermostable DNA polymerase and delayed extraction MALDI-TOF mass spectrometry. Genome Res 7:378–388, 1997.

24. P Ross, L Hall, I Smirnov, L Haff. High level multiplex genotyping by MALDI-TOF mass spectrometry. Nat Biotechnol 16:1347–1351, 1998.

25. WE Evans, MV Relling. Pharmacogenomics: translating functional genomics into rational therapeutics. Science 286:487–491, 1999.

26. D Schmalzing, N Tsao, L Koutny, D Chisholm, A Srivastava, A Adourian, L Linton, P McEwan, P Matsudaira, D Erlich. Toward real world sequencing by microdevice electrophoresis. Genome Res 9:853–858, 1999.

27. K Tang, DJ Fu, JD Braun, CR Cantor, H Köster. Chip-based genotyping by mass spectrometry. Proc Natl Acad Sci USA 96:10016–10020, 1999.

28. H-P Chou, H Spence, A Scherer, S Quake. A microfabricated device for sizing and sorting DNA molecules. Proc Natl Acad Sci USA 96:11–13, 1999.

12

Multiplex Genotyping by Specialized Mass Spectrometry

Philip L. Ross, Laura Hall, and Larry Haff
Applied Biosystems, Framingham, Massachusetts

Alex Garvin
Biocenter of the University of Basel, Basel, Switzerland

1 INTRODUCTION

A number of efforts, both public and privately funded, aim to unravel the complete sequence of the human and other genomes. This sequence data will serve as a reference point for a new generation of pharmacogenomic discovery. In addition to raw sequence information, these efforts will provide comparative data for a number of individuals from which to identify regions of genomic sequence variation, including single-nucleotide polymorphisms (SNPs). It is estimated that 3 million SNPs will be derived from comparison of genomic sequence from individuals among several populations [1]. These variants can be used as an important tool in association studies or linkage disequilibrium mapping to elucidate the genetic foundation of multifactorial disorders. Other than its genomic location, the most important attributes of an SNP are its frequency in various populations and the correlation between its inheritance and any phenotypes such as a disease trait. Since the number of putative SNPs is so large, and each must ultimately be evaluated in a population, the throughput requirement is so large that new analytical methods are required. Hence, future pharmacogenomics efforts making use of SNPs will have, at the center, a robust, automated, cost-effective analytical technology for the collection and processing of laboratory data.

Historically, mass spectrometry has been used to precisely determine molecular weights and structures of labile molecules. Recent technological breakthroughs have fostered the evolution of mass spectrometry into a biomolecule analysis tool. In particular, the development of matrix-assisted laser desorption/ ionization time-of-flight mass spectrometry (MALDI-TOF MS) [2] combined with delayed-extraction (DE) time-of-flight technology [3,4] has allowed mass spectrometry to become a highly precise and accurate tool for routine, high-throughput characterization of polypeptides and nucleic acids. In MALDI-TOF MS, a sample is combined with a large excess of a "matrix" molecule, typically an organic molecule with a good UV absorption cross section, and spotted onto a stainless-steel target. After drying, the sample is placed into a vaccuum chamber which houses ion extraction optics and a detector. By a gas-phase energy transfer process, the matrix enables desorption and subsequent ionization of intact biomolecules following absorption of UV radiation from a pulsed laser. The ions produced travel toward the detector with a velocity inversely proportional to the square root of the exact molecular weight of the analyte species. By simple electrostatic relationships, exact molecular weight is calculated from the arrival time of the ions at the detector. The separation and detection of biological molecules in this fashion is intrinsically fast; from a single laser pulse ($\sim$5 nsec) a spectrum is recorded in a few microseconds. Typically, data from several laser pulses is collected and averaged to yield a mass spectrum; hence, an analysis is complete in several seconds. High-throughput analysis is accomplished by spotting samples onto the MALDI target in an arrayed fashion of 96,384 or more spots, in which case samples are analyzed sequentially by rastering the target across the laser path on a precision X-Y translation stage.

As a high-throughput tool for analysis of nucleic acids, MALDI-TOF MS exhibits a number of desirable features. As illustrated above, the processes of separation and detection are very rapid. Since analysis is based on an intrinsic property, exact molecular mass, nucleic acids can be identified without the requirement of fluorescent or radioactive labels. Over a given mass range, MALDI-TOF MS supports high-resolution analysis capable of resolving two components differing by substitution of a single DNA base; therefore a large number of species can be separated and detected in a single sample. Finally, the processes of preparing samples on a MALDI target, scanning an array of samples in the MALDI-TOF instrument, and recording and interpreting data can all be automated. Hence, MALDI-TOF MS represents an ideal end-detection system for a large-scale SNP analysis effort.

2   DNA ANALYSIS BY MALDI-TOF MS

The chronology of DNA analysis by MALDI-TOF MS has been the subject of a number of reviews [5,6], so in this discussion representative works demonstrating a specific capability are cited. The reader can refer to references within [5,6] for a thorough progression of earlier developments in mass spectrometry of nucleic acids. The successful detection of mixed-base nucleic acids by MALDI-TOF was first demonstrated routinely as recently as the early 1990s [5,6]. The real promise of MALDI-TOF MS as a legitimate genetic analysis tool came with the development of superior matrix formulations [7,8] which enabled enzymatic sequencing of oligonucleotides [9,10], direct analysis of PCR products harboring sequence variations [11,12], and a number of probe-based post-PCR assays [13,14]. With the resolution and sensitivity enhancement brought about by delayed extraction, MALDI-TOF-based genotyping in formats compatible with routine, high-throughput settings were developed. Concurrent with instrument hardware improvements, appropriate sample-handling methodologies can carry MALDI-TOF MS from laborious "one-at-a-time" analysis to rapid serial analysis of large numbers of parallel processed samples.

Two limitations of DE-MALDI-TOF MS that influence the design of assays and subsequent sample handling are the decrease in sensitivity and resolution with increasing oligonucleotide size, and the intolerance of the MALDI-TOF process to salts, detergents, and other typical enzymatic reaction components. As a general guideline, the most useful genotyping approach is one where the molecular size of the informative reaction product is minimized, and where this product can be easily isolated following reaction.

2.1   Single-Nucleotide Primer Extension Assay

There are an increasing number of reported SNP genotyping methods and applications based on mass spectrometry, including MALDI-TOF MS, which have been covered in recent review articles [15,16]. To a newcomer, the most straightforward approach may appear to be direct analysis of short PCR products. To routinely resolve base substitutions, PCR products must typically be shorter than 35 bases, which imposes a significant limitation on PCR primer design. Thus, strategies based on post-PCR assays offer greater versatility and ultimately appear to be more amenable to automated analysis. One such general format will be highlighted here as an illustration of the advantages and limitations of MALDI-TOF MS–based SNP genotyping in post-genome-era pharmacogenomics. In this format, SNP genotypes are determined by mass spectral analysis of single-nucleotide primer extension assays [17,18]. The essential features of this assay are displayed in Figure 1. After PCR amplification, PCR products are treated with Exonuclease I and shrimp alkaline phosphatase to remove residual PCR primers and deoxy-

The Sequazyme™ PinPoint Assay

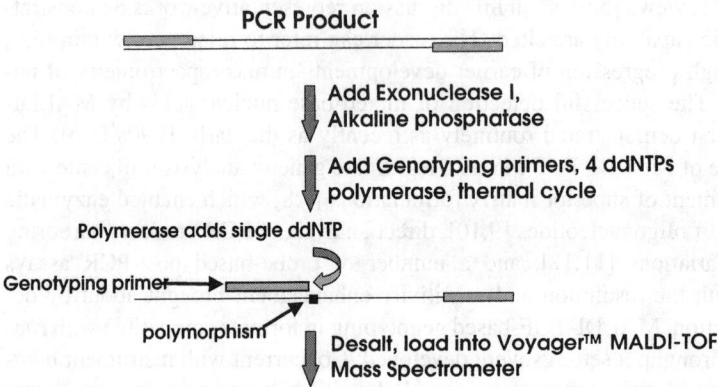

PCR Product

Add Exonuclease I,
Alkaline phosphatase

Add Genotyping primers, 4 ddNTPs
polymerase, thermal cycle

Polymerase adds single ddNTP

Genotyping primer

polymorphism

Desalt, load into Voyager™ MALDI-TOF
Mass Spectrometer

Alleles determined from accurate mass signatures of extended primers

FIGURE 1 Schematic illustration of the Sequazyme-Pinpoint single nucleotide
primer extension assay.

nucleotide triphosphates (dNTPs), respectively. Then, one or more genotyping
primers are added directly to the solution containing treated PCR products along
with a reaction buffer containing all four dideoxynucleotide triphosphates
(ddNTPs), and a suitable DNA polymerase. The reaction buffer is designed to
promote a high specific activity for ddNTP incorporation by the added DNA
polymerase. As illustrated in Figure 1, the genotyping primer is designed to anneal directly to the 3' side of the polymorphic site. The reaction mixture is then
subjected to several rounds of thermal cycling, during which the genotyping primers are extended by a single base corresponding to the variable target base. After
the reaction is complete, it is necessary to isolate nucleic acid reaction products
in a form that is free of salts, detergents, ddNTPs, and other buffer components.
The approach most compatible with a high-throughput environment makes use
of 96- or 384-well filtration microplates, where reaction products are adsorbed
onto a solid phase, washed, and eluted with an appropriate buffer into MALDI
matrix. The isolated oligonucleotide reaction products are then arrayed onto the
MALDI target and analyzed.

The information derived from the mass spectra of such an assay is depicted
in Figure 2. For every primer in the reaction mixture, the spectrum will show
peaks corresponding to one or more extension products as well as unextended
primer. The mass difference between the extended and unextended primer corre-

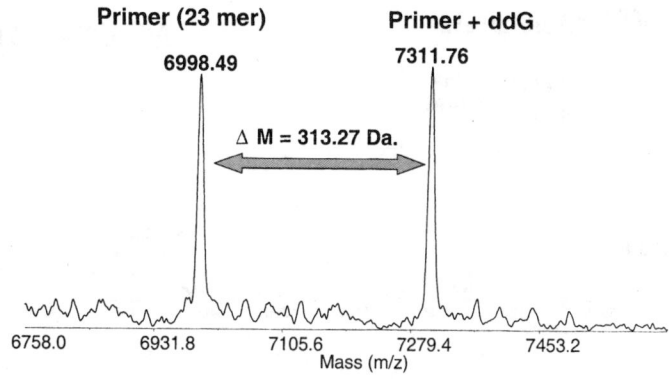

Primer (23 mer)   Primer + ddG
6998.49   7311.76

Δ M = 313.27 Da.

6758.0   6931.8   7105.6   7279.4   7453.2
                              Mass (m/z)

Formulae and Exact Mass of Dideoxy and Deoxy Nucleotide Bases

Dideoxy Base	Formula	Mass	Deoxy Base	Formula	Mass
ddC	$C_9H_{12}N_3O_5P$	273.155	dC	$C_9H_{12}N_3O_6P$	289.184
ddT	$C_{10}H_{13}N_2O_6P$	288.196	dT	$C_{10}H_{13}N_2O_7P$	304.195
ddA	$C_{10}H_{12}N_5O_4P$	297.210	dA	$C_{10}H_{12}N_5O_5P$	313.209
ddG	$C_{10}H_{12}N_5O_5P$	313.209	dG	$C_{10}H_{12}N_5O_6P$	329.208

Figure 2 Illustration of DE MALDI-TOF mass spectrum obtained from a single-nucleotide primer extension assay. Mass assignments of extended and unextended primer are used to calculate ΔM, as labeled. Inset table displays exact masses of the dideoxy and deoxy nucleotide monophosphates.

sponds very precisely to the mass of one of the four dideoxy nucleotide mono-phosphates (ddNMP), so the genotype is determined unambiguously.

2.2 Advantages of MALDI-TOF Primer Extension Approach

There are numerous advantages of this approach over virtually all other SNP-genotyping approaches, MS-based or otherwise. Both the mass spectrometry platform and the single-tube, solution-phase nature of this approach impart distinct advantages. First of all, since the molecular weight of each of the four ddNMPs is distinct, genotypes can be unambiguously determined without the use of fluorescent labels. The inset table in Figure 2 lists exact molecular-weight data for the four ddNMPs and dNMPs. The mass of any given ddNMP differs by at least 9 Da from each of the other ddNMPs; hence, all possible genotypes and heterozygous combinations at a particular site can be resolved using a single primer.

Examples of various heterozyote combinations are illustrated in Figure 3. The smallest mass difference (9 Da) occurs with an A/T heterozygote, which

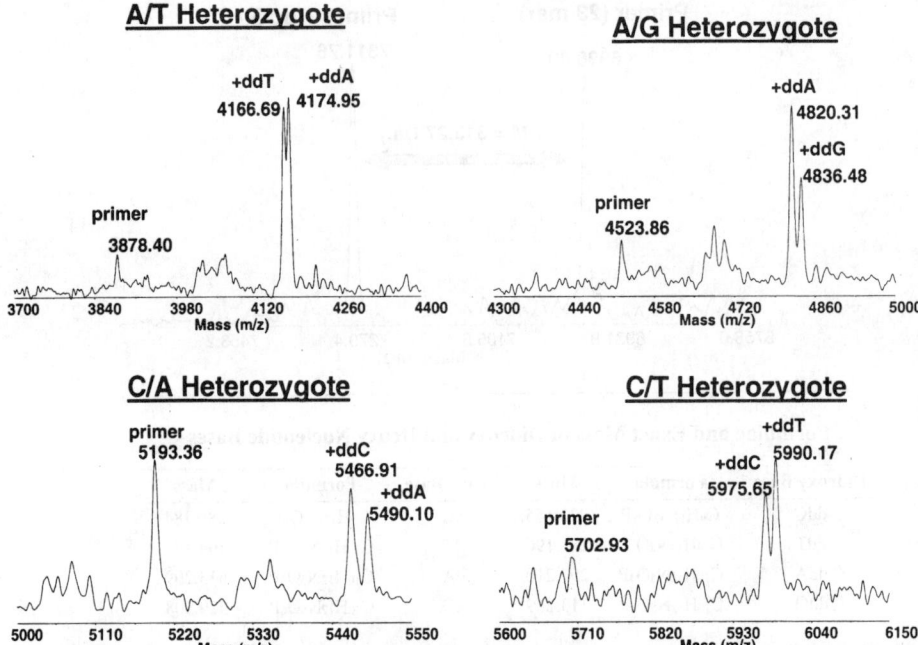

FIGURE 3 Illustrations of DE MALDI-TOF mass spectra obtained from SNP assays of various heterozygote combinations.

can be routinely resolved for genotyping primers up to 20 bases in length. In addition to unlabeled ddNMPs, the assay uses a single unlabeled oligonucleotide primer at each site, thus conveying a significant economic advantage over other formats in terms of cost per genotype. The assay is not strictly limited to single-base substitutions; localized deletion/insertion mutations can be addressed with a single primer in much the same fashion as simple substitutions. An example of this is shown in Figure 4 which shows typical results from genotyping the common cystic fibrosis transmembrane conductance regulator (CFTR) ΔF508 3-base insertion/deletion mutation. In most such cases, it is a straightforward matter to design a primer whose extension products unambiguously reflect the possible sequence variants at any given locus. For more complex polymorphisms, combinations of forward and reverse primers can usually be designed to determine all possible genotypes. The assay is easily multiplexed by using primers with different lengths and/or molecular weights in a single reaction (see Sect. 3). The use of size standards can be avoided since the mass spectrometer measures the intrinsic molecular weight of the analyte species.

Wild type sequence 5'- GCACCATTAAAGAAAATATCAT CTT TGGTGTT

Δ 508 deletion carrier 5'- GCACCATTAAAGAAAATATCATTGGTGTT

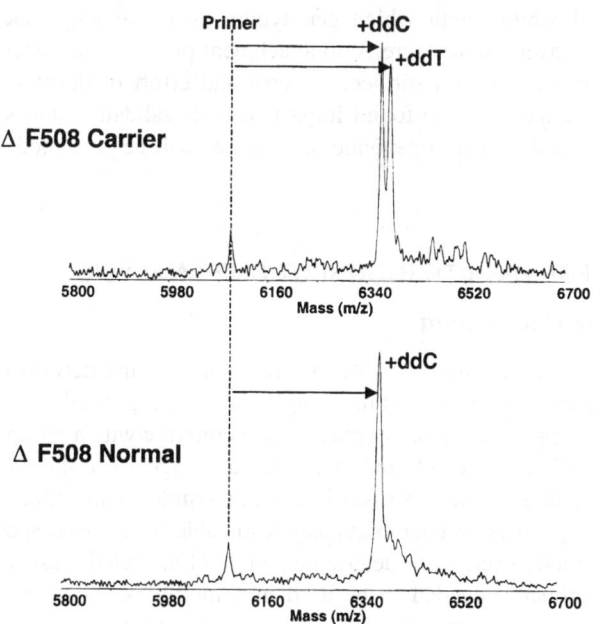

FIGURE 4 Demonstration of Sequazyme-Pinpoint assay performed on CFTR gene for an individual carrying the Δ508 mutation and a wild-type individual. Underlined sequence information shows the sequence used for the genotyping primer, and the 3-base deletion is boxed.

The solution phase assay format depicted in Figure 1 gives way to a host of beneficial aspects, irrespective of the mass spectrometry platform. Linear amplification of the extension product is achieved by using an excess of genotyping primer, a thermostable polymerase, and a thermal cycling protocol in the assay, so there is a sensitivity enhancement over direct PCR product analysis or use of hybridization probes. The use of a thermal cycled protocol eliminates the requirement of generating single-stranded material following PCR. The assay format performs efficiently with no offline purification, preconcentration, or precipitation of the target PCR products; the use of well-characterized, heat-labile enzymes allows an in situ, single-step treatment of the target DNA. Furthermore, the target PCR products remain double stranded, thus allowing confirmatory genotyping from both DNA strands, or alternatively, flexibility in assay design in cases where interfering secondary structures may be present in one strand.

Perhaps the most overwhelming advantage inherent to solution-phase single-base extension, in contrast to technologies based on surface arrays, is the simplicity and flexibility with which genotyping assays at any scale can be designed and deployed. Since there is no attachment of a predetermined ensemble of probes or primers to a surface, the cost and effort of development are minimized. This aspect has profound impact in both validation and screening phases of SNP-based pharmacogenomic research, as will be presented in a later section.

3   FORMAT FOR HIGH-THROUGHPUT SNP ANALYSIS

3.1   Multiplex Genotyping

A uniquely powerful capability enabled by the assay format described here is that of multiplexing SNP tests within a single sample. In general, multiplexing is performed by supplying the genotyping reaction mixture with a group of primers, each with a different length and/or molecular weight. The most important guideline in designing a multiplex assay is that all possible combinations of primers and extended primers be unambiguously resolvable in the mass spectrum. It is a simple arithmetic exercise to determine a table of expected masses for a set of genotyping primers intended to be used in a multiplex assay, from which adjustments to primer sequence can be made to achieve the necessary separation to ensure unambiguous mass spectral results. There are considerations governing both minimum and maximum primer length which impact the design of a multiplex assay. A minimum primer length of 12–14 bases is necessary to ensure specificity, succesful annealing to target during thermal cycling, and recognition of the annealed primer by the DNA polymerase in the reaction. A maximum length of 30 bases is recommended so that there is adequate sensitivity and resolution of the MALDI-TOF instrument for extension products from heterozygotes.

The simplest approach to primer design is to use primers that differ by 2 bases (e.g., 14, 16, 18, 20, 22, 24); therefore it is virtually assured that all primers and dideoxy extension products will not overlap in the mass spectrum. The length can be varied merely by using target sequence, or by using 12 or more bases from the target sequence and then making use of nontemplated 5′ tails to reach the desired length. Using entirely template sequence may increase annealing temperature and perhaps specificity. The use of nontemplated 5′ bases, particularly a poly(dT) tail, may have beneficial effects in terms of mass spectral performance since it is well established that deoxythymidine bases are more resistant to degradation during the MALDI process than other DNA bases [19]. Since typical annealing temperatures of 37°C are used during thermal cycling, 12–14 bases of template sequence is sufficient to allow annealing and subsequent extension of the primer.

A somewhat more sophisticated approach to designing multiplex primers makes more efficient use of the molecular-weight resolution afforded by DE-MALDI systems. This approach draws attention to the exact molecular weight of primers and extended primers to ensure that no overlaps occur. Basically, primers of equal length can be used together provided they differ by at least 50 Da from each other. This spacing is required to accommodate the four possible single-base extension products, which lie in a 40-Da mass window. Using a process termed mass tuning in our laboratory, judicious placement of a few appropriate 5′ bases, nontemplated or otherwise, allows primers and extension products to be separated adequately for successful mass spectral readout. For example, if two 20-mer primers have identical or very similar mass, the corresponding primer extension products will overlap, thereby confounding genotype scoring. However, if two 5′ bases of each primer are replaced by dCdC on one and dGdG on the other primer, a molecular weight spacing of up to 80 Da will be imposed, thereby allowing sufficient resolution of all possible genotypes. The implementation of this approach is illustrated in Figure 5, where 12 primers are used simultaneously to genotype 12 SNP loci. Although such spectra become visually complex, all genotypes are easily read with signal-to-noise ratios of 25 or greater and 50% baseline resolution of heterozygotes.

3.2 Multiplex PCR

In principle, multiplex analysis of 15–20 SNP loci per sample can be accomplished using the mass-tuning approach described above. At this point, there is considerably greater difficulty in successfully performing multiplex PCR on a routine basis. Even to observe adequate yields of all products in a 5-fold multiplex PCR requires careful design of PCR primers, optimization of thermal cycling conditions, and optimization of reaction mixture composition. Although this is portrayed as a limitation or even a disadvantage of PCR, there are approaches to PCR which allow much greater multiplexing with little or no optimization of the PCR itself. This form of PCR [20], which can be viewed as a two-step PCR process, is illustrated in Figure 6. The reaction uses hybrid primers which contain a 20-base common, or "universal," tail on the 5′ end of the target-specific PCR primer sequence. In the first stage, the reaction is supplied with low concentrations of each pair of the hybrid primers, and thermal cycling generates low concentrations of product from each locus containing a common 5′ motif on forward and reverse strands. This common motif serves as the priming site for the universal primer, and all PCR amplicons are further amplified to high levels at essentially the same rate.

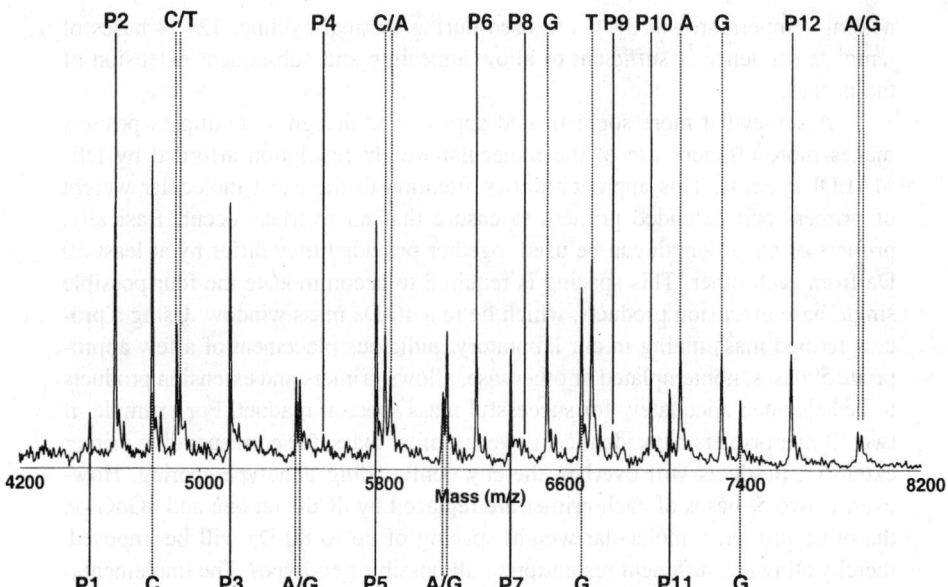

FIGURE 5 Illustration of mass spectrum obtained from a 12-fold multiplex PCR-SNP assay of common polymorphisms. Primer masses were optimized using a combination of 5′ poly(dT) tails and mass tuning using nontemplated 5′ bases, as described in Section 3.1. The PCR reaction used to simultaneously amplify 12 separate loci was performed according to the approach described in Figure 8 and Section 3.2. (From Ref. 18.)

Performing PCR in this manner virtually eliminates the need for optimization of primer concentrations, annealing temperature, or magnesium ion concentration. In our lab, this two-step PCR process has been used to simultaneously amplify up to 12 loci without any preliminary optimization. The use of a two-step procedure appears to add extra time and perhaps reagent cost to the genotyping operation; however, these factors are offset by eliminating optimization costs.

There are some guidelines that increase the chances of success in implementing this form of PCR. The product lengths should be kept to within a few hundred bases; in general, shorter amplicons will give better yield. To avoid primer dimer formation, a "hot-start" PCR reaction should be used. It will also be beneficial to use a DNA polymerase with a wide optimal magnesium ion range, such as Stoffel fragment of Taq DNA polymerase. Finally, it is possible to condense the above procedure to a single step by including both target-specific and universal primers at once. In this case, thermal cycling could be carried out such that the first series of cycles uses an optimal annealing temperature for the

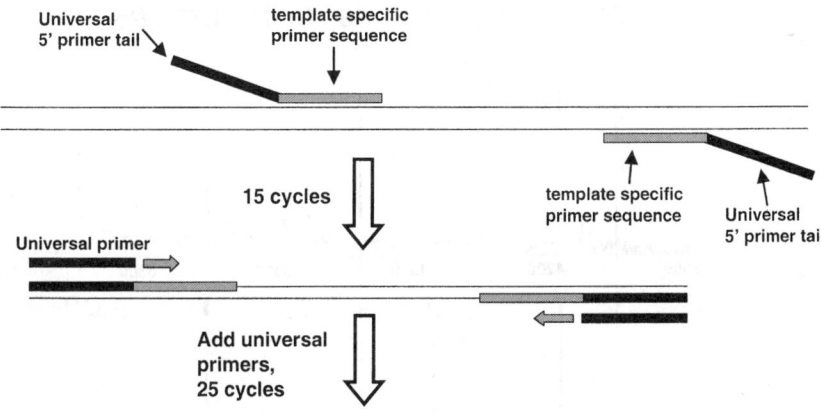

Similar Concentrations of each PCR Product

FIGURE 6   Schematic description of a two-step generic approach to multiplex PCR. The first step uses low concentrations of hybrid primer pairs containing a common 5′ motif of 20 bases. The common 5′ sequence then serves as a priming site in the second round, which employs high concentrations of one or two "universal" primers. The result of the process is generation of high levels of each amplicon with little or no optimization.

target-specific primers, followed by a number of rounds at a second, lower annealing temperature favored by the outer universal primers.

3.3   Applications of MALDI-TOF-Based Genotyping

Within the context of pharmacogenomics, the approaches described here have value in both large-scale validation and refinement of SNP markers, and in large-scale, clinic-based genotyping of patient DNA samples. The most compelling aspects of the MALDI-TOF-based approach described here—throughput, cost-effectiveness, and flexibility—make this the ideal follow-up technology to large-scale genomic sequencing. For a particular set of candidate genes, putative SNP sites are quickly validated by analysis of a small number of representative samples to determine allele frequency. Since the Sequazyme-Pinpoint format uses a very simple chemistry, the validation component of SNP-based gene discovery can be carried out immediately after candidate SNPs are identified, the only delay in the process being the time required to synthesize genotyping primers. Typical data from this form of validation study are displayed in Figure 7, where five SNP loci reported in the Whitehead Institute SNP database (wi.mit.edu) are evaluated across a panel of individuals. Primers for the 5-plex PCR were designed as described in the previous section, and SNP primers ranging from 13 to 21 bases

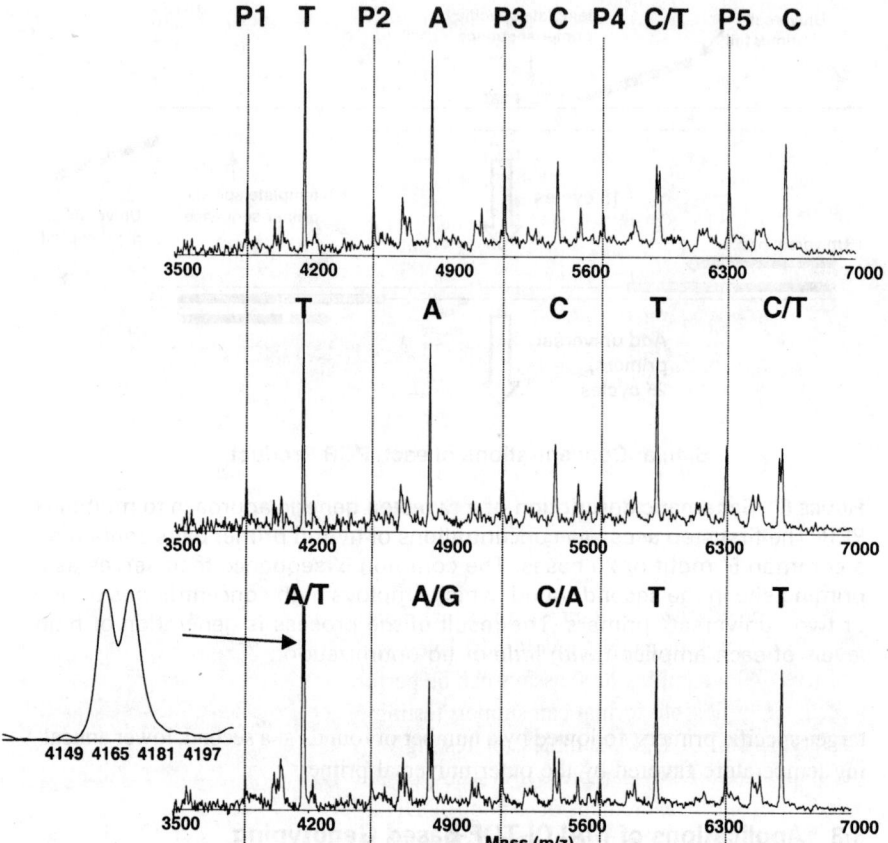

FIGURE 7 Mass spectra obtained from automated analysis of a validation panel of five database SNP loci (www.genome.wi.mit.edu) amplified in a multiplex PCR.

were utilized without further optimization of reaction conditions. Analysis of a panel of individuals clearly shows a high degree of heterozygosity at each of these loci.

The general operational format of MALDI-TOF-based SNP analysis is depicted in Figure 8. All reaction components, from PCR to primer extension, can be assembled directly in the thermal cycler by direct addition of reagents to each tube. Therefore, SNP reactions ready for desalting and MALDI analysis can be prepared using standard automated liquid handlers. Parallel, semiautomated desalting of (one or more) 96- or 384-well sample plates is carried out using centri-

Process Configuration for High-Throughput Genotyping

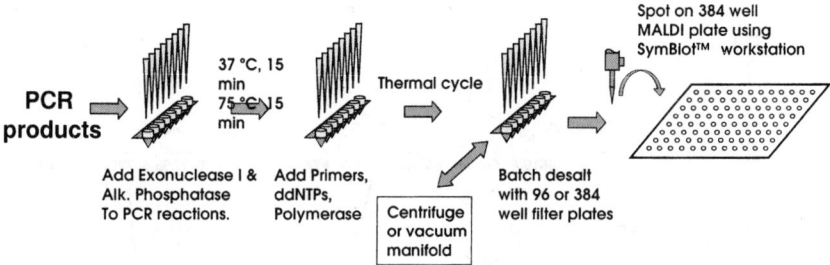

FIGURE 8 Schematic diagram of standard configuration for performing SNP analysis using the Sequazyme-Pinpoint approach. All reaction steps can be carried out by direct addition of reagents into PCR tubes held in a thermal cycler. Semiautomated sample desalting prior to MALDI-TOF analysis is accomplished by centrifugation of 96- or 384-well filtration plates, thereby allowing parallel processing of multiples of 96 or 384 samples.

fugation, and the resultant samples are automatically arrayed onto 384-well MALDI plates in nanoliter volumes. Even with a modest level of multiplexing of five SNPs/sample, 9600 assays can be performed in 8 hours of operation. The completely flexible format can support testing of a small number of SNPs across a large panel of DNA samples, or testing of a large panel of SNPs for a few representative DNA samples. It is also possible to directly obtain an allele frequency from measurement of a pool of DNA samples, as will be described in the final section of this report. As a result of the flexible format, the same MALDI-TOF-based genotyping laboratory can support analysis of large numbers of patient samples to establish correlations between genotype and responsiveness to treatment, often using the same genotyping primers designed for the validation phase of the project. As an illustration, Figure 9 shows data obtained from a survey panel containing several common disease loci, including polymorphisms in cytochrome P450 2D6, low-density lipoprotein receptor, and neurofibromatosis genes. A number of publications also illustrate clinical applications of methodologies similar to those presented here [21,22]

3.4 Automated Genotype Scoring

Commercial MALDI-TOF instruments are equipped with automated sample analysis, data-recording, and processing capabilities. Data from single-base extension assays as described here are easily handled by genotype scoring software. Figure 10 illustrates the basic software format for automated interpretation of SNP assays. The only required input is the sequences of each genotyping primer sup-

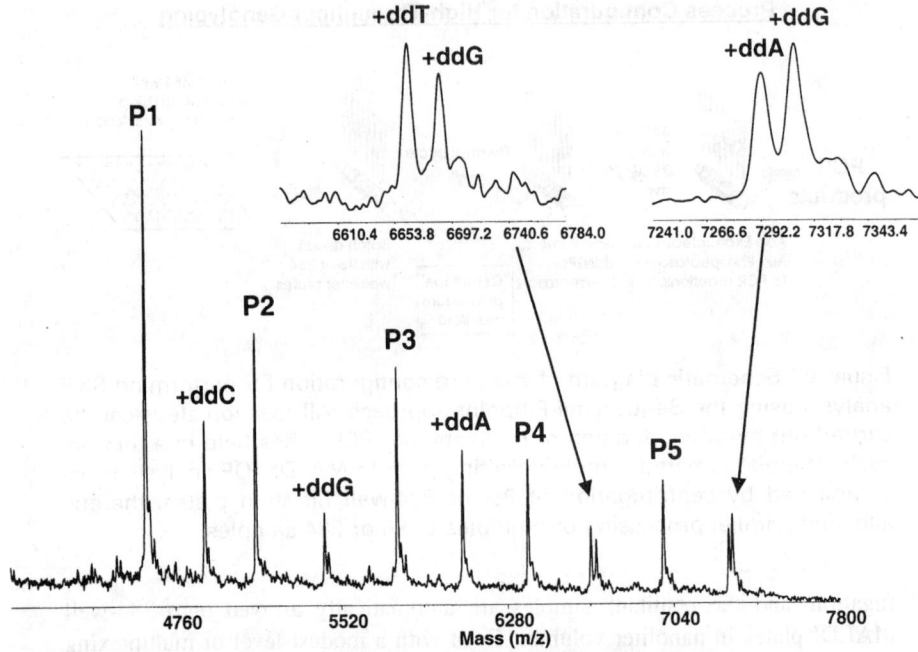

FIGURE 9 Illustration of mass spectrum obtained from 5-fold multiplex SNP assay. Primer lengths range from 15 to 23 bases and employ 5′ poly(dT)tails to space the primers 2 bases apart. The PCR and genotyping primers are designed to genotype common polymorphic loci found on the cytochrome P450 2D6, low-density lipoprotein receptor, and neurofibromatosis genes.

plied to each reaction. The sequence allows calculation of the exact mass of primers and all possible extension products, thus generating a comparison table for incoming raw data. During automated spectrum acquisition, raw mass spectra are first calibrated by simply using one or more of the genotyping primer masses as an internal calibrant. Spectra are then reduced to a peak table by treatment with a specific set of peak detection parameters. This table is then compared to the table of expected masses, and a second set of user-definable peak detection parameters is applied. This second set of parameters allows the user to accept or reject a heterozygote call based on relative peak areas, and to define narrow mass windows in which to detect peaks, thereby improving the stringency of automated interpretation. The quality of genotype scores can be rated based on a number of measurable properties of the data, which include signal-to-noise ratios of the relevant extension products, absolute peak areas, and area ratios

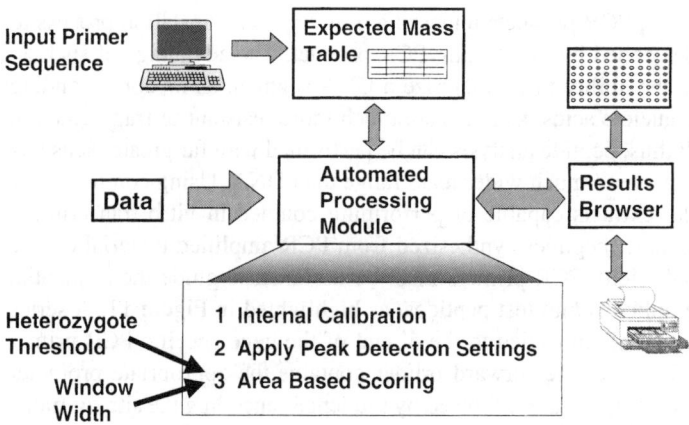

FIGURE 10   Schematic diagram of process involved in software for automated genotyping of mass spectral data from automated SNP assays.

between extended and unextended primer. In our lab, the accuracy of this scoring model approaches 99% using data spanning a range of applications.

4   FUTURE DIRECTIONS

Clearly, the emphasis of this report is on the strengths of routine MALDI-TOF-based SNP genotyping. As demonstrated here, routine, high-throughput analysis of known SNPs is ideally suited to this platform. It is perhaps preliminary to considering MALDI-TOF as a niche technology, particularly with regard to continually evolving tools of molecular biology which may serve to expand the range of tractable genomic applications.

4.1   Screening/Discovery of Unknown Mutations

In general, the early phase of pharmacogenomic discovery is the process of screening unknown regions for potentially useful sequence variants. Discovery of unknown variations in a region of double-stranded DNA by MALDI-TOF (or any form of mass spectrometry) is considerably more challenging than analysis of known SNPs, owing primarily to the precipitous decrease in sensitivity and resolution for DNA longer than 100 bases. Fortunately, the MALDI-TOF MS platform itself is a flexible and highly versatile tool, limited only by the design of various molecular assays that are supplied to the instrument. An alternative assay format has been recently described [23] which essentially circumvents the size limitation encountered in MALDI-TOF analysis of DNA. In this assay, depicted in Figure 11, PCR products undergo a transcription/translation process to generate peptides coded by the starting PCR product. The advantage of such an approach lies in the ability to characterize a DNA segment as its corresponding peptide. Unlike nucleic acids, peptides are much more resistant to fragmentation during MALDI; thus, peptide analysis can be performed with far greater sensitivity and resolution over a much wider mass range than DNA. Using commercially available cellular extracts capable of performing coupled in vitro transcription and translation, intact peptides synthesized from PCR amplified material can be recovered in high yield. PCR primers must be designed to guide the sequential processing of amplicons into test peptides, as highlighted in Figure 11. A series of sequence motifs are appended to the 5′ end of the gene-specific PCR primer sequence. The 5′ end of the forward primer contains the appropriate promoter sequence for RNA polymerase, followed by sequences encoding the site for translation initiation, and finally, a sequence region encoding a peptide tag sequence. Test peptides are isolated and desalted on affinity gel by affinity-based capture via the peptide tag. Matrix is then added to the bound peptides and MALDI-TOF analysis is performed.

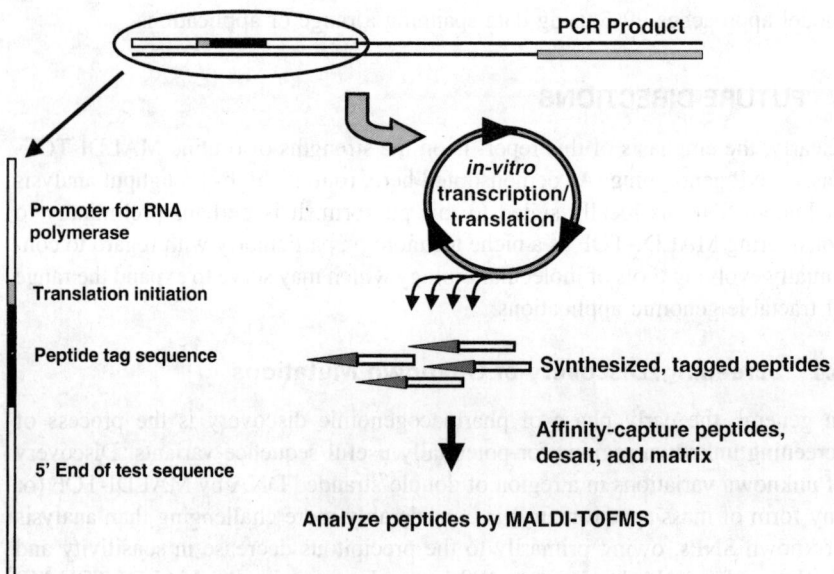

FIGURE 11 Schematic diagram of DNA mutation screening assay using coupled in vitro–synthesized peptides. The leftmost region highlights the sequence motifs carried by the forward PCR primer to support transcription and translation of PCR product into peptides.

An illustration of this assay (Fig. 12) using PCR products generated from the cytochrome P450 2D6 gene demonstrates high-accuracy analysis of the resultant peptides and the capability for multiplexing the assay. In the example shown, two test peptides are synthesized from the corresponding PCR products, one of which contains the 1934 G-A splice site mutation [24]. Analysis of a carrier sample shows that an additional peptide whose mass corresponds precisely (expected Δmass = 99.13 Da) to the expected glycine-to-arginine substitution is generated in the assay. Thus, it is not only possible to detect all possible coding mutations with this approach; by judicious design of PCR primers to facilitate

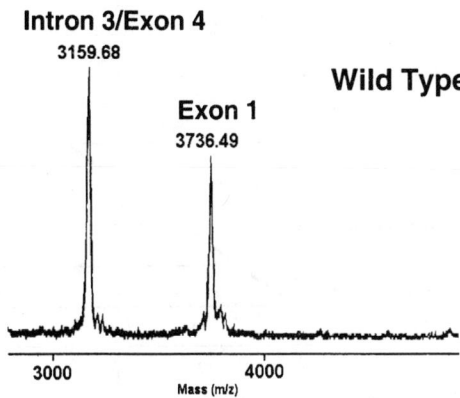

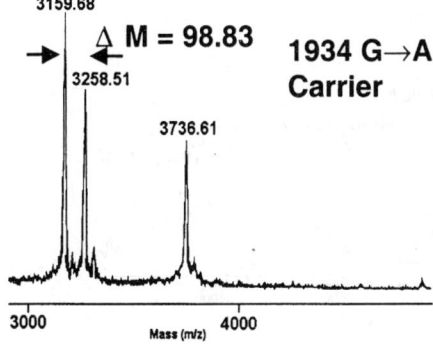

FIGURE 12 Mass spectra obtained from screening test peptides generated from amplified regions within cytochrome P450 2D6 gene. The spectrum from the wild-type sample shows the two expected peptides, while for the carrier sample, an additional peptide, corresponding to the mass of a Gly-Arg substitution, is observed.

in-frame extension of coding sequence, mutations within promoter and splice site regions can also be screened. The available MALDI-TOF mass range of this assay should allow multiplex screening of segments of 200 or more bases in length in multiplex fashion.

4.2 Quantitative Genotyping

The application of MALDI-TOF MS in a more quantitative role has remained relatively unexplored within the context of genetic analysis. Of particular interest in pharmacogenomics is the ability to quantify the amount of a particular allele in a collection of DNA samples. As highlighted above, analysis of a series of

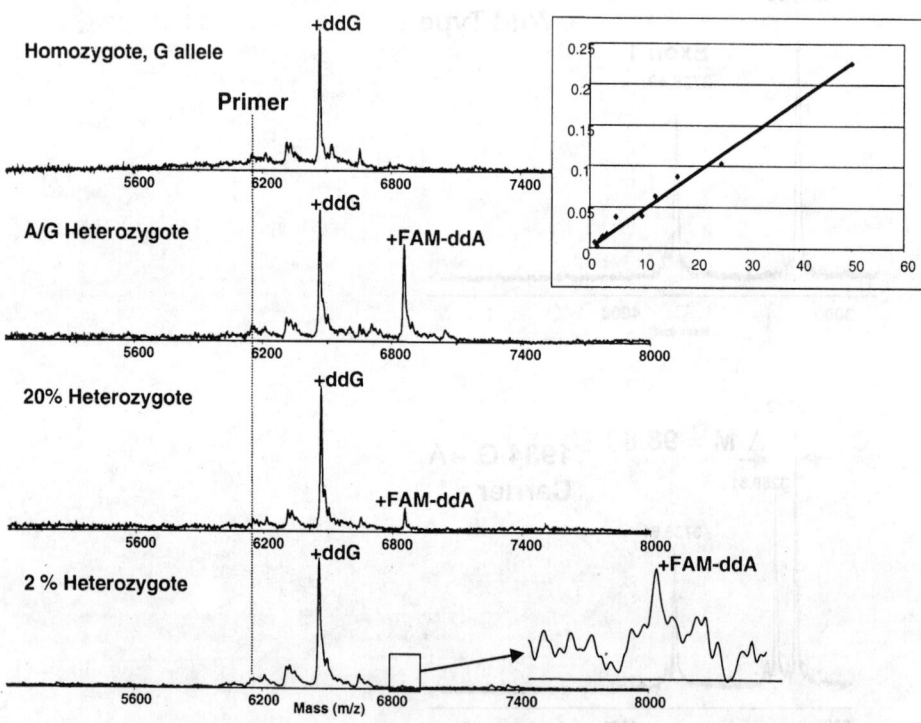

FIGURE 13 Demonstration of preparation of standard curves for MALDI-based SNP allele frequency measurement. The assay uses a primer extension mixture containing ddG, ddC, ddT, and FAM-labeled ddA, with all other aspects of the assay remaining identical to Figure 1 and Figure 8. Data are plotted from peak measurements obtained from an average of 5 mass spectra at each data point.

samples at known SNP sites can reveal common variations in a small number of experiments. It is often sufficient, if not more desirable, to obtain an allele frequency for a given population of DNA samples, as would be done in a large-scale association (linkage disequilibrium) study.

Figure 13 illustrates how such an application would be implemented. Although the single-base extension format detailed in this report does convey quantitative information between alleles of a heterozygote sample, the quantitative accuracy and sensitivity are limited. This limitation is imposed by difficulty in accurately measuring (or even detecting) peaks that are not fully resolved and have potentially widely varying relative areas. A slight modification of the approach, where the reaction mix contains one deoxy (typically corresponding to the expected low intensity allele) and three dideoxy nucleotides, allows separation of alleles by approximately 300 Da rather than 9–15 Da. Alternatively, supplying the reaction mixture with at least one mass-tagged ddNTP allows a similar separation of alleles. The result of this assay modification is spectra displaying alleles peak that are well separated and easily quantitated.

Initial investigations (Fig. 13) reveal that quantitation of alleles in mixtures of PCR products representing a range of allelic populations can be performed succesfully [25]. The limit of quantitation of such an approach was found to be 2–5%, although the limit of detection can be as low as 1% of a particular allele. With this approach, it is observed that a 1:1 heterozygote does not give equal peak intensities, presumably due to unequal amplification or dideoxy incorporation efficiency between alleles. Therefore a quantitative analysis requires the use of a known mutant or heterozygote sample to determine a relative response factor between alleles. The overall benefit of utilizing the approach described here is to reduce the time and cost of analysis for routine validation of common SNPs or association-based genetic linkage. This method has sufficient accuracy and quantitative capacity to determine allele frequency in large DNA pools and may ultimately become more attractive than genotyping each individual in a study.

4.3 Outlook

At present, MALDI-TOF is one of many tools currently utilized to perform routine SNP analysis. The capabilities introduced in this section, quantitative SNP analysis in DNA pools and screening/discovery of unknown polymorphisms, extend the utility of MALDI-TOF technology into numerous phases of the pharmacogenomic workflow. As illustrated here, screening targeted polymorphic regions for important genetic variants can have tremendous impact for clinical analysis. However, since a large proportion of SNPs occur in coding regions (c-SNPs) of DNA [26], this approach will allow a drastic reduction in the amount of DNA sequencing required for large-scale discovery of c-SNPs. Only those genetic regions harboring a sequence variant as discovered by MALDI-TOF analysis will then undergo sequencing to confirm the identity of the polymorphism. Following high-throughput validation of SNPs as described in the bulk of this report, allele frequency measurements in various populations or clinical pools can be performed. The quantitative capacity described in the previous section may give rise to MALDI-TOF-based gene expression analysis. The vision for the near future is therefore one in which c-SNP discovery, validation, and population-based quantitation, followed by targeted gene expression analysis, is performed using a devoted laboratory equipped with an integrated network of automated MALDI-TOF mass spectrometers.

REFERENCES

1. DG Wang, JB Fan, CJ Siao, A Berno, P Young, R Sapolsky, G Ghandour, N Perkins, E Winchester, J Spencer, L Kruglyak, L Stein, L Hsie, T Topaloglou, E Hubbell, E Robinson, M Mittmann, MS Morris, N Shen, D Kilburn, J Rioux, C Nusbaum, S Rozen, TJ Hudson, ES Lander. Large-scale identification, mapping, and genotyping of single-nucleotide polymorphisms in the human genome. Science 280:1077–1082, 1998.
2. M Karas, F Hillenkamp. Laser desorption ionization of proteins with molecular masses exceeding 10,000 daltons. Anal Chem 60:2299–2301, 1988.
3. ML Vestal, P Juhasz, SA Martin. Delayed extraction matrix-assisted laser desorption time-of-flight mass spectrometry. Rapid Commun Mass Spectrom 8:865–868, 1995.
4. P Juhasz, MT Roskey, IP Smirnov, LA Haff, ML Vestal, SA Martin. Applications of delayed extraction matrix-assisted laser desorption/ionization time-of-flight mass spectrometry to oligonucleotide analysis. Anal Chem 68:941–946, 1996.
5. MC Fitzgerald, LM Smith. Mass spectrometry of nucleic acids: the promise of matrix-assisted laser desorption-ionization (MALDI) mass spectrometry. Annu Rev Biophys Biomol Struct 24:117–140, 1995.
6. E Nordhoff, F Kirpekar, P Roepstorff. Mass spectrometry of nucleic acids. Mass Spectrom Rev 15:67–138, 1996.
7. YF Zhu, CN Chung, NI Taranenko, SL Allman, SA Martin, L Haff, CH Chen. The study of 2,3,4-trihydroxyacetophenone and 2,4,6-trihydroxyacetophenone as matrices for DNA detection in matrix-assisted laser desorption/ionization time-of-flight mass spectrometry. Rapid Commun Mass Spectrom 10:383–388, 1996.
8. KJ Wu, A Steding, CH Becker. Matrix-assisted laser desorption time-of-flight mass spectrometry of oligonucleotides using 3-hydroxypicolinic acid as an ultraviolet sensitive matrix. Rapid Commun Mass Spectrom 4:99–102, 1993.
9. U Pieles, W Zurcher, M Schar, HE Moser. Matrix-assisted laser desorption ionization time-of-flight mass spectrometry: a powerful tool for the mass and sequence analysis of natural and modified oligonucleotides. Nucleic Acids Res 21:3191–3196, 1993.
10. IP Smirnov, MT Roskey, P Juhasz, EJ Takach, SA Martin, LA Haff. Sequencing oligonucleotides by exonuclease digestion and delayed extraction matrix-assisted

laser desorption ionization time-of-flight mass spectrometry. Anal Biochem 238:19–25, 1996.

11. NI Taranenko, KJ Matteson, CN Chung, YF Zhu, LY Chang, SL Allman, L Haff, SA Martin, CH Chen. Laser desorption mass spectrometry for point mutation detection. Genet Anal 13:87–94, 1996.

12. PL Ross, PA Davis, P Belgrader. Analysis of PCR products from conventional and microfabricated thermal cyclers using delayed extraction MALDI-TOF mass spectrometry. Anal Chem 70:2067–2073, 1998.

13. A Braun, DP Little, H Koster. Detecting CFTR gene mutations using primer oligo base extension and mass spectrometry. Clin Chem 43:1151–1158, 1996.

14. LA Haff, IP Smirnov. Single nucleotide polymorphism identification assays using a thermostable DNA polymerase and delayed extraction MALDI-TOF mass spectrometry. Genome Res 7:378–388, 1997.

15. PF Crain, JA McCloskey. Applications of mass spectrometry to the characterization of oligonucleotides and nucleic acids. Curr Opin Biotechnol 9:25–34, 1998.

16. TJ Griffin, LM Smith. Single nucleotide polymorphism analysis by MALDI-TOF mass spectrometry. Trends Biotechnol 18:77–84, 2000.

17. LA Haff, IP Smirnov. Multiplex genotyping of PCR products with mass tag-labeled primers. Nucleic Acids Res 25:3749–3750, 1997.

18. P Ross, L Hall, I Smirnov, L Haff. High level multiplex genotyping by MALDI-TOF mass spectrometry. Nat Biotechnol 16:1347–1351, 1998.

19. K Schneider, BT Chait. Increased stability of nucleic acids containing 7-deazaguanosine and 7-deaza-adenosine may enable rapid DNA sequencing by matrix-assisted laser desorption mass spectrometry. Nucleic Acids Res 23:1570–1575, 1995.

20. P Belgrader, MA Marino, M Lubin, FA Barany. A multiplex PCR-ligase detection reaction assay for human identity testing. Genome Sci Technol 1:77–87, 1996.

21. A Harksen, PM Ueland, H Refsum, K Meyer. Four common mutations of the cystathionine beta-synthase gene detected by multiplex PCR and matrix-assisted laser desorption/ionization time-of-flight mass spectrometry. Clin Chem 45:1157–1161, 1999.

22. DP Little, A Braun, B Darnhofer-Demar, H Koster. Identification of apolipoprotein E polymorphisms using temperature cycled primer oligo base extension and mass spectrometry. Eur J Clin Chem Clin Biochem 35:545–548, 1997.

23. AM Garvin, KC Parker, L Haff. MALDI-TOF based mutation detection using tagged in-vitro synthesized peptides. Nat Biotechnol 18:95–97, 2000.

24. D Marez, M Legrand, N Sabbagh, JM Guidice, C Spire, JJ Lafitte, UA Meyer, F Broly. Polymorphism of the cytochrome P450 CYP2D6 gene in a European population: characterization of 48 mutations and 53 alleles, their frequencies and evolution. Pharmacogenetics 7:193–202, 1997.

25. PL Ross, L Hall, L Haff. Quantitative approach to single-nucleotide polymorphism analysis using MALDI-TOF MS. Biotechniques 29:620–628, 2000.

26. M Cargill, D Altshuler, J Ireland, P Sklar, K Ardlie, N Patil, CR Lane, EP Lim, N Kalayanaraman, J Nemesh, L Ziaugra, L Friedland, A Rolfe, J Warrington, R Lipshutz, GQ Daley, ES Lander. Characterization of single-nucleotide polymorphisms in coding regions of human genes. Nat Genet 22:231–238, 1999.

13

Serial Analysis of Gene Expression
Transcriptional Insights into Functional Biology

Stephen L. Madden, Clarence Wang, and Greg Landes

Genzyme Corporation, Framingham, Massachusetts

1 INTRODUCTION

Understanding biology at the molecular level requires the development and implementation of technology platforms that can identify biochemical and genetic networks present within any cell type or tissue of interest. As a first step toward this understanding, we must first determine which genes or gene products are expressed and quantify their level of expression. Enabling technologies will generate transcriptomes and proteomes representing expressed gene and gene product profiles, respectively. These profiles not only provide the functional capabilities of the cell/tissue at the time of analysis but also yield valuable molecular insights into the phenotypic differences between cell types and tissues that differ spatially, temporally, or pathophysiologically. For the purpose of this monograph, we will limit the discussion to gene expression profiling in general and serial analysis of gene expression (SAGE), specifically.

Gene expression-profiling technologies can be classified into open and closed systems. Open systems are those platforms that can detect and quantify the expression of both known and novel genes. Novel genes in this instance are those genes that have been neither cloned nor sequenced. In contrast, closed systems, exemplified by cDNA microarrays and oligonucleotide chips, quantify the expression of known genes based on the design features of the microarray/chip. Open-system expression-profiling technologies are comprehensive and provide global gene expression profiles of interrogated cells and tissues while closed systems yield gene expression results for specific genes. SAGE is one of several open systems for gene expression profiling. Others include restriction enzyme analysis of differentially expressed sequences [1], amplified fragment length polymorphisms [2], total gene expression analysis [3], and gene calling [4]. The disadvantages of the open-system architecture are that throughput is moderate at best, with respect to the number of samples analyzed, and accordingly, costs per sample are higher. Not surprisingly, the open-system weaknesses are the advantages of the closed-system approach although, as discussed above, the gene expression information is limited to the gene content present on the chip, which will be incomplete for the first-generation commercial arrays.

2 THE SAGE PROCESS

2.1 Original Method for Library Construction

SAGE, developed by Velculescu, Vogelstein, and Kinzler at Johns Hopkins University, is a sequence-based approach that identifies which genes are expressed and quantifies their level of expression [5]. This catalog of gene expression for a given cell type or tissue is defined as the "transcriptome." To generate comprehensive and representative transcriptomes requires exacting transcript identification and accurate quantification using unbiased and highly efficient molecular processes. SAGE was developed to satisfy these functional requirements using three founding principles (Figs. 1–3). First, SAGE utilizes a short contiguous sequence of 10–11 bp, derived from a defined location within each transcript

SAGE Principle (1)

A short oligonucleotide sequence from a defined location within a transcript, a "tag", encodes sufficient complexity to identify an expressed gene.

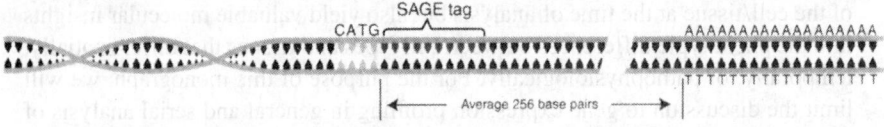

FIGURE 1   SAGE principle 1: Representation of a typical 3′ end of a cDNA molecule denoting the ultimate N1aIII site (CATG) and the adjacent SAGE tag.

and unique to each tag, to identify individual mRNAs (Fig. 1). SAGE tags are used not only for gene identification, but are also used to measure the relative abundance of their cognate transcripts within the mRNA population based on the number of occurrences of a given SAGE tag within a SAGE sequencing project. Second, to overcome throughput limitations associated with sequencing-based approaches, SAGE employs serial processing such that 25–50 transcripts (or SAGE tags) are analyzed on each lane of an automated DNA sequencer while continuing to use parallel processing with multiple sequencing lanes and sequencers operating simultaneously (Fig. 2). Finally, SAGE uses a PCR step like many of the contemporary expression analysis methods, but SAGE differs from these in that it has devised a mechanism for recognizing and eliminating amplification bias from the expression profile (Fig. 3). Consequently, individual transcript representation is maintained when analyzing complex natural mixtures of mRNA.

Each mRNA population to be analyzed by SAGE requires the construction of a library of clones whose inserts represent concatenated SAGE tags. Library generation has been described previously [5] but will be briefly reviewed here (Figs. 4–8). As in all gene expression-profiling methods, mRNA is converted to double-stranded cDNA using oligo(dT) to prime first-strand synthesis (Fig. 4). In this instance, the oligo(dT) primer contains a 5′ biotin moiety to enable recovery of 3′ cDNA fragments. The resulting double-stranded cDNA is digested with the restriction enzyme NlaIII (anchoring enzyme), which recognizes and cleaves

SAGE Principle (2)
A combination of serial and parallel analysis maximizes throughput.

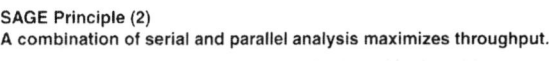

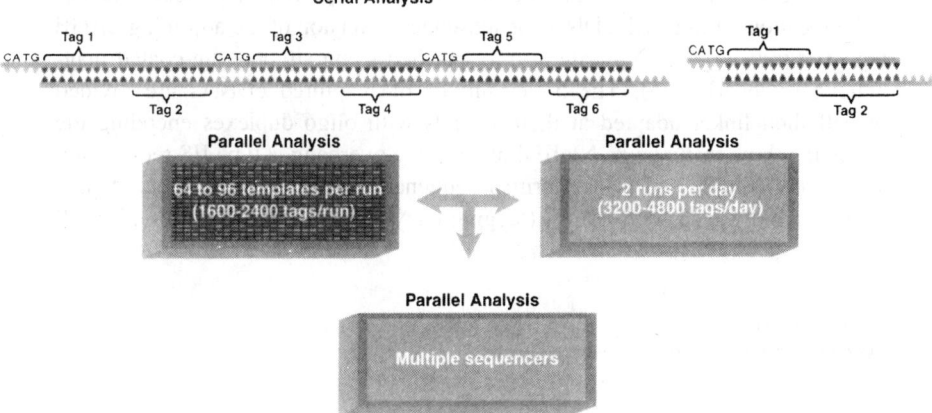

FIGURE 2 SAGE principle 2: Concatenation of multiple gene-specific tags within individual clones allows serial detection of tags. Multiple lanes and sequencers allow parallel processing of serially aligned SAGE tags.

SAGE Principle (3)
Minimize, recognize and eliminate PCR-mediated amplification bias.

Defer PCR until amplicons are ~equivalent in size (100 pb) and composition (~70% adaptors)

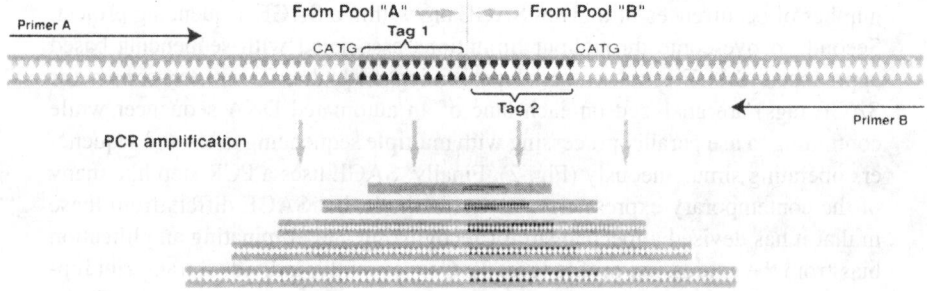

Recognize and eliminate residual amplification bias by using each ditag sequence once per project

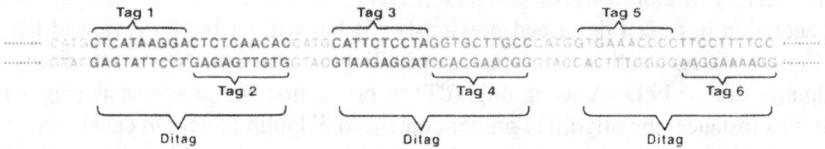

FIGURE 3 SAGE principle 3: Random association of any given tags to form ditag PCR templates.

DNA immediately 3′ of the sequence CATG. This digestion step creates the defined location within each cDNA for subsequent excision of the adjoining SAGE tag. Biotinylated 3′ cDNAs are affinity purified using streptavidin-coated magnetic particles (Fig. 5). The 5′ termini of the captured cDNAs are divided in half then linker adapted at their 5′ ends with oligo duplexes encoding the following three features: an NlaIII 4 nt cohesive overhang, a type IIS recognition sequence (BsmFI), and a PCR primer sequence (primer A or B). The adapted cDNAs are digested with BsmFI (tagging enzyme), which cleaves 14–15 bp 3′

SAGE Method (a)
Synthesis of biotinylated double-stranded cDNA.

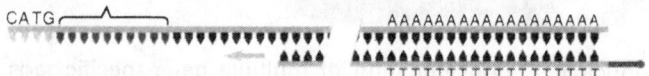

FIGURE 4 The SAGE method: Synthesis of ds-cDNA.

SAGE Method (b)
Restriction enzyme digestion of cDNA and capture of 3' most NlaIII cDNA fragment.

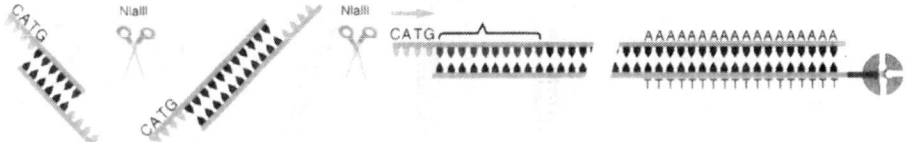

FIGURE 5 The SAGE method: Restriction enzyme digestion of cDNA and capture of 3' cDNA fragments.

of its recognition sequence, releasing the linker adapted SAGE tag from each cDNA (Fig. 6). BsmFI cleaves 15 bp downstream of its recognition sequence sites ~80% of the time while the remaining cleavage sites are 14 bp downstream of its recognition sequence. The linker-adapted SAGE tags from each pool are repaired with DNA polymerase (Klenow), mixed together, and then ligated with T4 DNA ligase. The resulting linker-adapted ditags are amplified by PCR using primers A and B, digested with NlaIII to release the primer-adapters, and the SAGE ditags are purified (Fig. 7). The SAGE ditags are polymerized using T4 DNA ligase, size selected and then cloned into a high-copy plasmid vector. Each cloned insert is organized as a concatenated series of ditags of ~20–22 bp in length, separated by the 4-bp recognition sequence for the anchoring enzyme NlaIII (Fig. 8).

The complexity of each SAGE library is ~2 × 10⁶ SAGE tags (or transcripts) based on 5 × 10⁴ cfu per library on average with cloned insert sizes of ~500 bp (40 SAGE tags per clone). For most projects, about 2000 individual SAGE clones are sequenced to yield ~50,000 SAGE tags. Standard sequencing chemistries and platforms are used with the resulting sequence outputs analyzed by custom software (below).

2.2 Methodological Improvements

As is the case for other types of cloned DNA libraries, each step in SAGE library construction needs to be performed efficiently to ensure that the entire process will result in a high-complexity, unbiased collection of cloned SAGE tags. To this end, several improvements to the original published procedure have been reported that can enhance the efficiency of specific steps in library construction and thereby increase the robustness of the entire process. These modifications are reducing the amount of starting mRNA required and creates opportunities to analyze transcriptomes from biological systems that have previously resisted

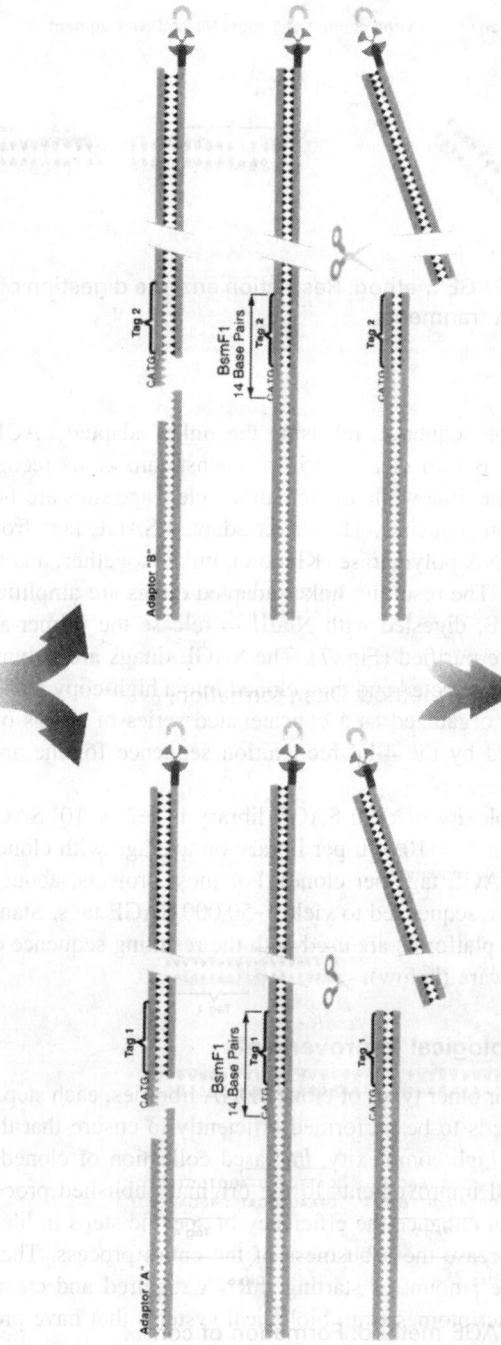

FIGURE 6 The SAGE method: Adaptor modification and excision of tags.

SAGE Method (d)
Formation of ditags, amplification, and removal of adaptors.

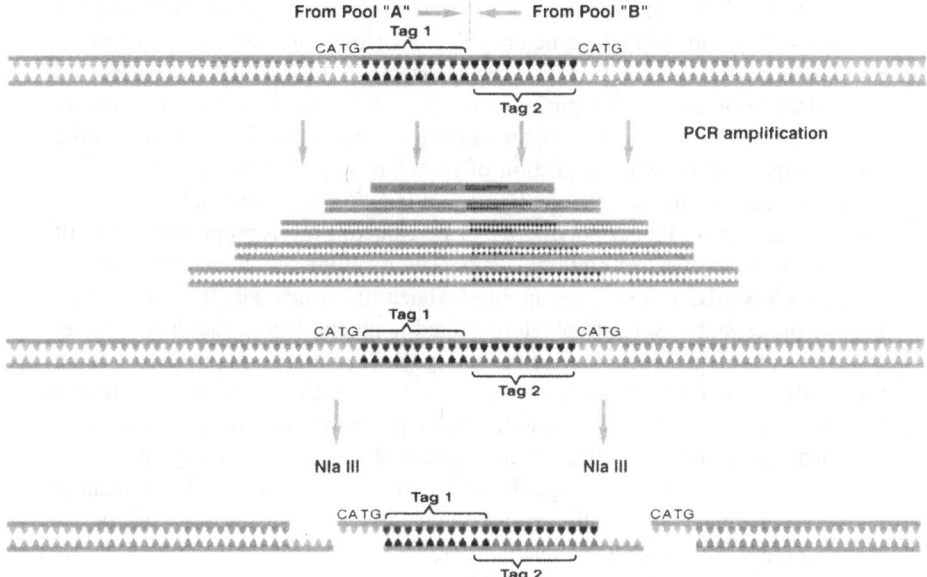

FIGURE 7   The SAGE method: Ditag formation, amplification, and adaptor removal.

SAGE Method (e)
Formation of concatamers and sequencing.

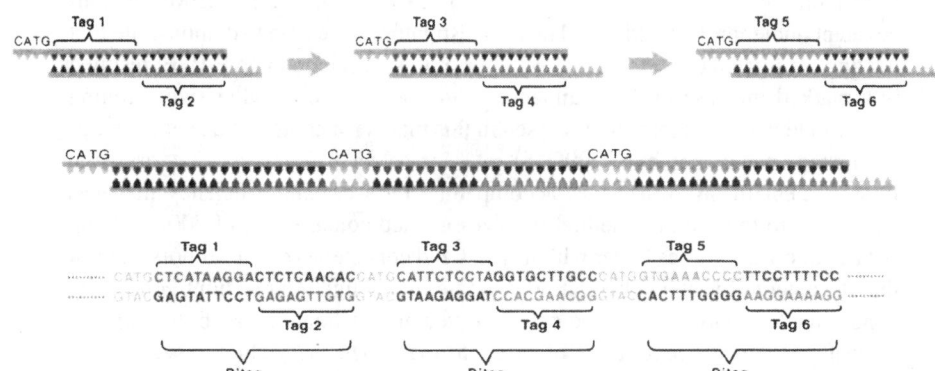

FIGURE 8   The SAGE method: Formation of concatemers and sequencing.

characterization due to insufficient quantities of starting mRNA. Included in this set are biopsies, tissue punches, and even single-cell preparations.

One of the first methodological improvements was described by Powell [6] and focused on improving the efficiency of concatemer formation (Fig. 8). Powell reasoned that the efficiency of this crucial step is a function of the purity and concentration of ditags. The purity of ditags is influenced by the effectiveness of gel purification of ditags and the accompanying removal of contaminating linker-adapters after NlaIII digestion of the PCR amplified ditags. Any linker-adapter molecules that remain can ligate to ditags forming dead-end products on one end that can no longer polymerize or be cloned. Powell proposed the use of biotinylated amplimers to amplify ditags. The resulting amplicons could be digested with NlaIII, to dissociate the biotinylated linker-adapters from the ditags. Further processing, using streptavidin-coated magnetic beads, facilitates the recovery of unbound ditags while eliminating the haptenated components. Using this strategy, four SAGE libraries were constructed. Compared to the original method, Powell's modification resulted in the generation of a minimum of twice as much ditag, and when ligated and cloned, the number of ditags per clone was increased by 43% on average. Therefore, this improvement can significantly enhance the quality of the library and concomitantly elevate the yield of sequenced tags per lane of a sequencing gel.

Kenzelmann and Muhlemann [7] also modified the protocol to improve concatemer formation. In contrast to Powell's modification [6], they addressed the observation that the cloning of size-selected contamers resulted in clones whose average insert size was significantly smaller than that expected from gel purified DNA. They hypothesized that size-selected DNA consisted of both DNA concatemers of the expected size as well as a substantial population of contaminating smaller concatemers that had aggregated. Aggregated concatemers could result from annealing of complementary overhangs in the presence of high concentrations of Mg^{2+} present in the ligation reaction and the formation of non-covalent nucleoprotein adducts. These investigators were able to demonstrate that heating the ligated concatemers to 65°C prior to size selection on PAGE, resulted in a marked increase in the abundance of concatemers of smaller size. Cloning of size-selected concatemers processed in this manner increased the average number of tags per clones by ~200% for all size selected fractions. This dramatic improvement in insert size was accompanied by a cloning efficiency that was equivalent to the original method for size-selected concatemers of 700–1000 bp but became 1.5–2 times lower with larger-sized concatemers. The authors suggest that the extent of vector self-ligation is greater in the ligation reactions containing concatemers of larger size. The extent of vector self-ligation can be minimized by using higher concentrations of insert to maximize the yield of vector-insert linear products early in the ligation reaction. Subsequently, the ligation reaction can be diluted 5- to 10-fold and allowed to proceed such that all of the linear products can circularize and become clonable. The modification of Powell (above) will yield significantly larger amounts of ditag and concatamer and, when coupled with the suggestions of Kenzelmann and Muhlmann for concatemer purification, should result in libraries whose clones have larger inserts while potentially enabling less starting mRNA to be used since ditag generation is improved.

In contrast to the above concatemer-specific improvements, the modifications proposed by both Datson et al. [8] and Virlon et al. [9] focused on steps prior to the formation of ditags and concatemers (Figs. 4, 5, and 6). Each of these groups proposed the use of a single reaction tube for performing a series of steps beginning with mRNA isolation and continuing through the generation of linker-adapted tags. This strategy maximizes the generation of linker-adapted SAGE tags by minimizing the loss of intermediates that normally occur during their purification at each individual step. In fact, Virlon and colleagues demonstrated a fourfold improvement in cDNA yield followed by a 400-fold increase in the recovery of cDNA after digestion the anchoring enzyme NlaIII. The single-tube modification of Datson and coworkers enabled them to construct "micro-SAGE" libraries from 0.3-mm punches of 325-μm-thick tissue sections of the dentate gyrus of the rat hippocampus. They estimated that the tissue punches used for library construction contained no more than 1×10^5 cells or $\sim$1–5 ng of mRNA. An additional reamplification of excised ditags of 8–15 cycles was necessary to generate a sufficient mass of ditags for library construction. Because Datson et al. [8] were operating at the limits of mRNA amounts needed for library construction, they were unable to validate the robustness of their modifications by comparison to the original method. Furthermore, only 1497 ditags were sequenced. Future studies need to validate these modifications using readily available tissue sources so that libraries can be made in parallel using the original and modified protocols.

Virlon et al. [9] constructed "SAGE adapted for downsized extract" (SADE) libraries from murine kidney using their single tube modification and either 250 or 0.5 mg of tissue. The resulting libraries were compared to a library made using the original SAGE protocol and starting with 500 mg of tissue. The authors were able to demonstrate a significant correlation ($r = .88$) between the abundance of the same tags in the two SADE libraries based on sequencing 1200 tags per library. Furthermore, the extent of differential expression between the profiles from the original SAGE library and the 0.5-mg SADE library was not significantly different ($P < .05$ by Monte Carlo analysis) than that between two SAGE libraries from the same tissue. These findings, however, are based on only 1200 tags and need to be reevaluated at the $\sim$100,000 tag level. Nevertheless, these results suggest that the single-tube modifications do not appear to cause tag bias and are likely to be more robust while enabling libraries to be constructed from minute quantities of tissue. These single tube improvements along with those that enhance the yield and quality of both ditags and concatemers [6,7] offer the possibility of characterizing the expression of homogenous cell types in primary tissues/organs as a function of temporal, spatial, or physiological state.

The most demanding application of SAGE with respect to starting mRNA was that of Nielson and colleagues, who reported the transcriptome of human oocytes using nine GV-stage oocytes based on a method called PCR-SAGE [10]. Rather than modifying the SAGE protocol, these investigators amplified the starting cDNA by PCR (29 cycles). A similar strategy was developed by Peters et al. [11] although the preparation of cDNA for PCR amplification utilized the intrinsic template switching activity of reverse transcriptase to deploy universal primer sequences at the termini of cDNA. In both cases, the resulting material was then used for standard library construction. Neilson et al., estimated that each oocyte contained about 100 pg of mRNA, so less than 1 ng of mRNA was used for library construction. The starting RNA used by Peters and colleagues was derived from 1- to 2-mm tissue biopsies and contained <100 ng of total RNA or <2 ng of mRNA.

It is unclear whether the collective improvements described above would have circumvented the need for PCR amplification of cDNA prior to library construction. Nevertheless, the resulting oocyte library was sequenced to a level of $>50,000$ tags, which represented the expression of 27,073 different transcripts. Approximately 75% of the SAGE tags corresponded to known cDNAs or ESTs. Nielson et al. [10] were very concerned about distortion of the transcript populations due to the necessity of PCR prior to library construction. They suggested that if amplification bias occurred, it did not have a marked effect on transcript abundances based on two observations. First, the resulting oocyte transcriptome was complete with respect to expressed sequences that are known to be present in human oocytes or those of other mammalian species while being deficient in transcripts known to absent in a variety of mammalian species. Second, by comparison to the representation of β- and γ-actin sequences in a murine oocyte cDNA library and the larger volume of the mouse oocyte compared to its human counterpart, the authors claimed that the 0.073% abundance of the human actins in the GV-stage oocyte was in good agreement with the volume adjusted findings of 0.085% in the murine oocyte [12].

In the SAGE-lite method of Peters et al. [11] 22 cycles of PCR was determined to be optimal in that sufficient cDNA for library construction was generated while the cDNA complexity did not appear to be biased based on monitoring the abundance of five different transcripts. Subsequently, SAGE-lite libraries were made from minute surgical samples (1–2 mm) of the saccular dilatation of the intracranial artery (ICA) and the superficial temporal artery (STA). ICA and STA library sequencing was to a level of 11,495 and 7297 tags, respectively, which represented 4924 and 3552 unique transcripts. Several transcripts predicted by SAGE-lite to be differentially expressed, were confirmed by dot blot hybridization.

As was the case with the micro-SAGE and SADE procedures, future PCR-SAGE and SAGE-lite studies should include additional validation of the modified methods by comparison to the standard protocol. Comparisons between multiple libraries, each sequenced to levels of 50,000–100,000 tags, would go along ways towards acceptance of these changes while encouraging their use in new discovery applications in multiple biological settings.

3 SAGE BIOINFORMATICS

SAGE, being a sequence-based expression-profiling platform, utilizes DNA sequence as its underlying bioinformatic currency. This is a major strength of SAGE from a bioinformatic standpoint but to take full advantage of this feature requires efficient computational tools for data generation, management, and analysis. The custom tool for these tasks is the SAGE software, a Windows-based application designed to handle processing and analysis of tag data from an individual SAGE library or multiple libraries [5].

The core functions of the SAGE software are (1) extraction and tabulation of tag sequences and counts from raw sequence files; (2) comparison of tag abundances between projects; and (3) matching of tags to reference sequences in other databases. The tag extraction function involves the reading of concatenated ditag sequences from text files generated from sequencing of library clones. The sequence is parsed for ditags punctuated by the anchoring enzyme recognition site. Ditags that pass minimum and maximum length criteria are checked against a running list of ditags, and discarded if previously observed in that project. This constraint of allowing only unique ditags within a SAGE project minimizes PCR-induced bias in the SAGE analysis. The allowed ditags are dissected for their component tags, which are tabulated in separate look-up lists for each project. These lists are used for the second core function, the generation of a report comparing the expression profile of a project against one or more others.

The third key function of the SAGE software is the matching of experimentally observed tags to a species-specific database of reference sequences. The software constructs this database in advance by parsing a text file containing multiple sequences in GenBank format. Each sequence is scanned for the 3'-most anchoring enzyme site and its adjacent SAGE tag, which is collected and stored along with abbreviated annotation in a tag-indexed database file. Matching a list of observed tags against this file reveals the corresponding known genes.

Figure 9 summarizes the data analysis procedure for a typical SAGE experiment. As sequencing of SAGE clones is initiated and progresses, the newly obtained sequence is processed with the software in order to confirm the tag content of the project clones, and to monitor the depth of the tag library. Even at this early stage, matching of the most abundant observed tags to an appropriate reference sequence database may suggest potentially informative functional relationships.

SAGE Data Analysis

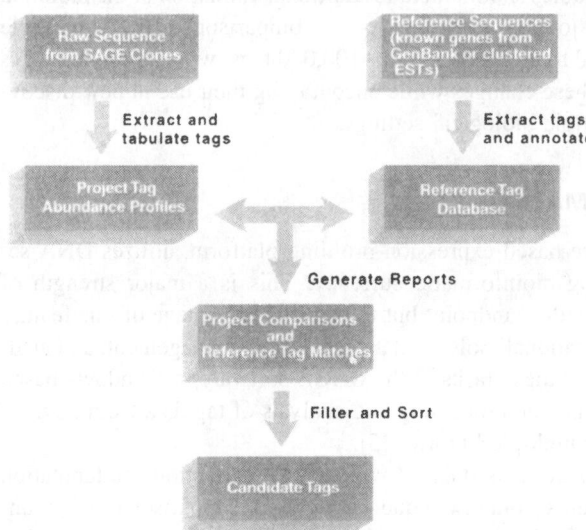

FIGURE 9   SAGE data analysis. Transcript abundance profiles are generated from sequencing of tags in SAGE clones. Observed tags are matched to reference sequences from various sources. Sorting and filtering of tags based on differential expression reveals candidates for further investigation.

When sequencing is complete, the final tag processing is done, and various reports can be generated. In a simple study, for example, there may be two samples, representing a test condition and a control. A report comparing the two projects tabulates all of the observed tags with their normalized abundances in each sample. The tags are then matched to a reference sequence database containing tag entries from known transcripts for the source species.

SAGE tags that are not readily ascribed to a known, characterized transcript may be further investigated in a number of gene expression databases accessible via the Internet. These databases have been generated by similarity clustering algorithms applied to large collections of transcript fragments called expressed sequence tags (ESTs). The resulting subsets of ESTs, or clusters, each represent a single transcript, or a family of related transcripts. The UniGene database at the National Center for Biotechnology Information [13–15] and the Sequence Tag Alignment and Consensus Knowledgebase at the South African National Bioinformatics Institute (SANBI) [16] offer Web-based querying of their respective cluster datasets. Querying with a SAGE tag sequence (4 nt NlaIII site + 10 nt tag) in these databases may return EST hits constituting one or more such clusters of homologous sequences. Alternatively, a SAGE tag query in the Human Gene Index at the Institute for Genome Research [17] or the SANBI Sanigene database [16] may hit to a consensus sequence representing an entire cluster. Since such searches do not take into account the number or location of NlaIII sites in the clusters, hits from these databases must be screened to ascertain which of the represented transcripts contains the query tag at its 3′-most anchoring enzyme site. Further examination of the resulting candidate sequences may provide clues to function for a potentially novel transcript, extended sequence information, as well as a physical source for the actual clone.

Lal et al. have recently described SAGEmap, a public repository of human SAGE data accessible via the Internet (http://www.ncbi.nlm.nih.gov/SAGE) [18]. As part of the Cancer Genome Anatomy Project at the National Cancer Institute, this online resource provides tools for viewing and analyzing tag data from a compilation of >40 SAGE libraries. These data have been posted by a number of laboratories investigating gene expression in human cancer. Web query forms allow one to search for expression levels of individual genes or tags, and to view comprehensive comparisons between multiple SAGE libraries.

A key feature of SAGEmap is its systematic approach to mapping of SAGE tags to UniGene EST clusters. Rather than simply matching SAGE tags across all NlaIII sites in the sequence clusters, SAGEmap incorporates EST frequency, location, and orientation information, plus a correction for sequencing error, to refine the mapping of tags to genes. This mapping represents a "best guess" for the matching of observed tags to expressed sequences in the public database.

We have expanded on the basic functions of the SAGE software with the goals of streamlining the production and analysis of SAGE data, enhancing the sharing of project data and annotation among researchers, and linking the tags to a variety of external data sources (unpublished results). To this end, we have compiled tag abundance data and annotations from all of our internal SAGE projects (comprising ~4 million tag counts) into a centralized relational database. With a common, shared storage location, researchers throughout the company have access to consistent, up-to-date SAGE data at all times.

The interface to the our SAGE database is a custom Windows application with a number of features supporting flexible, yet detailed analysis of SAGE data. Researchers can compare transcript profiles from different projects in multiple combinations. In a simple example, expression profiles from several samples of normal tissue can be merged into a "virtual profile" which may then be compared to that of one or more disease tissue samples. Such a comparison highlights the potentially disease-specific differences in gene expression, while deemphasizing sample-specific variations. The investigator may construct additional comparison scenarios at will, combining and comparing various experiments, with the option to save both analysis schemes and results for later review.

The database interface provides built-in sorting and filtering functions, permitting the user to apply relative abundance, ratio, or significance cut-offs to the data. In this manner, a full set of tens of thousands of observed tags may be winnowed down to a more manageable set of several hundred of the most interesting differentially expressed tags from a given group of experiments.

In addition to storing experimental tag data, the SAGE database also serves as the repository for reference sequence information extracted from external sources, such as GenBank and Unigene. The interface application supports searching and retrieval of this prefiltered information, and also provides an integrated web-browser for interactively linking tags or reference sequences to the original databases.

Researchers may also add their own custom tag-specific annotations to the database. Thus, investigators conducting independent analyses may conveniently share observations and insights regarding tags of mutual interest. The opportunity for such ''cross-fertilization'' maximizes the integration of SAGE data into our research knowledge base.

Finally, we are implementing a SAGE pipeline that automates the process of producing tag data. A series of utility programs run on a network server collects raw sequence files, parses them for tag abundance data, and updates the relevant tables in the SAGE database. Automation of these steps increases not only the efficiency of generating new SAGE data, but also the consistency and integrity of the database itself. Continued development of the SAGE database and interface application is focused on enhancing the links between tag data and diverse downstream data sources, such as high-throughput screening databases and signaling pathway schemes.

4   SAGE APPLICATIONS

4.1   Gene Discovery

One of the major benefits of open system gene expression profiling platforms like SAGE is the global assessment of the expression of both known and novel transcripts in cells or tissues of interest. This data set complements in several ways the genomic sequencing efforts being performed at multiple human genome sequencing centers in both the corporate and academic sectors. First, SAGE and other open system platforms can significantly contribute to the annotation of known and novel genes by providing quantitative spatial expression information for organ systems and the different cell types that comprise each organ. Obviously, the technological improvements described above for SAGE [6–11] will have a great impact on enabling the transcriptomes of individual cell types to be determined. Second, the expression of novel transcripts as revealed by SAGE can contribute dramatically to annotating novel genomic segments whose coding potential had not been suspected previously, or possibly only predicted based on gene finding algorithms.

The compilation of published SAGE-derived transcriptomes is shown in Table 1. The tissues and cell types that have been profiled are presented along with the number of tags sequenced and the number of unique tags represented. Fifty-four different SAGE libraries have been described in the literature (see references in Table 1), consisting of 39 human, 10 rodent, 4 yeast, and 3 rice transcriptomes. An additional 19 libraries are described by Lal et al. [18], but unfortunately were not included in the table because the information relating to SAGE tags sequenced and unique SAGE tags per library was not provided. The sequencing efforts have focused predominantly on the human libraries yielding greater than 2.5 million SAGE tags when the efforts of Lal et al. [18] are included with those described in Table 1.

While the cumulative sequencing depth of the human SAGE libraries listed in Table 1 is significant, this compilation does not address the number of transcripts encoded by the human genome. To begin to answer this question, four laboratories combined their data sets derived from sequencing >3.5 million SAGE tags from 84 independent human SAGE libraries [19]. To account for sequencing errors that occurred, it was required that each unique tag sequence occur two or more times in the pooled data set. In addition, for some transcripts with high cumulative expression, multiple redundant sequencing errors may have occurred in a given tag sequence. In these instances, if the observed expression level of a tag did not exceed its expected incidence due to redundant errors by a factor of 5, it was assumed to be the result of a repeated sequencing error. Applying these accounting factors resulted in the identification of 134,135 unique transcript tags. Fifty-four percent of these transcripts matched known genes or ESTs while the remainder corresponded to previously uncharacterized expressed sequences. Almost 1000 genes were expressed in all cell types and tissues analyzed while very few genes were expressed exclusively in any one cell or tissue type. An important comparative result from this large collection of transcriptomes from tumors and their normal counterparts was the identification of 40 genes that were consistently overexpressed in cancer. Studies such as these provide important insights into the expression potential of the entire genome, the extent of the genome expressed in any one cell or tissue type, and finally a demonstration of the programmatic expression changes that accompany the cancer phenotype in a wide variety of tumor types.

4.2 Pathway Elucidation

The applications for high-throughput transcript profiling technologies are seemingly ever expanding. Underlying these applications is the unprecedented opportunity to view phenotypic responses within the context of global transcriptional

TABLE 1　SAGE-Derived Transcriptomes

Organism	Tissue/cell type	Number of libraries	SAGE tags sequenced	Unique SAGE tags	References
Human	GV-stage oocyte	1	50,684	27,073	10
Human	Liver	1	30,982	8,596	33
Human	Liver myofibroblast	1	10,562	5076	34
Human	Skeletal muscle	1	53,875	12,000	35
Human	Normal breast epithelium	2	108,288	27,790	30
Human	Breast tumor cell line 21PT	1	59,537	16,187	
Human	Breast tumor cell line 21MT	1	60,827	14,368	
Human	Normal colon epithelium	2	62,148	14,721	28
Human	Colon tumors	2	60,878	19,690	
Human	Tumor-derived colon cell lines	2	60,378	17,092	
Human	Pancreatic tumors	2	61,592	20,471	
Human	Tumor-derived pancreatic cell lines	2	58,695	14,247	
Human	Colon cancer cell line DLD-1 + Ad-lacZ	1	51,853	7,202	21
Human	Colon cancer cell line DLD-1 + Ad-p53	1	53,022	—	
Human	Colon cancer cell line HCT116	1	5,266		22
Human	γ-irrad. colon cancer cell line HCT116	1	55,429	20,291	
Human	Colon cancer cell line HT29-βGal	1	55,846	14,346	24
Human	Colon cancer cell line HT29-APC	1	51,622		
Human	Bronchial tracheal epithelium	2	118,158	24,924	29
Human	Squamous cell lung cancer	2	108,718	27,676	
Human	Saccular dilatation, intracranial artery	1	11,495	4,924	11
Human	Superficial temporal artery	1	7,297	3,552	
Human	T-cell line MOLT-4	1	71,147	24,472	36
Human	HIV-infected MOLT-4	1	71,462	24,872	

Organism	Description				Ref.
Human	Quiescent arterial endothelial cells	1	6573	5,448	25
Human	Activated arterial endothelial cells	1	6148	collectively	
Human	Monocytes	1	57,560	35,037 collectively	27
	GM-CSF macrophages	1	57,463		
	M-CSF macrophages	1	55,856		
Human	Monocyte-derived dendritic cells	1	58,540	17,000	26
Mouse	Whole kidney (500 mg of tissue)	1	12,154	4,800	9
	Whole kidney (250 mg of tissue)	1	1,200	764	
	Whole kidney (0.5 mg of tissue)	1	1,200	820	
	Nephron segment: ascending limb Henle's loop	1	7,500	—	
	Nephron segment: outer medullary collecting duct	1	7,500	—	
Mouse	Microglial cell line	1	10,000	6,013	37
Rat	Dentate gyrus of hippocampal brain slice	1	2,200	1,242	8
Rat	Embryo fibroblasts with ts-p53^{Val135} (permissive temperature)	1	30,386	9,950	20
	Embryo fibroblasts with ts-p53^{Val135} (nonpermissive temperature)	1	30,313	9,240	
	Embryo fibroblasts with p53^{Phe132} (permissive temperature)	1	10,519	5,119	
Yeast	Log phase (glucose as carbon source)	1	20,184	4,665	38
	S-phase arrested	1	20,034	collectively	
	G2/M-phase arrested	1	20,415		
Yeast	Sole carbon source: oleate	1	10,366	1,700	39
Rice	Seedlings from aerobic conditions	1	10,122	5,921	40
	Seedlings from aerobic conditions	1	2,094	1,496	
	Seedlings from anaerobic conditions	1	2,205	1,551	

changes ongoing in cell populations. Within the foundation of these comprehensive views of transcriptional responses will be distinct pathways and cascades previously unrecognized. It is the identification of these distinct pathways, ultimately forming a network correlating phenotypic response with transcriptional changes, that will allow for the functional assignment to specific gene products involved in these pathways.

SAGE is heralded as an unbiased and comprehensive high-throughput transcript profiling technology and is therefore ideally suited for novel pathway elucidation. As is the case with any attempt at pathway elucidation utilizing transcript profiling, biological samples with isogenic backgrounds generally exhibit few transcriptional changes and therefore the data output is more readily interpreted. SAGE has been applied in this way towards elucidating the transcriptional manifestations within cells harboring functional or nonfunctional p53. p53 pathway elucidation utilizing SAGE was applied both in a well-characterized rat model system where the endpoint phenotype compares growth versus growth arrest [20] and to a human system, where cells expressing functional p53 progress to an apoptotic endpoint [21]. The growth arrest rat p53 model system demonstrated the utility of SAGE for identifying a large number of previously identified p53-regulated genes, including induced genes such as MDM2, WAF1, Cyclin G, BAX, CGR11, CGR19, EGR1, Shabin 80, and Shabin 123. SAGE was also able to identify an additional 40 differentially expressed genes, comprised of both known and novel genes, that had not been previously known to be regulated by p53.

The human p53 SAGE study was more rewarding in the sense that a large fraction of the p53-induced genes revealed by SAGE could be clustered into a family of genes whose function could explain the apoptotic phenotype at the molecular level. Eight of the top 14 genes induced by p53 were previously implicated in either generating or responding to oxidative stress (Table 2), a pathway documented to play a role in apoptosis [21 and references therein]. As with the rat p53 SAGE study, the human apoptotic system also revealed novel genes highly differentially expressed with respect to p53 status. Having this SAGE-derived immortal p53 database as an archive proved to be extremely useful in subsequent SAGE experiments on γ-irradiated colorectal cancer cells [22]. SAGE studies on these colorectal cancer cells revealed overlaps with the pre-existing p53 differential SAGE data [21]. By pooling SAGE data sets and determining commonalties from different experiments, the *14-3-3* σ gene was shown to be important in responding to γ irradiation in a p53-dependent manner.

The utility of applying global transcript profiling for pathway elucidation was further demonstrated by SAGE transcript profiling of cells expressing or not expressing the tumor suppressor gene *APC* (adenomatous polyposis coli), which functions to monitor cell growth in the intestinal mucosa [23]. It was demon-

TABLE 2 Genes Induced by p53 in a Human Epithelial
Cell Apoptosis Model

ROS Effect*	Induced gene	Known gene, function, or homology
Induced by ROS	P21	CDK inhibitor
	PIG4†	Serum amyloid A
	PIG7	TNFα-induced mRNA
	PIG8	Etoposide-induced mRNA
	PIG12	GST homolog
Generator or enhancer of ROS	PIG3	Quinone oxidoreductase homolog
	PIG1	Galectin 7
Redox effector	PIG6	Proline oxidase homolog

* The relationship between the genes induced by p53 and the generation of or response to reactive oxygen species (ROS).
† p53 induced genes (PIG).

strated prior to this study that APC affects cell growth, in part, by altering the activity of the β-catenin/Tcf-4 transcription factor complex. SAGE transcript profiles were able to define a subsequent step in the APC cascade by delineating a transcriptional effect on the *c-Myc* oncogene, which, as it turns out, is directly regulated by β-catenin/Tcf-4. Thus, this novel pathway elucidation allowed for the intriguing functional convergence of the tumor suppressor *APC* and the oncogene *c-Myc* [24].

Another isogenic application of SAGE was described by de Waard et al., using resting and activated human vascular endothelial cells (HUVECs) to discern changes in steady-state mRNA levels that accompany atherogenesis [25]. SAGE libraries were made from resting (untreated) HUVECs and HUVECs activated for 6 hours. To focus on gross changes, sequencing of the respective libraries was relatively shallow, ~6000 tags/library, but did reveal the expression of almost 5500 genes collectively between the two libraries. A comparison of the resulting transcriptomes from resting and activated endothelial cells revealed that ~1% of the genes were differentially expressed by fivefold or more. SAGE predicted elevated gene expression of recognizable activation markers such as IL8, MCP1, VCAM1, PAI1, Gro-α, and E-selectin. SAGE also identified transcripts induced in activated HUVECs encoding proteins not known to be associated with activated endothelial cells. Included in this set is activin $β_A$, a member of the TGFβ superfamily. Subsequent verification studies were performed by Northern blot analyses using RNAs derived from HUVECs activated for 1.5–16 hours.

The RNA blots confirmed the SAGE predictions of the activation markers and activin β_A, while highlighting the induction kinetics of these atherogenic transcripts.

Hashimoto et al. utilized SAGE to identify the transcriptomes of human monocytes and monocytes that were differentiated in vitro to macrophages or dendritic cells [26,27]. The studies were initiated using purified preparations of monocytes (>99%) that were either untreated or treated with either M-CSF or GM-CSF for 7 days in culture to represent two different populations of macrophages. Alternatively, purified monocyte preparations were incubated with GM-CSF, IL-4, and TNF-α for 5 days to promote differentiation into dendritic cells. RNA was isolated from the monocyte population along with the differentiated progeny and used to make SAGE libraries. More than 55,000 tags were sequenced for each SAGE library. The combined transcriptomes for monocytes, GM-CSF differentiated macrophages and M-CSF differentiated macrophages represented an expression repertoire of 35,012 genes. Combining the transcriptomes of monocytes, GM-CSF differentiated macrophages and monocyte-derived dendritic cells gave a very similar transcript complexity of 36,605 expressed genes.

The transcriptomes of the monocytes and the differentiated macrophages populations were compared. Both of the macrophage transcriptomes showed >300 transcripts with significant expression differences ($P < .01$) when compared to the monocyte transcriptome. The GM-CSF macrophage transcriptome contained 201 repressed transcripts and 153 induced transcripts when compared to the monocyte transcriptome. The M-CSF macrophage transcriptome contained 157 repressed genes and 157 induced genes when compared to the monocyte transcriptome. In contrast to the macrophage-monocyte comparisons, a comparison between the two macrophage transcriptomes showed only 117 genes that were differentially expressed with high significance ($P < .01$); 57 genes were overexpressed in GM-CSF macrophages, while the remaining 60 genes were overexpressed in the M-CSF macrophages. Not surprisingly, these results show that the macrophage transcriptomes are more similar to each other than to that of the monocytes.

Many of the GM-CSF macrophage genes whose expression was induced or repressed when compared to the monocyte transcriptome showed a similar response in the transcriptome of M-CSF macrophages. Examples of this include a tag frequency for hc-gp39 of 0, 288, and 182 tags in the monocyte, GM-CSF, and M-CSF macrophages transcriptomes, respectively, with similar associations for apolipoprotein C1 of 6, 1515, and 1261 and apolipoprotein E of 6, 1044, and 657. Genes whose expression were repressed in both macrophage transcriptomes include a tag frequency for MRP-8 of 287, 0, and 13; for IL-8 of 97, 0, and 5; and for ficolin-1 of 244, 3, and 13 for monocyte, GM-CSF macrophages, and M-CSF macrophage transcriptomes, respectively.

Known genes that were differentially expressed between the two macrophage transcriptomes include overexpression in GM-CSF macrophages of RING6, GA733-1, MDC, prostaglandin D synthetase, and TGF-β while the M-CSF macrophage transcriptome showed overexpression of legumain, CD48, lysosomal sialoglycoprotein, and MRP-8. However, the identity of most of the genes that were differentially expressed between the two types of macrophages remains unknown. The identification of known and novel genes that are differentially expressed in the two macrophage populations should provide insight into the expression changes that accompany macrophage development while defining the functional capabilities of different macrophage lineages.

SAGE analysis of the immature DCs was performed to a level of 58,540 tags which represented the expression of 17,000 different genes [26]. Not surprisingly, MHC class I/II transcripts were highly expressed as were transcripts encoding gene products with cellular roles in the cytoskeleton. A transcriptome comparison between the parental resting monocytes and the immature dendritic cell progeny showed that the expression of most genes did not change significantly. However, 313 genes were differentially expressed between the two cell populations based on statistical criteria ($P < .01$); 180 transcripts were induced in dendritic cell while 132 transcripts were repressed. Genes whose expression was induced or repressed in DCs when compared to monocytes showed a similar pattern of differential expression in GM-CSF macrophages. Overexpressed transcripts in DCs included those that encoded proteins involved with cell structure, lipid metabolism, and chemokines while repressed transcripts could be categorized as those that encoded proteins in the complement pathway, transcription factors, and cell surface markers. Differentially expressed genes that were unique to DCs compared to other monocyte-derived cell types included induced genes TARC, HAI-2, Factor XIII, CD23, MCP-4, and metalloproteinase, and repressed genes MRP-14, MIP-1α, CD14, α1 antitrypsin, HLA-B, and transketolase. Collectively, these data indicate that the differentiation of monocytes into immature DCs is accompanied by a gene expression program that enables greater cellular plasticity and mobility along with the production of chemokines that specifically attract Th2 cells.

4.3 Expression Analysis of Complex Systems

The relatively simple transcript profiles resulting from plus/minus treatment regimens, as just described, have great value in sorting out biological function. However, it is a more daunting challenge for transcript profiling to reveal previously unrecognized or novel pathways important in complex diseases such as cancer. To begin to unravel complex disease pathways, SAGE was used to elucidate normal versus disease transcriptomes for gastrointestinal cancers [28], non-small-cell lung cancer (NSCLC) [29], and breast cancer [30]. Relative to the isogenic SAGE comparisons described above, the disease transcriptomes identified many more differentially regulated genes (Fig. 10). With these complex disease transcriptomes, revelations concerning functional pathways involved in disease progression are not immediately apparent, although several individual genes previously implicated in cancer progression were observed.

The dilemma that has evolved from many large complex disease transcriptome analyses is that further verification efforts are necessary to limit the pool of potential interesting candidate genes. The verification process becomes extremely important when using SAGE or other open-system gene expression platforms to identify potential targets or markers for the development of novel therapeutics and diagnostics, respectively. The wealth of potential disease-specific genes that have been revealed by SAGE in the cancer arena necessitates a verification platform to aid in limiting the time-consuming functional work downstream from data generation. cDNA microarrays are currently being formulated by utilizing SAGE data to design the target array which will ultimately be interrogated by additional samples. This approach is more advantageous than using prefabricated cDNA or oligomer arrays where one is restricted to interrogating only previously defined cDNAs while omitting novel genes that could be relevant to the specific disease being investigated. SAGE tags that do not correspond to known genes or ESTs, and which therefore could represent novel genes, can be used effectively to amplify additional sequences from cognate cDNAs. This facilitates the integration of potentially novel cDNAs into the design of SAGE-defined microarrays.

Using this strategy of SAGE for primary discovery and custom microarrays for verification, we were able to identify several genes that were differentially expressed in primary and metastatic breast cancer [30]. Some of the SAGE-predicted known genes that were overexpressed in tumor samples as determined by hybridization to microarrays included MUC-1, HER2/neu, Zinc α2-glycoprotein, and Claudin-7; their repressed counterparts included Plakophilin-1, Integrin α6, PRSS1, ATM, and CCND2. Several differentially expressed ESTs from the SAGE analysis were also confirmed to be differentially expressed by microarray analysis.

4.4 Diagnostic Applications

The functional elucidation of critical pathways involved in disease progression often requires large resource commitments of time and money. Relatively rapid utilization of the SAGE-archived database without necessarily integrating functional characterization has been demonstrated for the prognostic and diagnostic evaluation of cancer. In the case of squamous NSCLC, several genes observed with SAGE to be differentially induced in squamous cell carcinoma with respect

10 Fold or Greater Induction in COLON Cancer

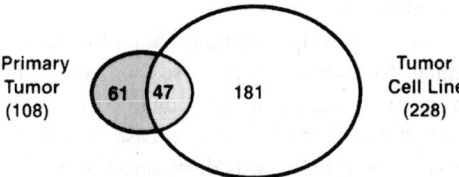

10 Fold or Greater Induction in BREAST Cancer
2 normal vs. 2 tumors

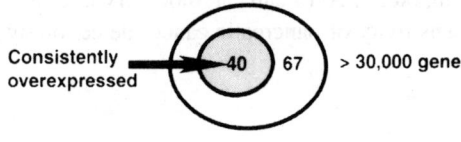

10 Fold or Greater Induction in LUNG Cancer
2 normal vs. 2 squamous carcinomas

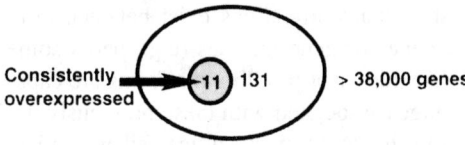

FIGURE 10 Genes induced in cancer. (Upper) A comparison of genes induced at least 10-fold in colon cancer as measured using primary tumors and tumor-derived cell lines against normal colon epithelium. (Middle) Genes induced at least 10-fold in breast cancer as measured using cell lines derived from both primary and metastatic tumors and compared to normal mammary epithelium. Forty genes are induced in both of the tumor lines and 27 genes are induced in only one of the two tumor cell lines. Over 30,000 unique genes contributed to this analysis. (Lower) Genes induced at least 10-fold in breast cancer as measured using cell lines derived from non-small-cell lung cancer tumors and compared to normal lung epithelium. Over 38,000 genes are included in this analysis.

to normal cells were evaluated for their expression in additional cell lines and clinical tumor samples [31]. This verification effort yielded a subset of genes that showed consistent overexpression in squamous lung cancer cells. PGP9.5, a ubiquitin carboxy-terminal hydrolase, was particularly valuable in this effort in that expression of this gene product not only correlates with the presence of lung cancer, but has prognostic value in showing ever-increasing expression as the disease progresses to more advanced stages.

Through the use of SAGE and other transcript profiling technologies, expanded pools of genes or gene products for diagnostic purposes will likely be identified. SAGE has already shown utility in adding an additional marker onto a previous diagnostic screen for pancreatic cancer [32]. In this case, the tissue inhibitor of metalloproteinase (TIMP-1) gene product was discovered by SAGE to be specifically overexpressed in pancreatic tumor samples and not in normal or cancerous colon samples. This TIMP-1 marker by itself was inadequate for diagnosis of pancreatic cancer. However, TIMP-1 in conjunction with the previously characterized pancreatic cancer markers CA-19 and carcinoembryonic antigen (CEA) was able to increase the sensitivity of pancreatic cancer detection by >10%.

4.5 Toxicological Profiling

One of the most significant perceived added values transcription profiling brings to drug development efforts is the enormous potential to reduce costly and time-consuming drug development work by assessing drug toxicity early on in the evaluation process. It is well established that correlations exist between drug toxicity and the expression of certain genes or gene families (e.g., peroxisome proliferation). Certainly SAGE and other transcript profiling platforms are capable of deciphering gene expression changes associated with these previously defined toxicity-related genes. Importantly, however, many drugs fail in clinical trials both due to the inability to evaluate toxicity early on in drug development and simply because the drug may be acting to alter gene expression directly or indirectly within biological pathways.

The affected biological pathways may be unknown or known but not anticipated for certain clinical indications. Thus, even though a drug may not be toxic per se, its effects on certain biological pathways could prevent or limit its therapeutic use. Awareness of these pathway effects early in the drug development process can provide a more rigorous basis for advancing candidates that do not elicit these effects or for optimizing the chemistry of lead compounds to eliminate or minimize these effects. In either case, gene expression profiling can monitor a drug candidate's direct and indirect effects on biochemical pathways. Fulfilling the enormous potential for the molecular classification of drug effects relies on analytical approaches that are accurate and comprehensive. This is particularly difficult with certain transcript-profiling technologies but noticeably when their are extended to evaluating model organism transcriptomes. Since elucidation of drug toxicity and biological pathway is usually assessed initially in animals such as mouse and rat, the ability to profile gene expression changes in these model systems is vital for the application of transcript profiling to drug toxicology assessment. The limited genomic information currently available for mouse and rat model organisms as compared to human restricts the utility of technologies that rely exclusively on prior transcript identification. Since SAGE does not require this prior knowledge, it has the power to extract much more information from these model organisms for toxicological studies.

4.6 Identification of Targets for Therapeutic Development

Disease management facilitated by comprehensive and sensitive diagnostic tools and early drug evaluation utilizing toxicological transcript profiling are certainly ventures that ultimately reduce cost and potentially increase efficacy of lead drug candidates. A seemingly greater challenge is to use SAGE transcript profiles to discover or facilitate the discovery of novel therapeutics. This challenge is necessarily greater due to the wealth of information obtained and the functional characterization required in evaluating a good therapeutic lead. Thus, the real challenge is to design clever data analysis strategies whereby the results reveal valid therapeutic candidates based on functional characterization.

In this regard, SAGE has been employed to profile cells and tissues that either exhibit or lack a specific phenotype of therapeutic interest. By initially stratifying samples based on phenotype, expression profiles can be performed on the most appropriate samples (extreme phenotypes, intermediate phenotypes, and different genetic backgrounds). This approach is most powerful with a quantitative phenotypic assay and access to sufficient numbers of different cell and tissue samples to adequately cover the phenotypic spectrum. An expression comparison between transcriptomes derived from cells/tissues of known phenotypes rapidly reveals the strongest candidates from a large pool of differentially expressed genes, while enhancing the likelihood of being able to correlate phenotype to genotype at the cDNA level. This strategy is currently being employed at Genzyme and Genzyme Molecular Oncology to identify a number of expressed genes that can be tested for their ability to confer a phenotype of therapeutic value (unpublished data).

Providing efficacious therapies requires the ability to administer a therapeutic to the appropriate location in the body. This attribute is particularly important in the case of gene therapy to maximize efficacy and safety by limiting expression to defined cell or tissue types. The ability of SAGE to define specific transcriptomes will aid in the development of gene therapies whereby cell- or tissue-specific promoters and genes can be utilized to appropriately express and deliver a given therapy.

The identification of more therapeutic targets of higher quality is a necessary step in improving the drug development process. SAGE provides a robust platform for discerning relevant drug targets in a comprehensive fashion, based on differential gene expression in diseased cells or tissues. SAGE alone or in combination with either closed-system gene expression platforms or, alternatively, with proteomic approaches such as protein expression profiling and protein network screens, should accelerate the identification of high-quality drug targets and catalyze the development of high-throughput screens to reveal the next generation of therapeutic products.

5 CONCLUSION

The use of the SAGE technology over the past 5 years has increased progressively. The method has evolved from requiring large amounts of mRNA, 2-5 µg, to robust processes using 10–100 ng of total RNA with preliminary reports of compelling studies resulting from as little as 900 pg of mRNA. The methodological developments open the possibility of analyzing transcriptomes in a variety of biological samples that have not been studied due to limitations in sample size. Furthermore, the pooling and sharing of transcriptomes between multiple laboratories exemplifies the uniformity and portability of the data sets while accelerating our understanding of the molecular differences in biological systems that vary spatially, temporally, or physiologically. Finally, the application of SAGE to the study of human disease has begun to identify markers and targets that may lead to the next generation of diagnostic and therapeutic products.

ACKNOWLEDGMENTS

We recognize and thank our colleagues in the Gene Expression and Analysis group and the Bioinformatics group at Genzyme Molecular Oncology for their expertise, contributions, and dedication. A special thanks to Mardi Landes for the graphics used in this publication.

REFERENCES

1. Y Prashar, SM Weissman. READS: a method for display of 3′-end fragments of restriction enzyme-digested cDNAs for analysis of differential gene expression. Methods Enzymol 303:258–272, 1999.
2. CW Bachem, RS van der Hoeven, SM de Bruijn, D Vreugdenhil, M Zabeau, RG Visser. Visualization of differential gene expression using a novel method of RNA fingerprinting based on AFLP: analysis of gene expresion during potato tuber development. Plant J 9:745–753, 1996.
3. JG Sutcliffe, PE Foye, MG Erlander, BS Hilbush, LJ Bodzin, JT Durham, KW Hasel. TOGA: an automated parsing technology for analyzing expression of nearly all genes. Proc Nat Acad Sci USA 97:1976–1981, 2000.
4. RA Shimkets, DG Lowe, JT Tai, P Sehl, H Jin, R Yang, PF Predki, BE Rothberg, MT Murtha, ME Roth, SG Shenoy, A Windemuth, JW Simpson, JF Simons, MP Daley, SA Gold, MP McKenna, K Hillan, GT Went, JM Rothberg. Gene expression

analysis by transcript profiling coupled to a gene database query. Nat Biotechnol 17:798–803, 1999.

5. VE Velculescu, L Zhang, B Vogelstein, KW Kinzler. Serial analysis of gene expression. Science 270:484–487, 1995.

6. J Powell. Enhanced concatemer cloning-a modification to the SAGE (serial analysis of gene expression) technique. Nucleic Acids Res 26:3445–3446, 1998.

7. M Kenzelmann, K Muhlemann. Substantially enhanced cloning efficiency of SAGE (serial analysis of gene expression) by adding a heating step to the original protocol. Nucleic Acids Res 27:917–918, 1999.

8. NA Datson, J van der Perk–de Jong, MP van den Berg, ER de Kloet, E Vreugdenhil. MicroSAGE: a modified procedure for serial analysis of gene expression in limited amounts of tissue. Nucleic Acids Res 27:1300–1307, 1999.

9. B Virlon, L Cheval, JM Buhler, E Billon, A Doucet, JM Elalouf. Serial microanalysis of enal transcriptomes. Proc Nat Acad Sci USA 96:15286–15291, 1999.

10. L Neilson, A Andalibi, D Kang, C Coutifaris, JF Strauss III, JL Stanton, DPL Green. Molecular phenotype of the human oocyte by PCR-SAGE. Genomics 63:13–24, 2000.

11. DG Peters, AB Kassam, H Yonas, EH O'Hare, RE Ferrell, AM Brufsky. Comprehensive transcript analysis in small quantities of mRNA by SAGE-lite. Nucleic Acids Res 27:e39, 1999.

12. JL Rothstein, D Johnson, JA DeLoia, J Skowronski, D Solter. Gene expression during preimplantation mouse development. Genes Dev 6:1190–1201, 1992.

13. GD Schuler. Pieces of the puzzle: expressed sequence tags and the catalog of human genes. J Mol Med 75:694–698, 1997.

14. GD Schuler, MS Boguski, EA Stewart, LD Stein, G Gyapay, K Rice, RE White, P Rodriguez-Tome, A Aggarwal, E Bajorek, S Bentolila, BB Birren, A Butler, AB Castle, N Chiannilkulchai, A Chu, C Clee, S Cowles, PJ Day, T Dibling, N Drouot, I Dunham, S Duprat, C East, TJ Hudson. A gene map of the human genome. Science 274:540–546, 1996.

15. MS Boguski, GD Schuler. ESTablishing a human transcript map [news]. Nat Genet 10:369–371, 1995.

16. RT Miller, AG Christoffels, C Gopalakrishnan, J Burke, AA Ptitsyn, TR Broveak, WA Hide. A comprehensive approach to clustering of expressed human gene sequence: the sequence tag alignment and consensus knowledge base. 1999.

17. J Quackenbush, F Liang, I Holt, G Pertea, J Upton. The TIGR gene indices: reconstruction and representation of expressed gene sequences. Nucleic Acids Res 28: 141–145, 2000.

18. A Lal, AE Lash, SF Altschul, V Velculescu, L Zhang, RE McLendon, MA Marra, C Prange, PJ Morin, K Polyak, N Papadopoulos, B Vogelstein, KW Kinzler, RL Strausberg, GJ Riggins. A public database for gene expression in human cancers. Cancer Res 59:5403–5407, 1999.

19. VE Velculescu, SL Madden, L Zhang, AE Lash, J Yu, C Rago, A Lal, CJ Wang, GA Beaudry, KM Ciriello, BP Cook, MR Dufault, AT Ferguson, YH Gao, TC He, H Hermeking, SK Hiraldo, PM Hwang, MA Lopez, HF Luderer, B Mathews, JM Petroziello, K Polyak, L Zawel, W Zhang. Analysis of human transcriptomes. Nat Genet 23:387–388, 1999.

20. SL Madden, EA Galella, J Zhu, AH Bertelsen, GA Beaudry. SAGE transcript profiles for p53-dependent growth regulation. Oncogene 15:1079–1085, 1997.

21. K Polyak, Y Xia, JL Zweier, KW Kinzler, B Vogelstein. A model for p53-induced apoptosis [see comments]. Nature 389:300–305, 1997.

22. H Hermeking, C Lengauer, K Polyak, TC He, L Zhang, S Thiagalingam, KW Kinzler, B Vogelstein. 14-3-3 sigma is a p53-regulated inhibitor of G2/M progression. Mol Cell 1:3–11, 1997.

23. AB Sparks, PJ Morin, B Vogelstein, KW Kinzler. Mutational analysis of the APC/beta-catenin/Tcf pathway in colorectal cancer. Cancer Res 58:1130–1134, 1998.

24. TC He, AB Sparks, C Rago, H Hermeking, L Zawel, LT da Costa, PJ Morin, B Vogelstein, KW Kinzler. Identification of c-MYC as a target of the APC pathway. Science 281:1509–1512, 1998.

25. V de Waard, BM van den Berg, J Veken, R Schultz-Heienbrok, H Pannekoek, AJ van Zonneveld. Serial analysis of gene expression to assess the endothelial cell response to an atherogenic stimulus. Gene 226:1–8, 1999.

26. S Hashimoto, T Suzuki, HY Dong, S Nagai, N Yamazaki, K Matsushima. Serial analysis of gene expression in human monocyte-derived dendritic cells. Blood 94:845–852, 1999.

27. S Hashimoto, T Suzuki, HY Dong, N Yamazaki, K Matsushima. Serial analysis of gene expression in human monocytes and macrophages. Blood 94:837–844, 1999.

28. L Zhang, W Zhou, VE Velculescu, SE Kern, RH Hruban, SR Hamilton, B Vogelstein, KW Kinzler. Gene expression profiles in normal and cancer cells. Science 276:1268–1272, 1997.

29. K Hibi, Q Liu, GA Beaudry, SL Madden, WH Westra, SL Wehage, SC Yang, RF Heitmiller, AH Bertelsen, D Sidransky, J Jen. Serial analysis of gene expression in non-small cell lung cancer. Cancer Res 58:5690–5694, 1998.

30. M Nacht, AT Ferguson, W Zhang, JM Petroziello, BP Cook, YH Gao, S Maguire, D Riley, G Coppola, GM Landes, SL Madden, S Sukumar. Combining serial analysis of gene expression and array technologies to identify genes differentially expressed in breast cancer. Cancer Res 59:5464–5470, 1999.

31. K Hibi, WH Westra, M Borges, S Goodman, D Sidransky, J Jen. PGP9.5 as a candidate tumor marker for non-small-cell lung cancer. Am J Pathol 155:711–715, 1999.

32. W Zhou, LJ Sokoll, DJ Bruzek, L Zhang, VE Velculescu, SB Goldin, RH Hruban, SE Kern, SR Hamilton, DW Chan, B Vogelstein, KW Kinzler. Identifying markers for pancreatic cancer by gene expression analysis. Cancer Epidemiol Biomarkers Prev 7:109–112, 1998.

33. T Yamashita, S Hashimoto, S Kaneko, S Nagai, N Toyoda, T Suzuki, K Kobayashi, K Matsushima. Comprehensive gene expression profile of a normal human liver. Biochem Biophys Res Commun 269:110–116, 2000.

34. W Boers, C Linthorst, PH Reitsma. Identification of expressed genes from transformed human stellate cells associated with liver fibrosis. Cells Hepatic Sinusoid 7: 171–172, 1999.

35. S Welle, K Bhatt, CA Thornton. Inventory of high-abundance mRNAs in skeletal muscle of normal men. Genome Res 9:506–513, 1999.

36. A Ryo, Y Suzuki, K Ichiyama, T Wakatsuki, N Kondoh, A Hada, M Yamamoto,

N Yamamoto. Serial analysis of gene expression in HIV-1-infected T cell lines. FEBS Lett 462:182–186, 1999.

37. H Inoue, M Sawada, A Ryo, H Tanahashi, T Wakatsuki, A Hada, N Kondoh, K Nakagaki, K Takahashi, A Suzumura, M Yamamoto, T Tabira. Serial analysis of gene expression in a microglial cell line. Glia 28:265–271, 1999.

38. VE Velculescu, L Zhang, W Zhou, J Vogelstein, MA Basrai, DE Bassett, Jr., P Hieter, B Vogelstein, KW Kinzler. Characterization of the yeast transcriptome. Cell 88:243–251, 1997.

39. AJ Kal, AJ van Zonneveld, V Benes, M van den Berg, MG Koerkamp, K Albermann, N Strack, JM Ruijter, A Richter, B Dujon, W Ansorge, HF Tabak. Dynamics of gene expression revealed by comparison of serial analysis of gene expression transcript profiles from yeast grown on two different carbon sources. Mol Bio Cell 10: 1859–1872, 1999.

40. H Matsumura, S Nirasawa, R Terauchi. Transcript profiling in rice (*Oryza sativa* L.) seedlings using serial analysis of gene expression (SAGE). Plant J 20:719–726, 1999.

A. Yamamoto serial analysis of gene expression in HIV infected T cell lines. FEBS Lett 361:153-156. 1999.

32. H. Hou, Ja. Sawada, Ka. Kato, H. Tanahashi, T. Wada, Ishi, A. Hada, M. Kodash, K. Nagashid, X. Fukushima, A. Sugimura, M. Yamamoto, et al. Serial analysis of gene expression data in multiplet cell lines. Genes 2:165-271 1999.

33. V. Vossbeck, T. Zhang, W. Zhou, J. Yee, Isein, M.A. Basrai, Ph. Bassin, 1997. Hinton, V. Velculescu, K.W. Kinzler, Quantitation of the yeast transcriptome. Cell 88:243-251. 1997.

34. A.F.M. Al Saadi, Isai, Veld, V. Beaux, V. Velculescu, M.D. Keraghan, K. Adelmann, S. et al. Th. Birgan, A. Richter, B. Fuson, W. A. Singe, Ph. Tanka. Dynamics of gene expression revealed by comparison of serial analysis of gene expression from cerebral cells from yeast grown on two different carbon sources. Mol Biol Cell 10:1859-1872. 1999.

35. H. Matsumura, S. Nirasawa, K. Terauchi. Transcript profiling in rice (Oryza sativa L.) seedlings using serial analysis of gene expression (SAGE). Plant J 20:719-726. 1999.

14

Proteomics

Frank A. Witzmann

Indiana University–Purdue University, Columbus, Indiana

1 INTRODUCTION

The overall goals of pharmacogenomics are (1) to improve our understanding of the nature of complex diseases and drug effects, (2) to discern the impact of polymorphisms on therapeutic susceptibility and safety, and (3) to ultimately develop personalized therapeutics with high efficacy in the absence of toxicity. These goals underscore the need for tools capable of analyzing interindividual variations based on genotype, and equally important based on phenotype. The ultimate significance of linking genotypic data to their phenotypic counterparts has become increasingly evident as we reach the so-called "end of the genome era." As this chapter is written, >93% of the human genome has been sequenced or is in draft form [1]. Its completion by public sector efforts is expected by 2002 [2], and private efforts at Celera involve annotating their sequenced genome. A principal consequence of this genomic revolution is the ever-increasing availability of reliable open reading frames (ORF) that represent protein-coding exons. As a result, a new era called "functional genomics" has begun and is rapidly gaining prominence. Functional genomics comprises approaches to study globally the mRNA and protein products expressed by the genome and to correlate expression profiles with specific effects of disease and (altered) function.

Ironically, it is also the inadequacy of genomics that underlies the rapid growth of functional genomics. Genomic information alone is static and does not reveal the dynamic features of a cell such as metabolic, structural, and signaling activities. While the genome is identical in each individual cell of an organism, gene expression is specific for each cell type and is altered quantitatively and qualitatively in cellular dysfunction, injury or disease, following administration of pharmaceuticals or xenobiotics, or due to other epigenetic phenomena. Functional genomics at the level of mRNA gene transcripts (the "transcriptome") has been shown to correlate poorly with corresponding profiles at the protein level [3–7]. This strongly suggests that mRNA degradation, alternative splicing, co- and posttranslational modification, and posttranscriptional regulation of gene expression are essential cellular processes that make it difficult to extrapolate from mRNA to protein profiles and cellular function. Consequently, there is growing evidence that protein profiling of the expressed genes in tissues and individual cells is more likely to lead to a better understanding of cellular regulation and to give insights into disease and the molecular effects of xenobiotics and drugs.

There is no better example of this movement than that found in "*proteomics*," the study of the expressed genome, e.g. the "*proteome*." The proteomics approach has made the separation, quantification, and identification of proteins a practical matter. This is a direct result of recent technical developments in protein separation, detection, mass spectrometric analysis of protein digests, and protein sequence information now available in readily accessible public databases.

The term proteome was first introduced by Wilkins in 1995 [8]. Proteomics has since been defined more aptly by Anderson [9] as "the use of quantitative protein-level measurements of gene expression to characterize biological processes (e.g., disease processes and drug effects) and decipher the mechanisms of gene expression control." The principal core of protein separation still lies in the two-dimensional electrophoretic (2DE) separation of the complex mixture of thousands of proteins represented in a living cell.

In fact, rather than a new development, 2DE has been around for quite some time. Its history has been reviewed eloquently by the pioneers of large-scale, high-throughput protein analysis, Norman and Leigh Anderson [10]. The analysis of protein expression profiles using a 2DE approach combining separation by isoelectric focusing and denaturing sodium dodecyl sulfate electrophoresis, was first published in 1975 independently by Klose [11], O'Farrell [12], and Scheele [13]. The utility of 2DE in global protein analysis was postulated early the next decade [14,15] and technical improvements making it a large-scale, quantitative and qualitative analytical tool have continued to the present [16–20]. There is an ongoing effort to replace the 2DE step with a more straightforward technology, but no promising alternative that renders *quantitative* protein expression data is imminent.

This chapter will address the various components of the proteomics approach, the state of the art, and future trends with relevance to pharmacogenomics.

2 PROTEOMIC METHODS

At the core of proteomics is the separation and quantification of very complex protein mixtures, protein assortments characterized by enormous heterogeneity and conceivably composed of >10,000 different proteins. Whether these protein samples are obtained from organs, tissues, body fluids, isolated cells, or subcellular fractions, the quality of separation depends appreciably on sample preparation, e.g., protein solubilization. No single preparation technique suits all samples or all first-dimension separation systems, and thus numerous approaches to sample preparation abound.

Likewise, there exist a variety of separation methodologies that are often adapted to specific sample types, isoelectric point ranges, and protein solubilities. Unlike nucleotides, however, proteins cannot be amplified by PCR-like techniques. Therefore detection methods are critical to visualize, if not accurately quantify, low-abundance proteins whose functional alterations are as significant as their high-abundance counterparts. Scanners and software programs to analyze and quantify 2DE protein profiles and to assess posttranslational modifications are numerous and diverse, as well.

All of the above, in one way or another, are essential aspects of proteomics and each must be optimized to enable the identification of separated proteins by immunological, sequencing, or mass spectrometric techniques and by mining the various protein bioinformatics databases. Two recent books [21,22] address the methodologies of all elements of proteomics in great detail.

The development of robotics systems like those now marketed by companies such as Genomic Solutions, ABiMED, or BioRad have catalyzed an integrated development of complete proteomics platforms that would enable a generalized proteomics approach like that shown in Figure 1. Unfortunately, only a few laboratories can address the development of each and every component of a proteomics platform. Thus advances in one technique often are made somewhat independently of others and these must then be incorporated by research laboratories as budgets and individual investigator preferences dictate. Because proteomics is not yet a uniform approach and involves individual variations of all of the technical approaches mentioned above, this section will address the variety of technologies used in each component of a typical proteomics platform.

2.1 Two-Dimensional Gel Electrophoresis

2DE protein separation typically resolves (depending on the sample and staining technique) 1000–2000 proteins in a single tissue sample [23] and up to 10,000

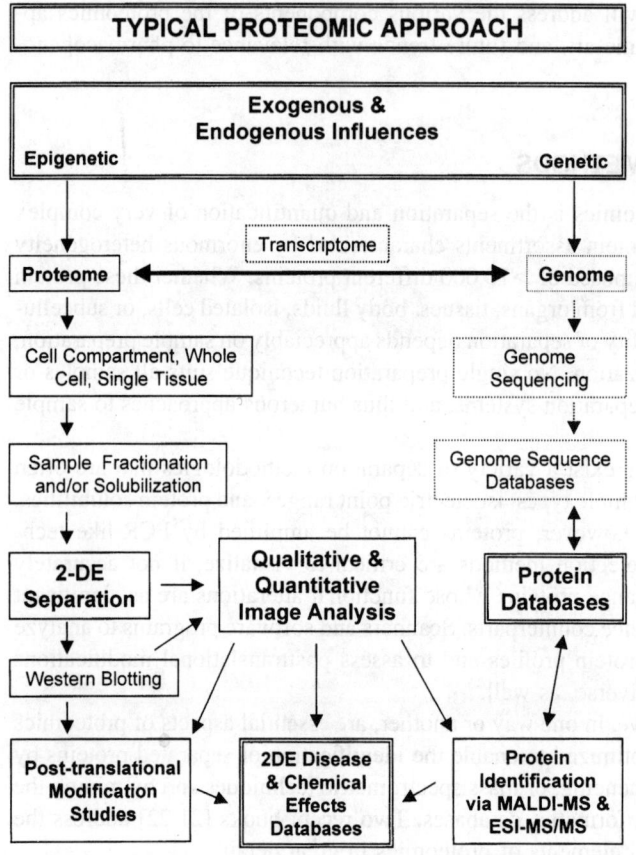

FIGURE 1   Typical elements of a proteomics approach that enables one to generate proteome profiles and identify proteins for inclusion in various databases.

on a large-format gel [24]. Proteins are separated based on their content of acidic and basic amino acids (isoelectric focusing; IEF) in the first dimension and then by molecular mass (sodium dodecyl sulfate–polyacrylamide gel electrophoresis; SDS-PAGE, or DALT) in the second dimension (Fig. 2). In combination, these two separation techniques produce a unique two-dimensional protein pattern representative of each separated sample. Each protein spot within a 2DE pattern is quantified by its optical density, and alterations in abundance, charge, and molecular mass can be detected relative to a standard pattern. Abundance changes suggest up- or downregulation of gene expression or altered protein turnover rates.

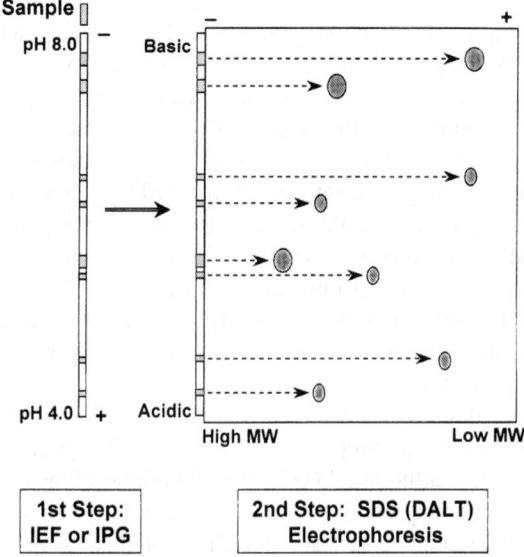

Two-dimensional Electrophoresis

FIGURE 2   Protein separation by two-dimensional electrophoresis (2DE). Protein samples (complex mixtures) are first separated based on individual protein charge by isoelectric focusing in gel tubes (IEF) or on immobilized pH-gradient (IPG) strips. The IEF/IPG separation is then placed on a polyacrylamide slab gel and proteins separated according to mass. The result is a unique 2D pattern of resolved protein spots whose coordinate positions are predicted by their physicochemical characteristics.

Charge and molecular mass modifications suggest either posttranslational protein modification such as phosphorylation, glycosylation, conjugation, adduct formation, genetic polymorphisms, or amino acid substitutions resulting from point mutations in the genome.

A well-resolved 2DE protein pattern, or proteome map, reflects most of the expressed cellular proteins and is thus a rich source of information regarding the cell/tissue's molecular phenotype and, if compared to an appropriate control pattern, its response to disease, pharmacotherapy, or toxic insult. The nature and number of proteins resolved and reproducibly detected in a typical proteome pattern are a function of protein detection sensitivity, range, stability of the first-dimension pH gradient, gel size, and protein solubility. This last characteristic relates the first important step in a comprehensive proteome analysis—sample preparation.

2.1.1   Sample Preparation

The importance of optimal sample solubilization cannot be understated [25], and great care to avoid unnecessary sample handling and artifactual alteration of the isolated proteins must be taken. Generally, a one-step solubilization technique is used that achieves both minimal sample handling and relatively complete solubilization. This involves the physical disruption of tissues/cells/organelles via ground-glass or Teflon homogenization or ultrasonication in a medium that simultaneously solubilizes, denatures, and reduces the sample proteins, breaking noncovalent interactions and disulfide linkages, removing interfering substances such as nucleic acids, and inhibiting the actions of intracellular proteases [26]. In this way, proteins can be separated as the nonmultimeric entities encoded by the genome while covalent post-translational modifications that typify certain proteins and cellular conditions remain unaltered.

A typical solubilization medium contains 7–9 M urea, 4% nonionic or zwitterionic detergent such as 3-[(3-cholamidopropyl)dimethylammonio]-1-propanesulfate (CHAPS), and 50–100 mM dithiotreitol (DTT) or tributylphosphine [27] as a reducing agent. In addition, some additives include buffering agents such as 40 mM Tris or high-pH range ampholytes (pH 10–12) to maintain high pH for acid protease inhibition and enhanced solubilization [28]. When immobilized pH gradient (IPG) strips are used for first-dimension separation (see Sect. 2.1.2.1), protein hydrophobicity becomes a problem. In this case, combining urea and thiourea in a two- to fourfold ratio during solubilization and IPG strip reswelling (Sect. 2.1.2.1.2) prevents protein adsorption to the IPG strip and loss of resolvable proteins [29].

Many proteins are present in very low copy numbers, are concentrated in specific subcellular fractions or compartments, or both. This creates problems for their detection on a 2D gel, amino acid sequencing, and for peptide mass detection as well (see Sect. 2.4.2). Prefractionating samples and thus increasing protein abundance in the sample applied to 2DE may be necessary in such cases. Two approaches to fractionation—differential centrifugation [30] or sequential extraction of cells and tissues with detergent-containing buffers [31]—serve two distinct purposes. First, low-abundance proteins become enriched in a specific compartment or fraction and thus become detectable on the gel as well as increasing the tryptic peptide molarity for mass spectrometric analysis. Second, knowledge of protein translocation (e.g., subcellular redistribution), particularly for proteins involved in cell signaling cascades detected by 2DE, can help to clarify a broad range of biological processes and changes therein [32]. Finally, microdissection [33,34] or chromatographic separation [35] of specific organ/tissue regions prior to solubilization and subsequent electrophoretic analysis may improve the sensitivity of 2DE and the specificity of the resulting 2D protein pattern [36].

2.1.2   Protein Separation

2.1.2.1   First-Dimension Separations.   After prefractionation and solubilization, protein samples are first separated according to charge by any one of three common techniques: isoelectric focusing in tube gels with low acrylamide concentrations; immobilized pH-gradient electrophoresis on gel strips; or nonequilibrium pH gradient electrophoresis in gel tubes for proteins with very alkaline isoelectric point (pI).

ISOELECTRIC FOCUSING (IEF).   Traditionally, 2DE separations have used IEF in the first dimension where denatured proteins are separated according to their charge [37,38]. In IEF, charge separation is accomplished by adding carrier ampholytes, a mixture of aliphatic polyaminopolycarboxylic acids with various pHs ranging from 2 to 11, to a low concentration polyacrylamide gel tube. This creates a relatively linear environment of increasing H^+ concentration in which a protein, placed at the basic end of the IEF gel, migrates until it reaches a pH where its surface charge equals 0 and its electrophoretic migration ceases. This is the isoelectric point, a unique characteristic of each protein that is solely dependent on amino acid composition and modifications therein. This powerful separation technique enables sharp resolution of complex protein mixtures but suffers from batch-to-batch variability, gradient instability that leads to significant inter- and even intralaboratory variation, poor resolution at basic pH due to cathodic drift and electroendosmosis [39], physical fragility, and an inability to adequately and reproducibly separate preparative loads of protein. However, at narrow ranges of pH (4–7) and moderate protein loading (100–200 μg), IEF remains an exceptional first-dimension separative tool.

IMMOBILIZED pH GRADIENT ELECTROPHORESIS (IPG).   In response to the limitations of IEF, dried gel strips copolymerized with Immobilines were developed. IPG strips consist of immobilized pH gradients [40,41] with several distinct advantages over conventional IEF. First, batch-to-batch reproducibility of IPGs has been shown to be good [42,43], though anecdotal evidence suggests some inconsistency among batches. In contrast to IEF separations for 2DE, IPG pI resolution up to 0.01 pH unit has been reported [40] in highly stable gradients where cathodic drift is minimal. Furthermore, narrow range IPGs can spread 1 to 2 pH units over a large distance (18 cm) achieving high resolution separations that enable the assembly of ''proteomic contigs,'' overlapping pH regions used to construct panoramic 2D images of global protein expression [44]. Because each IPG strip is cast with a GelBond backing, it has improved physical stability that simplifies handling and avoids gel breakage. Gel sample loading has also been optimized by taking advantage of the commercially available IPG strip shipped in dehydrated form. By rehydrating (reswelling) the IPG strip with sample buffer [45], sample precipitation at the application point is avoided, precise quantitative control of sample loading is facilitated, and >10 mg protein can be loaded to improve detection of low-abundance proteins. Recent improvements in pH range and alkaline stability have produced IPG strips with functional immobilized gradients of pH 3–12 [46]. However, despite reswelling techniques, protein precipitation and consequent quantitative reproducibility problems have been a recurrent problem according to anecdotal evidence (electronic discussion groups).

NONEQUILIBRIUM pH GRADIENT ELECTROPHORESIS (NEPHGE). Before the development of IPG technology, proteins with very alkaline pI could not be resolved reproducibly on IEF 2D gels, primarily due to the buffering effect of urea and cathodic drift. To study the expression of proteins with pI >7.0, a nonequilibrium approach was developed [47] to separate proteins by charge. Using a typical IEF system, NEPHGE gels can be run by simply applying the solubilized protein sample to the anodic end of the tube gel (rather than the cathodic end as in IEF) and allow the proteins to migrate in this nonequilibrium system until sufficiently separated. Subsequent second-dimension gel (NEPHGE-DALT) patterns do not lend themselves well to quantitative/qualitative image analysis because run to run reproducibility and resolution are problematic with this approach [39]. However, reasonably good charge separation of proteins with extremely alkaline pI can be attained and the proteins quantified with acceptable accuracy and later identified [46].

2.1.2.2 Second-Dimension SDS-PAGE. Following first-dimension separation, the IEF/NEPHGE gel or IPG strip is placed on a polyacrylamide gel slab (DALT) for separation by molecular mass, producing a 2D gel pattern (IEF-DALT, IPG-DALT, or NEPHGE-DALT). The procedures involved in SDS slab gel electrophoresis vary according to apparatus available. Most 2D systems are limited to 2–10 slab gels per run while some large-scale systems support 20 gels per run [48,49]. The latter systems significantly reduce gel-to-gel variability, improve gel imaging and quantitative/qualitative protein analysis, and are the foundation for the development of automated, large-scale, high-throughput proteomics systems [50].

As mentioned previously, SDS-PAGE or DALT gel electrophoresis is a method for separating polypeptides according to their molecular weights (MW). SDS is an anionic detergent that denatures proteins and forms anionic complexes with constant net negative charge/mass ratio. Thus, when proteins are treated with both SDS and a reducing agent like DTT, separations exclusively by molecular weight are possible. Most 2DE systems use a Tris-Glycine buffer system described by Laemmli [51]. Other buffer systems like Tris-Tricine system [52] for better and more accurate resolution of polypeptide molecular weight. Acrylamide

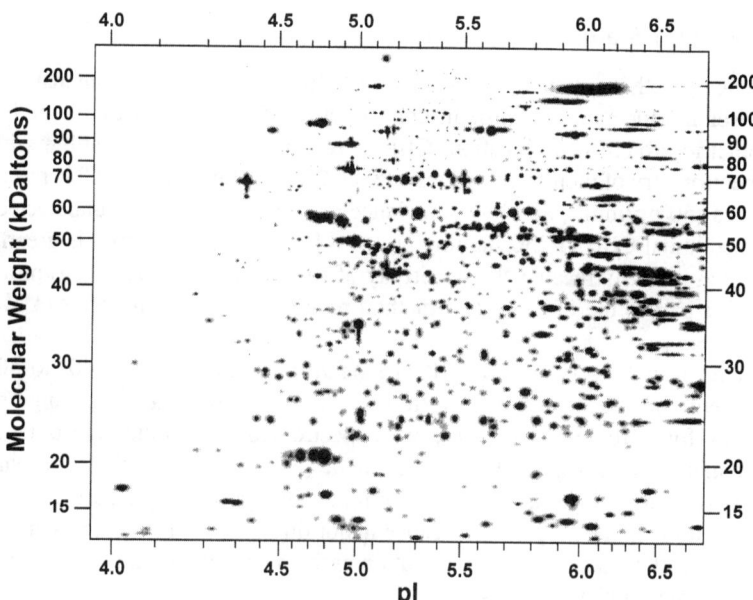

FIGURE 3 Representative proteome profile of mouse liver on a 2DE gel pattern. First-dimension separation was accomplished by IEF using pH 4–8 ampholytes, and second-dimension separation on a 1.5-mm-thick slab with an 11–17% polyacrylamide gradient. Proteins were visualized using colloidal Coomassie blue staining. Molecular weight and pI calibrations are estimates based on the calculated MW and pI of protein spots identified in the pattern (via EXPASY Compute pI/MW Tool, http://www.expasy.ch/tool/pi_tool.html).

concentration significantly affects protein mobility by means of its sieving effect [53], making it possible to alter acrylamide concentrations or incorporate acrylamide gradients [49] to optimize resolution of complex, heterogeneous mixtures of low-, high-, and intermediate-molecular-weight proteins. Completion of the 2D procedure results in a gel pattern illustrated in Figure 3.

2.2 Protein Detection Methods and Protein Quantification

Vital to a sound proteomics platform is reproducibly accurate and quantitative detection of the resolved protein pattern. A variety of methods are used for the staining/visualization/detection of proteins separated by 2DE and all have their limitations. Those amenable to automation will be the methods of greatest utility to proteomics in the future.

2.2.1 Protein Staining

The triphenylmethane dye Coomassie Brilliant Blue (CBB) staining intensity is linear over a wide range of protein concentration [54] and thus excellent for densitometric protein quantification. CBB-stained proteins are compatible with mass spectrometry of their tryptic digests (Sect. 2.4.4.1), but CBB R-250 is rather insensitive (50 ng/mm^2), and low-abundance proteins are often left undetected. Using a colloidal CBB G-250 staining protocol [55], protein detection is greatly improved as it nearly reaches the sensitivity of silver stain (e.g., 0.5–1 ng) probably due in part to the fact that this method requires no destaining prior to MS analysis.

Silver stain is very sensitive (0.04 ng/mm^2) and linear over a 40- to 50-fold concentration range (up to 2 ng/mm^2) [56] compared to a linear range of 10–200 ng for CBB [57]. However, mass spectrometry of tryptic digests from silver-stained proteins reportedly is problematic [57] and requires the additional step of silver removal (destaining) [58] with potential protein loss. Furthermore, slight variations in the reagents can cause major differences in staining intensity and background, thus creating quantification problems in large-scale experiments with very large numbers of gels.

Other staining techniques that are more amenable to mass spectrometry yet sensitive and rapid are reversible metal chelate stains [59] and imidazole-zinc negative stain [60]. Unlike CBB and silver stains, zinc-imidazole protocols require no in-gel protein fixing, and thus subsequent protein elution from the gel is simplified. Similarly, fluorescent dye staining of 2DE protein patterns via SYPRO Orange and SYPRO Red protein gel stains [61,62] requires no protein fixation, is as sensitive as silver stain, and the protocols are quite rapid. However, due to these stains' dependence on protein-SDS saturation, quantitative results are not uniform across all proteins in the gel. The development of spot-cutting robotic systems compatible with both visible and fluorescent detection and the need for high-throughput in proteomics makes SYPRO staining even more advantageous.

Another sensitive detection technique involves the colloidal gold staining of electroblotted 2D patterns [63]. This approach is useful following immuno-staining for single-protein identification because the coordinate position of the identified protein can be ascertained relative to neighboring proteins in the complex pattern on the gel. While the colloidal gold stain is very sensitive [64], electroelution from the gel during blotting is more efficient for low-MW proteins than for high MWs, thus this approach is not very quantitative.

2.2.2 Radiolabeling

Detection and quantification of separated proteins by in vivo or in vitro radiolabeling and autoradiography, particularly with phosphor imaging, is very sensitive and flexible [65]. This approach not only enables the detection of resolved proteins but has the advantage of permitting double-label experiments in which various cellular/biochemical events can be identified simultaneously [66] using different radiolabels. Disadvantages of the radiolabeling approach involve the difficulties of working with, storing, and disposing of relatively large quantities of radioisotopes, the cost of phosphor imaging equipment, and the specificity of phosphor screens.

2.2.3 Protein Quantification

While optimized protein separation, detection, and identification methods are central to the proteomics approach, precise and reproducible quantification of individual protein spots is the critical step if one is to properly describe the dynamics of physiological and disease processes and to distinguish the magnitude of various drug effects. There is currently no practical approach to routinely and precisely measure the absolute amounts of each protein present in a typical 2D gel. However, accurate quantitation relative to a reference pattern is possible. Most proteomic investigations use CBB or silver staining, or both, for densitometric protein quantification which lend themselves reasonably well to computer-aided densitometry [67,68]. Consequently, relative protein abundance can be determined and quantitative differences in protein expression statistically compared using any one of a number of commercially available 2D gel analysis systems.

Most gel analysis systems address quantification and gel processing rather similarly, although individual algorithms vary greatly. Therefore, most 2D gel image analysis packages commonly consist of scanning a stained 2DE pattern via laser densitometry or photodiode array, digitizing the image, processing the image (e.g., background and streak subtraction and mathematical morphology operations to detect and optimize each spot), and creating a reference pattern to which all other patterns are then matched to create a set of essentially superimposable 2D protein patterns. Lists of protein spot abundances can then be subjected to statistical analysis to search for quantitative, qualitative, and positional (charge) alterations in the proteome patterns (see Fig. 4).

2.3 Protein Identification

Once the complex 2D protein pattern has been resolved and the constituent proteins detected, specific proteins in the gel pattern can be selected for identification. In large, proteomic projects, the goal is the identification of all expressed proteins [8], thus verifying the sequenced genome, linking it to the proteome and vice versa. Frequently, in less ambitious studies, only those proteins altered in response to some experimental manipulation/disease state or those detected in greatest abundance are earmarked for identification. Regardless of the scope of protein identification, it is possible for the investigator to select from a variety of identification techniques, traditional approaches that are slow and labor-

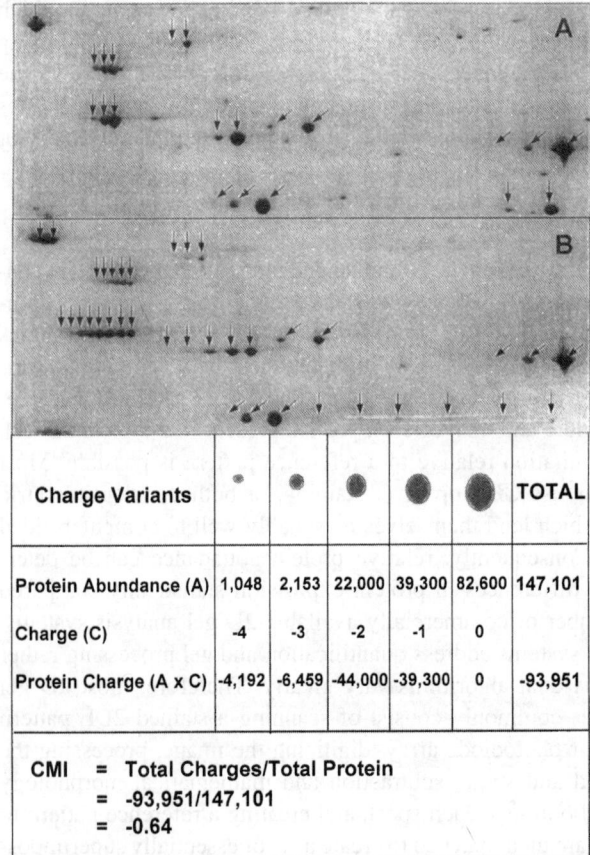

Charge Variants						TOTAL
Protein Abundance (A)	1,048	2,153	22,000	39,300	82,600	147,101
Charge (C)	-4	-3	-2	-1	0	
Protein Charge (A x C)	-4,192	-6,459	-44,000	-39,300	0	-93,951

CMI = Total Charges/Total Protein
    = -93,951/147,101
    = -0.64

Figure 4

FIGURE 4 Quantification of charge modification using the calculable charge modification index (CMI) [104]. Panel A illustrates a portion of a 2DE pattern from normal rat liver. Proteins indicated by arrows are those with posttranslational modifications (see Sect. 2.1), consequently resolved as charge heterogeneities (additional spots with more acidic pI). Panel B illustrates the same gel region but from a rat exposed to thioacetamide. The additional arrows indicate new charge variants on some proteins, presumably generated by reactive sulfone-adducts exclusively on endoplasmic reticular proteins. Using methods described in this chapter, the additional charge variants can be removed from the gel and the nature of posttranslational modification studied using MS/MS. This figure illustrates an important utility of proteome analysis, that is the quantification of protein modification via 2DE and image analysis.

intensive and contemporary techniques that are fast, less expensive, and amenable to high-throughput applications [69].

2.3.1 Immunoblotting

Perhaps the most traditional protein identification approaches involve Western blotting and immunostaining [70,71]. Proteins on 2DE gels are transferred electrophoretically onto a suitable membrane (e.g., nylon, nitrocellulose, or polyvinylidene fluoride [PVDF]). The membrane is probed with a primary antibody which binds to the desired membrane-bound protein, if it is present, and this reaction is detected by application of the secondary antibody incorporating either a radiolabel or enzyme yielding a colored product with the addition of an appropriate substrate. While this approach can be extremely precise, nonspecific binding of either primary or secondary antibodies can be misleading. Thus, this approach requires significant optimization for each protein. Furthermore, immunoblotting entails a search for known proteins for which antibodies are available, rather than attempting to globally and methodically identify all or a large subset of proteins in the pattern. Accordingly, this technique's greatest utility may relate to the use of antibodies whose epitopes recognize posttranslationally modified proteins such as phosphoproteins [72] or other covalent adducts [73] to characterize epigenetic phenomena.

2.3.2 Amino Acid (AA) Sequence Analysis

The quintessential identifying characteristic for a protein that is most related to the encoding genome is its AA sequence. Prior to the development of peptide mass fingerprinting, the traditional method for identifying or at least characterizing electroblotted proteins was (and still is, in some applications) automated N-terminal sequencing via Edman degradation [74]. This sensitive technique can help identify proteins from 2DE gels whose sequence is known, but contributes far less information for proteins not yet in a protein sequence database. Furthermore, even with automation, the technique is slow and labor-intensive, and the reagents are expensive. Due to the predominance of N-terminal blockage in biological systems, sequencing either is impossible or requires additional deblocking procedures [75]. Therefore, for high-throughput protein identification from 2DE gels, amino acid sequencing is impractical though it is still an important technique for those individual proteins that cannot be identified in any other way.

A practical approach for characterizing the N-terminally blocked protein is internal sequencing [76]. In this case, proteins are visualized in the gel by reversible staining, cut out, and digested in situ by proteolytic enzymes. The resulting peptide fragments can then be separated by reverse-phase HPLC, collected, and peptides N-terminally sequenced as above. The utility of internal sequencing for the characterization of individual, N-terminally blocked proteins is undeniable. Furthermore, multiple independent peptide sequences are generated which can be used to generate oligonucleotide probes for molecular cloning and/or to search sequence databases for related proteins. Nevertheless, the limitations of Edman-based sequencing mentioned above still apply with regard to throughput.

2.3.3 Amino Acid Composition Analysis

Amino acid composition is determined simply by the number of each AA present in a particular protein and thus represents a rather straightforward analysis. In essence, a protein's constituent amino acids are determined, expressed as ratios or percent of total. These data are compared to a theoretical amino acid composition database for known protein sequences. One approach involves radiolabeling of amino acids [77], but this is not suitable for high-throughput because of its labor-intensive nature. More recently, chromatographic analysis of amino acids resulting from protein hydrolysis has overcome the throughput limitations of amino acid analysis [78] and, in addition to providing compositional data, may be combined with other front-end analyses to extend the information gained from a separated protein.

In the case of an organism whose entire genome has been sequenced and the open reading frames are well known, this approach is efficient and robust [79]. Unlike protein sequencing, AA composition analysis is less expensive and faster, and allows higher sample throughput thus making it more attractive for inclusion in contemporary proteomics platforms. In clinical applications, this approach can be of significant value in direct protein disease-marker quantification [80]. With the completed sequences of numerous mammalian genomes on the near horizon, this approach may become even more popular.

2.3.4 Peptide Mass Fingerprinting

Two technical developments in the last decade have essentially relegated the identification techniques described above to complementary or ancillary status. First, large-scale genome sequencing projects began generating vast electronic protein sequence databases that now show all the signs of eventually containing all proteins coded by a broad variety of relevant organisms. Second, mass spectrometric techniques evolved to a level that enabled the routine analysis of proteins and peptides with extremely high sensitivity, excellent precision, and the potential for high throughput. The application of mass spectrometric analysis to 2DE-separated proteins has been reviewed elegantly by Patterson and Aebersold [81] and will be described here in an abbreviated format. In essence, proteins separated on a 2D gel are fragmented into their constituent peptides, peptide masses are detected by mass spectrometry, and the resulting masses are compared to a theoretically derived database of peptide masses generated by calculating all possible mass fragments (using a variety of fragmentation techniques) for all known protein sequences [82–86].

2.3.4.1 Preparation of Peptide Fragments. Whether one is interested in identifying only a few altered proteins from 2DE patterns or every spot on the gel, two distinct approaches for generating measurable peptides are possible. The first involves in-gel digestion using a suitable protease, typically trypsin. Trypsin is an endopeptidase that cleaves peptide bonds at the C-terminal side of lysine (K) or arginine (R) residues. Other proteases such as LysC, ArgC, AspN, GluC (bicarbonate), GluC (phosphate), and chymotrypsin also work well and peptide mass databases are designed to reflect each unique cleavage point. Nonenzymatic cyanogen bromide (CNBr) cleaves at the C-terminal side of methionine (M) and converts M into a modified amino acid called homoserine lactone (HSL). It avoids the K_m considerations, side reactions, and autolytic peaks associated with enzymatic cleavage, and has the advantage of being very amenable to automation [87]. Nevertheless, trypsin and Lys-C have been the preferred proteases for proteomic applications mainly because they generate peptides in the 800- to 2500-kDa range, optimal for contemporary mass spectometric techniques.

A detailed protocol of various peptide fragment preparation techniques (in-gel and on-membrane) in recipe form has been published [88]. Briefly, a gel plug no larger than the stained protein spot is excised from a 2D gel and can be macerated. The gel piece is washed to remove detergents and other confounding materials and a reduction and alkylation of cysteine residues is performed. The gel is dried completely and rehydrated by the addition of buffered protease, the protein is digested (often overnight), and the peptides are extracted from the gel piece(s) [89]. After extraction, the peptides can be concentrated, desalted, and eluted [90] using microcolumn chromatography such as the Zip Tip$_{C18}$ from Millipore. This in-gel approach is particularly advantageous to large-scale protein characterization in that every step is amenable to automation and thus high throughput.

Proteins electroblotted onto membranes are also applicable to proteolytic digestion and peptide recovery. Preferred membranes are the Immobilon-CD, a cationic, hydrophilic, charge-modified polyvinylidene fluoride (PVDF) membrane that helps eliminates detergent contamination; Immobilon-P^{SQ}, a hydrophobic PVDF membrane with a pore size of 0.22 μm; or Immobilon-NC membrane, a combination of nitrocellulose and cellulose acetate. Membrane sections containing the blotted protein spots visualized by reverse staining are cut into tiny pieces and protease is added. Peptide fragments generated are eluted and cleaned up on a microcolumn. Following the generalized steps presented above, the peptide mixture is ready for mass analysis.

2.3.4.2 Matrix-Assisted Laser Desorption/Ionization (MALDI) Mass Spectrometry. Perhaps the most relevant technical development that has occurred to advance proteomics is the rapid improvement in the performance of mass spectrometry (MS) [91]. The core of this approach relies on (1) the production of gas-phase ions from solid or liquid states, and (2) their accurate mass determination. Accordingly, improvements in both ionization technique (matrix-assisted laser desorption and nanoelectrospray) and mass analyzers (linear and reflection time-of-flight (TOF), various quadrupole configurations, and ion trap) have led this advance. The principles of ionization and mass analysis for peptide and protein analysis, and application of MALDI and electrospray ionization (ESI) to protein identification and sequencing have been presented previously in a concise yet thorough tutorial review [92]. This section will summarize the relevant aspects of these techniques.

In conventional MALDI-MS analysis, concentrated peptide sample mixtures are combined with a crystalline matrix (e.g., alpha-cyano-4-hydroxycinnamic acid) whose role is to segregate the peptides, absorb the laser light, and transfer the energy to the analyte molecules. The analytes (peptide masses) become ionized by simple protonation by the photoexcited matrix, leading to the formation of the typical $[M+X]^+$ type ion species in what is called a "soft ionization" mechanism that renders the peptides into the gaseous phase intact. Depending on the laser wavelength, a variety of matrices are used and the concentration of analyte relative to matrix must be kept low for efficient, uniform ionization [93] and sensitive detection with high mass accuracy (± 20 ppm). In linear instruments, once the peptides are ionized they are accelerated in a magnetic field down a time-of-flight tube, detected by a linear detector, and the flight time from ionization to detection is precisely calculated. Because the flight time is dependent solely on momentum, the root of mass/charge (m/z) with accurate calibration absolute analyte masses can be calculated easily. The resulting spectrum of masses (see Fig. 5A) can then be saved for online database searching (Sect. 3).

Though this powerful analytical tool generally provides excellent results, ambiguous identifications via MALDI-MSA are common and require peptide sequence information. When the MALDI instrument is fitted with an ion mirror (reflectron) called a curved-field reflector and laser power is adjusted to fragment

---

FIGURE 5 (A) As one example of mass spectrometric data used in proteome analysis, this MALDI-MS spectrum of a tryptic digest shows one dominant peak and several weaker ones. Although this particular mass map is typical of MALDI mass spectra obtained from tryptic digests, submission of these masses failed to identify the protein studied. As a result, PSD of the m/z 1475 peak following derivatization [94] was undertaken. (B) PSD spectrum of the above peptide following derivatization with chlorosulfonylacetyl chloride. A fairly simple spectrum consisting mainly of y-ions was obtained. Database searching with this result returned a single candidate protein (fetuin) demonstrating the utility of this approach. (Courtesy of Dr. T. Keough, Procter & Gamble Company, Cincinnati, OH).

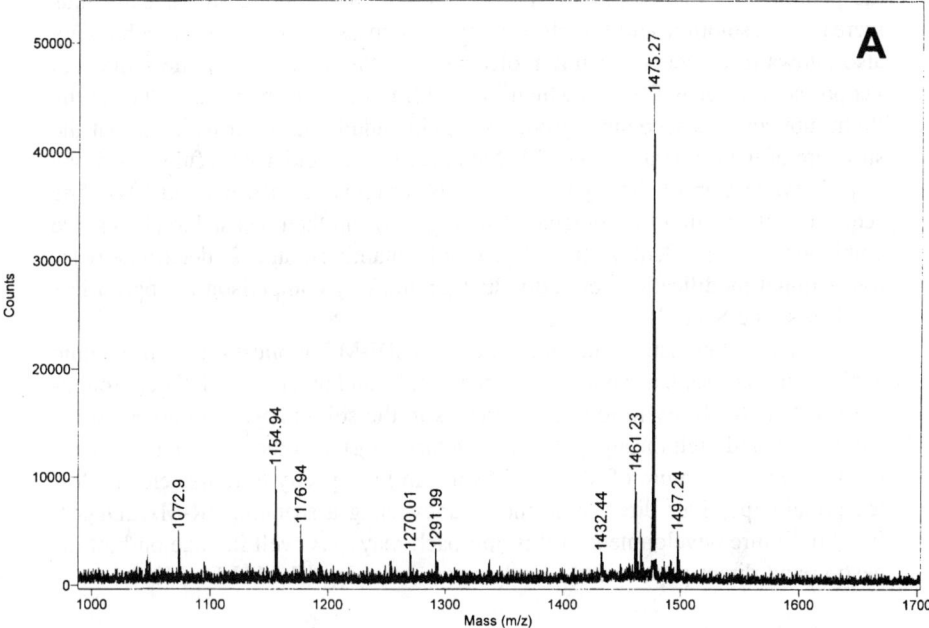

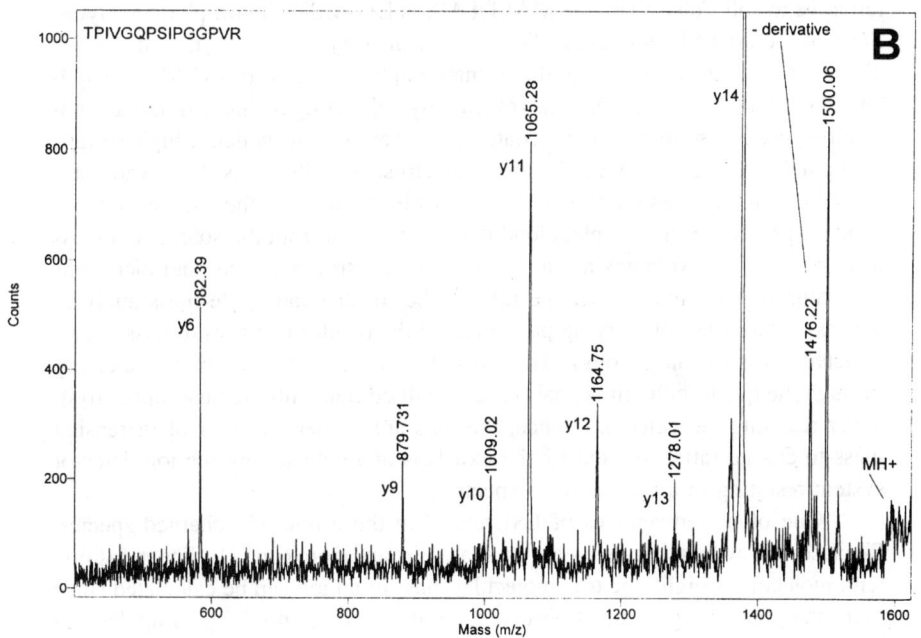

the peptides the reflectron effectively increases the TOF free-flight path, thus increasing resolution and therefore improving mass accuracy. This technology also allows researchers to study molecular structure of ions (peptide sequence) via postsource decay PSD, in which ionized fragments decompose further in the flight tube and the secondary products provide additional information about the structure of the original ion. The PSD approach is particularly useful when a one step derivatization of the tryptic peptide N-terminus is incorporated [94]. The sequence information thus obtained (see Fig. 5B) can then be used to (1) resolve ambiguous protein identification at picomole quantities, and (2) determine post-translational modifications on individual peptides by comparison to appropriate databases (see Sect. 3).

Some of the distinct advantages of MALDI-MS applications in proteomic analysis are its speed, accuracy, tolerance of salts and other potentially confounding substances, ability to ionize substances in the solid phase, and potential for automation and high throughput (multiple targeting). Another unique and potentially automated feature of MALDI-MS lies in its capacity to ionize electroblotted proteins/peptides directly on membranes using a scanning IR-MALDI-MS [95,96]. Future development of this approach may very well include on-blot digestion and direct peptide mass analysis via scanning IR-MALDI-MS.

2.3.4.3   Electrospray Ionization Mass Spectrometry (ESI-MS).   The alternative to solid-phase peptide MALDI-MS is ESI-MS of liquid-phase analytes. State-of-the-art ESI separation [97] is based on very low flow rates of peptide eluents from high-pressure liquid chromatography (HPLC) for LC/MS or capillary electrophoresis (CE) columns (essentially nebulizing the liquid) into a nanoelectrospray ion source, a metal-coated glass capillary to which a high voltage is applied creating an extremely strong electrostatic field. This then evaporates the solvent and creates multiply charged ions (depending on the number of basic residues present) in the droplet cloud that are directed from the source to a mass analyzer. Various voltages are applied to the electrodes to trap and eject ions according to their mass-to-charge ratios. The linear quadrupole mass analyzer acts as a mass filter by varying potentials on the quadrupole rods to pass only a selected mass-to-charge ratio. The ions that do not have a stable trajectory through the quadrupole mass analyzer and will collide with the quadrupole rods, never reaching the detector. Hence, the ions are ejected in order of increasing mass-to-charge ratio, focused by the exit lens and detected by the ion detector system resulting in a precise mass spectrum.

One of the advantages of ESI relates to these multiply charged species. Because the average charge state increases in an approximately linear fashion with molecular weight, the true molecular mass of an ion can be calculated since more than one charge state is observed. Furthermore, multiple quadrupoles can be added in tandem (MS/MS) to make multiple ion interpretation more robust and facilitate peptide sequence analysis. For instance, in a triple-quadrupole instrument, peptide ion masses are measured by the first quadrupole, a peptide of interest is sent to the second quadrupole where it is fragmented by collision-induced dissociation (CID), and the fragment masses measured at subpicomole levels in the third quadrupole known as the "sequence tag" method [98].

A third type of mass spectrometer, the quadrupole ion trap mass spectrometer, uses three electrodes to trap ions in a small volume in contrast to filtering the ions. The mass analyzer consists of a ring electrode separating two hemispherical electrodes. A mass spectrum is obtained by changing the electrode voltages to eject the ions from the trap. The advantages of the ion trap mass spectrometer include compact size, and the ability to trap and accumulate ions to increase the signal-to-noise ratio of a measurement. The high resolving power and efficiency of the ion trap allows for high resolution precursor ion selection and requires subsequent highly sensitive MS/MS analysis for peptide sequence analysis [99], but enables the investigator to "hold" the ions without losing them as one would in a multiple quadrupole instrument.

Various combinations of the ionization, filtering, trapping, and detection systems are possible. Combining ESI with a TOF to form a hybrid quadrupole-TOF spectrometer leads to a substantially greater precision of mass measurement. These instruments are now commercially available (e.g., Q-TOF from Micro-Mass; Mariner from PerSeptive Biosystems). ESI, ion trap, and TOF can also be combined [100] for speed and sensitivity of peptide mass analysis, but no such instrument is currently commercially available. At present, anecdotal evidence suggests that proteomic platforms optimized for sample throughput tend to use MALDI-MS, which, with multitarget arrays, can maximally generate masses from 30 samples per hour where as LC/ESI-MS is limited to 10 samples per hour. Further developments in robotics and automation make these numbers rather provisional.

Whatever the means, the resultant peptide masses and peptide sequences derived from the spectra are then amenable to database searching, identification, and characterization of post-translational modifications.

2.4 Detecting Posttranslational Modifications and/or Single-Nucleotide Polymorphisms (SNPs)

Before describing the databases available for protein identification, this section will briefly address the determination of posttranslational modifications (phosphorylation, glycosylation, prenylation, acetylation, adduct formation, etc.) and their relevance in proteomics [101].

The translation of mRNA to a polypeptide chain is frequently preceded by RNA splicing or followed by proteolytic cleavage such that the final protein product in no way resembles that predicted by the genome. Alternatively, a protein may be synthesized precisely as coded but specific amino acid residues in the chain may be chemically modified to transform its physicochemical characteristics in a way not necessarily predicted by the original gene sequence [102]. A good example of this lies in the alteration of pI (and frequently electrophoretic mobility in terms of mass) by chemical modification of a protein's constituent amino acids [103], alterations detectable and quantifiable by 2DE [104] (see Fig. 4) and identifiable by mass spectrometry [105–107].

Detectable in vivo posttranslational modifications are evidence of very natural cellular processes such as signaling systems, enzymatic regulation (activation/deactivation), intracellular translocation, structural associations and dissociations, etc. It has recently been postulated that more than half of all proteins are glycoproteins [108]. They are also the direct consequence of chemical intoxication (pharmaceutical or otherwise), frequently when normal conjugation systems are overwhelmed by huge exposures and reactive intermediates form protein adducts. The strength of proteomic analysis is its ability to detect, quantify, and identify such protein modifications (e.g., via databases such as FindMod [109], http://www.expasy.ch/tools/findmod) is a feature of great importance for pharmacogenomics research.

Along similar lines is the proteomic detection of genetic polymorphisms in general, and single-polynucelotide polymorphisms (SNPs) in particular. SNPs are heritable single-base changes in the genomic DNA sequence that may result in single amino acid substitutions in the coded protein. Proteins with single amino acid substitutions characteristically will have an atypical pI (negative or positive charge variant; see Fig. 4) [110,111] or mass [112] detectable by 2DE, MALDI-PSD, and ESI-MS/MS, and more importantly, the protein will have altered biological activity. Hence, SNPs generate genotypic fingerprints which may trigger individual variations of the phenotype (e.g. altered protein composition and function). Knowledge of SNPs and their potentially altered protein products could help pinpoint the genetic origins of diseases and be valuable in the development of the most appropriate drugs to treat disease.

3   PROTEIN BIOINFORMATICS

Annotated protein data in ever-expanding electronically and publicly accessible databases are the last crucial element in the proteomics approach. The bulk of protein data actually exists in two very different kinds of databases, both accessible to the public on the World Wide Web. The first includes 2DE protein patterns for interlaboratory comparisons and the second contains nonredundant translations of nucleic acid sequences in various formats for protein identification and characterization. This section will briefly summarize the characteristics and utility of these databases in proteomic applications.

3.1 2DE Databases

One of the early methods for tentative identification and characterization of proteins resolved on 2DE gels was the comparison of one's own 2DE patterns to those appearing in the published literature. However, due to significant gel-gel variation both within and between laboratories, this approach was not reliable, certainly not conclusive, and required confirmation by other means. Standardization of various aspects of 2DE technology, particularly with the introduction of IPGs (see Sect. 2.1.2.1.2), has improved gel-gel comparisons. Equally important was the introduction of Web-based 2DE protein patterns to a number of websites, a development that has improved interlaboratory comparison of 2DE patterns of similar samples (some are shown in Table 1). To overcome the subjectivity of Web-based protein pattern comparisons, Lemkin [113] developed a Flicker method of comparing two 2DE gel images of similar samples created in different laboratories to help identify or suggest protein spot identification [114]. Nonetheless, unambiguous identification of proteins on 2D patterns requires a more rigorous and reliable method (immunological, aa composition, aa seq., or peptide mass fingerprint).

Others have developed 2DE protein databases for intralaboratory comparisons of variable protein expression and documenting pattern alterations such as the Protein Disease Database [11,116], prototypical Molecular Effects Database [117], and Molecular Anatomy and Pathology (MAP) Database, and Molecular Effects of Drugs (MED) Database. The latter two are proprietary relational databases developed at Large Scale Biology Corp. as part of a proteomics platform that exemplifies the future of proteomics in what this group terms Pharmaceutical Proteomics. Other databases are accessible via the WWW such as: Protein Patterns in Human Epithelial Cells, University of Geneva, Switzerland; Human Astrocyte Cell Line, University of Geneva, Switzerland; Human Heart Protein Database, Imperial College, London, United Kingdom; Human CSF and Brain 2DE Protein Maps, University of Geneva, Switzerland.

3.2 Protein Sequence and Structure Databases

In high-throughput proteome projects where large numbers of protein spots must be analyzed and identified within a short period, the present identification method of choice seems to be peptide mass finger-printing via MALDI-TOF or ESI-MS, and/or MALDI-PSD or ESI-MS/MS sequence analysis. Peptide mass (spectral) and partial sequence data obtained from highly resolved protein spots are of little immediate use without relating them to known gene and protein sequences. To identify a 2DE protein spot unambiguously one must search all available, up-to-date peptide mass, MS/MS sequence tag, and/or MS/MS fragment-ion databases. These sources are all based on current protein sequence data contained in various

TABLE 1 Partial List of Web 2D Electrophoretic Gel Databases (http://www.lecb.ncifcrf.gov/EP/table2Ddatabases.html)

Material	Web location (URL)	Organization
Liver, plasma, HepG2, HepG2SP, RBC, lymphoma, CSF, macro-phage-CL, erythroleukemia-CL, platelet, yeast, E. coli, colorectal, kidney, muscle, macrophage-like-CL, pancreatic islets, epididymus, dictyostelium	http://www.expasy.ch/	ExPASy SWISS-2DPAGE
Mouse liver, human breast cell lines, pyrococcus	http://www.anl.gov/BIO/PMG/	Argonne Protein Mapping Group
Human: primary keratinocytes, epithelial, hematopoietic, mesenchymal, tumors, urothelium, amnion fluid, serum, urine, proteasomes, ribosomes, phosphorylations.	http://biobase.dk/cgi-bin/celis/	Danish Centre for Human Genome Research
Mouse: epithelial, newborn (ear, heart, liver, lung), human colorectal-CL, placental lysosomes	http://www.ludwig.edu.au/jpsl/jpslhome.html	Joint Protein Structure Lab
A375 melanoma cell line	http://rafael.ucsf.edu/2DPAGEhome.html	UCSF 2D PAGE
E. coli	http://pcsf.brcf.med.umich.edu/eco2dbase/	ECO2DBASE (in NCBI repository)

Yeast	http://www.proteome.com/	PROTEOME Inc (YPD-Yeast Protein DB)
Yeast	http://www.ibgc.u-bordeaux2.fr/YPM	Yeast 2D gel DB, Bordeaux
Human, rat, and mouse heart	http://www.harefield.nthames.nhs.uk/	HSC-2DPAGE, Heart Science Centre, Harefield Hospital
Human heart	http://www.chemie.fu-berlin.de/user/pleiss/	HEART-2DPAGE, German Heart Inst. Berlin
Human heart	http://www.mdc-berlin.de/~emu/heart/	HP-2DPAGE, MDC, Berlin
Rat neuronal	http://sunspot.bioc.cam.ac.uk/NEURON.html	Cambridge 2D PAGE
Embryonal stem cells	http://www.ed.ac.uk/~nh/2DPAGE.html	Immunobiology, Univ. Edinburgh
Rat, mouse, human liver, corn, wheat	http://www.lsbc.com/	Large Scale Biology Corp
Maize	http://moulon.moulon.inra.fr/imgd/	Maize Genome Database, INRA
Drosophila melanogaster	http://tyr.cmb.ki.se/	Karolinska institute
Bacillus subtilis	http://pc13mi.biologie.uni-greifswald.de/	Univ. Greifswald
Plasma, CSF, urine	http://www.lecb.ncifcrf.gov/PDD	NIMH-NCI Protein Disease Database (PDD)
Phosphoprotein, prostate, breast cancer drug screen, FAS (plasma). Cd toxicity (urine), leukemia	http://www.lecb.ncifcrf.gov/ips-databases.html	IPS/LECB, NCI/FCRDC

TABLE 1 Continued

Material	Web location (URL)	Organization
Rat: liver, kidney, serum, cerebrum Human: liver, serum. Bovine: testis	http://iupucbio1.iupui.edu/frankw/molan.htm	Molecular Anatomy Lab, Indiana U. Purdue U.
Human: inner ear	http://oto.wustl.edu/thc/innerear2d.htm	Washington Univ. Inner Ear Protein Database
Mouse: brain cerebellum, cortex, hippocammpus, striatum; *Arabidopsis thaliana* callus, leaf, seed, stem; *Oryza sativa* (rice) leaf, callus, germ, root, seed, stem	http://www.rs.noda.sut.ac.jp/~kamom/2de/2d.html	Res. Inst. for Biological Sci., Science Univ. Tokyo
Drosophila melanogaster	http://try.cmb.kl.se/	*Drosophila melanogaster* at the Karolinska Institute
Cyano2Dbase-*Synechocystis* sp. PCC6803	http://www.kazusa.or.jp/tech/sazuka/cyano/proteome.html	Protein Project of Cyanobacteria
Haemophilus influenzae and Neisseria meningitidis	http://www.abdn.ac.uk/~mmb023/2dhome.htm	2-D PAGE Aberdeen
Age-related proteome mapping of TIG-3	http://www.tmig.or.jp/2D/2D_Home.html	TMIG-2DPAGE—Tokyo Metro. Inst. Gerontology
Human leukemia cell lines	http://www-smbh.univ-paris13.fr/lbtp/biochemistry/biochimie/bque.htm	Lab. de Biochimie et Tech. des Proteines, Bobigny
Mycobacterium tuberculosis, vaccine strain *M. bovis* BCG	http://www.mpiib-berlin.mpg.de/2D-PAGE/	Max-Planck-Institut f. Infektionsbiologie

TABLE 2 Protein Sequence Databases for Peptide Mass, Sequence Tag, or Fragment Ion Comparison

Database	Bioinformatic content	URL
ATLAS	protein sequence	http://speedy.mips.biochem.mpg.de/mips/programs/atlas.html
BLAST	protein sequence	http://www.ncbi.nlm.nih.gov/BLAST/
FAST3	peptide sequence	http://www2.ebi.ac.uk/fasta3/
OWL	peptide sequence	http://www.bis.med.jhmi.edu/Dan/proteins/owl.html
EXPASY		
AACompIdent Tool	amino acid (AA) composition	http://www.expasy.ch/tools/aacomp/
MultiIdentTool	pI, MW, AA composition, sequence tag, peptide mass fingerprinting	http://www.expasy.ch/tools/multiident/
Peptident Tool	pI, MW, peptide mass fingerprinting	http://www.expasy.ch/tools/peptident.html
TagIdent	pI, MW, sequence tag	http://www.expasy.ch/tools/tagident.html
ProteinProspector		
MS-Fit	peptide masses	http://prospector.ucsf.edu/ucsfhtml3.2/msfit.htm
MS-Tag	MS/MS fragment ion	http://prospector.ucsf.edu/ucsfhtml3.2/mstagfd.htm
MS-Seq	MS/MS sequence tag	http://prospector.ucsf.edu/ucsfhtml3.2/msseq.htm
MS-Edman	peptide sequence	http://prospector.ucsf.edu/ucsfhtml3.2/msedman.htm
MOWSE	peptide masses	http://srs.hgmp.mrc.ac.uk/cgi-bin/mowse
PROWL	all of the above	http://prowl.rockefeller.edu/
PeptideSearch	all of the above	http://www.mann.embl-heidelberg.de/Services/PeptideSearch/
CombSearch	unified	http://cuiwww.unige.ch/~hammerl4/combsearch/

protein databases such as SWISS-PROT, PIR, PRF, PDB (115 databases are presented in the 2000 Database issue of Nucleic Acids Research). Currently, several such databases are accessible via the WWW. They appear in Table 2.

4   OTHER TECHNIQUES USED IN PROTEOMICS

Other separation techniques have been exploited recently, in advance of mass spectrometry and instead of 2DE, due to its labor-intensive nature. The advantages of chromatographic techniques such as sensitive and rapid quantification, automation, and myriad separation selectivities, along with recent technological developments, have brought these techniques to the forefront. For instance, high-throughput capillary isoelectric focusing (CIEF) linked to Fourier transform ion cyclotron resonance (FTICR) for mass detection provides a means for measuring reasonably large numbers of soluble proteins with greater sensitivity, speed, and mass accuracy than 2DE [118]. Similarly, direct identification of proteins in complex mixtures can be accomplished by solid-phase microextraction (micro-SPE)/multistep elution/capillary electrophoresis (CE)/tandem mass spectrometry (MS/MS) [119] or by combining a multidimensional liquid chromatographic separation prior to mass spectrometry for the identification of a limited population of proteins [120]. As a result of such technological developments, further optimization of these chromatographic separations will certainly render them complementary to electrophoretic approaches in proteomic systems in the near future.

Recent progress using isotope-coded affinity tags (ICATs) to quantify proteins expressed in yeast [121] may ultimately answer the quantification challenge (once sequence data for most proteins are available). This approach is based on stable isotope dilution techniques using chemical reagents called isotope-coded affinity tags (ICATs) combined with tandem mass spectrometry. The ICAT reagent consists of a biotin affinity tag (to isolate the peptides), a linker to incorporate stable isotopes, and a group that reacts with cysteines. In essence, the technique involves reacting cellular protein mixtures from different experimental conditions with light and heavy ICATs. The mixtures are combined, proteolytically digested to yield peptides; labeled peptides are isolated via biotin tag, peptides are separated and quantified by HPLC (relative quantification based on ratio of peptide pairs), and proteins are identified by MS/MS. Even very low-abundance proteins can thus be accurately quantified *and* identified in the same sample mixture.

5   APPLICATIONS OF PROTEOME ANALYSIS

Proteomics is well established as an enabling technology in a number of applied research areas. Numerous studies have documented the successful use of proteomics to analyze protein expression. A few of these recent applications include the study of plant proteomes [122] in which phenotypic traits of agricultural significance are identified; analysis of human and rodent organ/tissue proteomes in health and disease [123–128] (http://biobase.dk/cgi-bin/celis); the study of carcinogenesis [34,128–131]; the toxicity of xenobiotics [132–133]; and most importantly applications in pharmaceutical proteomics.

Pharmaceutical proteomics is the application of proteome profiling to the analysis of disease and drug effects on gene expression and this approach has become vital to drug discovery. The approach involves proteome profiling to identify and validate disease-specific proteins, identify and assign candidate targets, lead-compound identification and evaluation, mode of action assessment, and formal drug toxicology studies [134]. For instance, proteomics has been instrumental in discerning molecular mechanisms involved in cyclosporine A (CsA) nephrotoxicity [135,136] and the correlation of protein downregulation with immunosuppressant activity [137]. In addition, proteome profiling has been used effectively to determine protein markers indicative of therapeutic efficacy or toxicity and confirmed the utility of these markers for lead compound prioritization [138,139].

6 TRENDS AND OUTLOOK

Proteome analysis has gained a prominent place in modern biotechnology, not simply as an approach complementary to genomics but rather as a prospective strategic and comprehensive discipline that can reveal the molecular anatomy and physiology of a cell and cellular responses to disease, injury, and therapy. To maintain and improve this status and provide its demonstrated utility to the pharmaceutical industry and other life sciences, proteomics faces several technical challenges in virtually every aspect of its technology.

Though small-scale, focused applications of proteomics to specific research questions (by ''small'' laboratories) can be accomplished via access to suitably equipped ''biotechnology facilities,'' large-scale pharmaceutical application of proteomics requires reasonable cost, high throughput, precision, reproducibility, and above all comprehensiveness (e.g., identifying all resolvable proteins and thus completing the link between genome and proteome). To achieve these lofty objectives, innovative automation [140] and the incorporation of robotics into a ''proteomics platform'' [141] are necessary (such as the automation of protein identification developed by Genomic Solutions and BIO-RAD, or the completely automated 2DE system, ProGEx platform at Large Scale Biology Corporation).

Second, continued improvement and uniformity in separation technology is critical. The development of large-format (e.g., long) IPG first-dimension separation media with broad pH ranges and large-format slab gels (40 × 40 cm,

Proteomatron, Proteome, Inc., Beverly, MA) will improve resolution of proteomic separations. Increased sensitivity of protein detection is necessary and this must be matched by concomitant sensitivity of mass spectrometric techniques. Radioisotopically based differential display of proteins (developed by BioTraces, Inc., Fairfax, VA) is being developed that can attain subattomolar detection sensitivities so that a few copies of a protein expressed in a cell can be quantified. Improved fluorescent protein stains and prefractionation of cell/tissue samples by novel centrifugation techniques that ultrasubfractionate cellular compartments will lower the limits of protein detection and enhance the characterization of low-abundance and compartment specific proteins.

Protein chip technology [142], like that being developed by Ciphergen Biosystems (Palo Alto, CA) as the SELDI (surface-enhanced laser desorption/ionization) ProteinChip array, addresses issues of speed, cost, and sensitivity. On each chip, spots up to 1 mm in diameter can contain either a chemical (ionic, hydrophobic, hydrophilic, etc.) or biochemical (antibody, receptor, DNA, etc.) surface designed to capture proteins of interest. Application of a complex protein mixture onto the ProteinChip results in selected protein binding. This is followed by a wash step to remove unbound proteins, after which the chip is analyzed in a SELDI-TOF-MS instrument to determine the molecular weights of the bound proteins. It is claimed that this system enables the separation, quantification, identification, and characterization of previously characterized proteins at femtomole levels. However, because it is based on analysis of already characterized proteins, the ProteinChip is much like an ELISA (enzyme-linked immunosorbent assay), suffers from similar limitations, and thus is not a global analysis of protein expression.

The direct result of global proteomic analyses integrated with genomic data is a huge volume of quantitative and qualitative data that necessitates (1) data assembly into accessible archives, such as the BioKnowledge Library developed by Proteome Inc., and (2) systematic analysis of the protein expression in the context of genome and transcriptome to develop a better understanding of the functional design of biological systems [143].

The technological developments presented here, together with ample governmental and/or corporate support for continued refinement, will enable proteomics to reach its full potential and match or exceed the genomics revolution in scope and importance.

ACKNOWLEDGMENTS

The author wishes to thank Dr. Thomas Keough for providing the mass spectra, and Dr. Sandra Steiner and Dr. James Clack for their critical reading of the manuscript and their suggestions for its improvement.

REFERENCES

1. Human Genome Sequencing Progress: http://www.ncbi.nlm.nih.gov/genome/seq/
2. FS Collins. The human genome project and the future of medicine. Ann NY Acad Sci 882:42–65, 1999.
3. L Anderson, J Seilhamer. A comparison of selected mRNA and protein abundances in human liver. Electrophoresis 18:533–537, 1997.
4. I Humphery-Smith, SJ Cordwell, WP Blackstock. Proteome research: complementarity and limitations with respect to the RNA and DNA worlds. Electrophoresis 18:1217–1242, 1997.
5. PA Haynes, SP Gygi, D Figeys, R Aebersold. Proteome analysis: biological assay or data archive? Electrophoresis 19:1862–1871, 1998.
6. SP Gygi, Y Rochon, BR Franza, R Aebersold. Correlation between protein and mRNA abundance in yeast. Mol Cell Biol 19:1720–1730, 1999.
7. AO Gramolini, G Karpati, BJ Jasmin, Discordant expression of utrophin and its transcript in human and mouse skeletal muscles. J Neuropathol Exp Neurol 58: 235–244, 1999.
8. MR Wilkins, JC Sanchez, AA Gooley, RD Appel, I Humphery-Smith, DF Hochstrasser, KL Williams. Progress with proteome projects: why all proteins expressed by a genome should be identified and how to do it. Biotechnol Genet Eng Rev 13: 19–50, 1995.
9. NL Anderson, NG Anderson. Proteome and proteomics: new technologies, new concepts, and new words. Electrophoresis 19:1853–1861, 1998.
10. NG Anderson, NL Anderson. Twenty years of two-dimensional electrophoresis: past, present and future. Electrophoresis 17:443–453, 1996.
11. J Klose. Protein mapping by combined isoelectric focusing and electrophoresis of mouse tissues. A novel approach to testing for induced point mutations in mammals. Humangenetik 26:231–243, 1975.
12. PH O'Farrell. High resolution two-dimensional electrophoresis of proteins. J Biol Chem 250:4007–4021, 1975.
13. GA Scheele. Two-dimensional gel analysis of soluble proteins. Characterization of guinea pig exocrine pancreatic proteins. J Biol Chem 250:5375–5385, 1975.
14. BF Clark. Towards a total human protein map. Nature 292:491–492, 1981.
15. NG Anderson, L Anderson. The human protein index. Clin Chem 28:739–748, 1982.
16. JE Celis, R Bravo. Two-Dimensional Electrophoresis of Proteins: Methods and Applications. New York: Academic Press, 1984.
17. BS Dunbar. Two-Dimensional Electrophoresis, and Immunological Techniques. New York: Plenum Press, 1987.
18. MG Harrington. Two-Dimensional Gels. San Diego: Academic Press, 1991.
19. MJ Dunn. Quantitative two-dimensional gel electrophoresis: from proteins to proteomes. Biochem Soc Trans 25:248–254, 1997.
20. A Görg, G Boguth, C Obermaier, A Posch, W Weiss. Analytical IPG-Dalt. Methods Mol Biol 112:189–195, 1999
21. MR Wilkins, KL Williams, RD Appel, DF Hochstrasser. Preoteome Research: New Frontiers in Functional Genomics. Berlin: Springer-Verlag, 1997.

22. AJ Link, ed. 2-D Proteome Analysis Protocols. Totowa, NJ: Humana Press, 1999.

23. PZ O'Farrell, HM Goodman, PH O'Farrell. High resolution two-dimensional electrophoresis of basic as well as acidic proteins. Cell 12:1133–1141, 1977.

24. J Klose, U Kobalz. Two-dimensional electrophoresis of proteins: an updated protocol and implications for a functional analysis of the genome. Electrophoresis 16: 1034–1059, 1995.

25. B Herbert. Advances in protein solubilisation for two-dimensional electrophoresis. Electrophoresis 20:660–663, 1999.

26. T Rabilloud. Solubilization of proteins for electrophoretic analysis. Electrophoresis 17:813–829, 1996.

27. BR Herbert, MP Molloy, AA Gooley, BJ Walsh, WG Bryson, KL Williams. Improved protein solubility in two-dimensional electrophoresis using tributyl phosphine as reducing agent. Electrophoresis 19:845–851, 1998.

28. MN Horst, MM Basha, GA Baumbach, EH Mansfield, RM Roberts. Alkaline urea solubilization, two-dimensional electrophoresis and lectin staining of mammalian cell plasma membrane and plant seed proteins. Anal Biochem 102:399–408, 1980.

29. T Rabilloud. The use of thiourea to increase the solubility of membrane proteins in two-dimensional electrophoresis. Electrophoresis 19:758–760, 1998.

30. JM Graham, T Ford, D Rickwood. Isolation of the major subcellular organelles from mouse liver using Nycodenz gradients without the use of an ultracentrifuge. Anal Biochem 187:318–323, 1990.

31. ML Ramsby, GS Makowski, EA Khairallah. Differential detergent fractionation of isolated hepatocytes: biochemical, immunochemical and two-dimensional gel electrophoresis characterization of cytoskeletal and noncytoskeletal compartments. Electrophoresis 15:265–277, 1994.

32. WF Patton. Proteome analysis. II. Protein subcellular redistribution: linking physiology to genomics via the proteome and separation technologies involved. J Chromatogr B Biomed Sci Appl 722:203–223, 1999.

33. Y Sirivatanauksorn, R Drury, T Crnogorac-Jurcevic, V Sirivatanauksorn, NR Lemoine. Laser-assisted microdissection: applications in molecular pathology. J Pathol 189:150–154, 1999.

34. RE Banks, MJ Dunn, MA Forbes, A Stanley, D Pappin, T Naven, M Gough, P Harnden, PJ Selby. The potential use of laser capture microdissection to selectively obtain distinct populations of cells for proteomic analysis—preliminary findings. Electrophoresis 20:689–700, 1999.

35. K Karlsson, N Cairns, G Lubec, M Fountoulakis. Enrichment of human brain proteins by heparin chromatography. Electrophoresis 20:2970–2976, 1999.

36. FA Witzmann, CD Fultz, RA Grant, LS Wright, SE Kornguth, FL Siegel. Differential expression of cytosolic proteins in the rat kidney cortex and medulla: preliminary proteomics. Electrophoresis 19:2491–2497, 1998.

37. PG Righetti, JW Drysdale. Isoelectric focusing in gels. J Chromatogr 98:271–321, 1974.

38. PG Righetti. Isoelectric focusing as the crow flies. J Biochem Biophys Methods 16:99–108, 1988.

39. MJ Dunn. Isoelectric focusing. Gel Electrophoresis: Proteins. Oxford, England: Bios Scientific Publishers, 1993, pp 65–85.

40. B Bjellqvist, K Ek, PG Righetti, E Gianazza, A Gorg, R Westermeier, W Postel. Isoelectric focusing in immobilized pH gradients: principle, methodology and some applications. J Biochem Biophys Methods 6:317–339, 1982.

41. A Görg, G Boguth, C Obermaier, A Posch, W Weiss. Two-dimensional polyacrylamide gel electrophoresis with immobilized pH gradients in the first dimension (IPG-Dalt): the state of the art and the controversy of vertical versus horizontal systems. Electrophoresis 16:1079–1086, 1995.

42. JM Corbett, MJ Dunn, A Posch, A Görg. Positional reproducibility of protein spots in two-dimensional polyacrylamide gel electrophoresis using immobilised pH gradient isoelectric focusing in the first dimension: an interlaboratory comparison. Electrophoresis 15:1205–1211, 1994.

43. J Norbeck, A Blomberg. Two-dimensional electrophoretic separation of yeast proteins using a non-linear wide range (pH 3–10) immobilized pH gradient in the first dimension; reproducibility and evidence for isoelectric focusing of alkaline (pl > 7) proteins. Yeast 13:1519–1534, 1997.

44. VC Wasinger, B Bjellqvist, I Humphery-Smith. Proteomic 'contigs' of *Ochrobactrum anthropi*, application of extensive pH gradients. Electrophoresis 18:1373–1383, 1997.

45. JC Sanchez, V Rouge, M Pisteur, F Ravier, L Tonella, M Moosmayer, MR Wilkins, DF Hochstrasser. Improved and simplified in-gel sample application using reswelling of dry immobilized pH gradients. Electrophoresis 18:324–327, 1997.

46. A Görg, C Obermaier, G Boguth, W Weiss. Recent developments in two-dimensional electrophoresis with immobilized pH gradients: wide pH gradients up to pH 12, longer separation distances and simplified procedures. Electrophoresis 20:712–717, 1999.

47. Y Yamaguchi, SE Pfeiffer. Highly basic myelin and oligodendrocyte proteins analyzed by NEPHGE–two-dimensional gel electrophoresis: Recognition of novel developmentally regulated proteins. J Neurosci Res 56:199–205, 1999.

48. NG Anderson, NL Anderson. Analytical techniques for cell fractions. XXI. Two-dimensional analysis of serum and tissue proteins: multiple isoelectric focusing. Anal Biochem 85:331–340, 1978.

49. NL Anderson, NG Anderson. Analytical techniques for cell fractions. XXII. Two-dimensional analysis of serum and tissue proteins: multiple gradient-slab gel electrophoresis. Anal Biochem 85:341–354, 1978.

50. BJ Walsh, MP Molloy, KL Williams. The Australian Proteome Analysis Facility (APAF): assembling large scale proteomics through integration and automation. Electrophoresis 19:1883–1890, 1998.

51. UK Laemmli. Cleavage of structural proteins during the assembly of the head of bacteriophage T4. Nature 227:680–685, 1970.

52. WF Patton, N Chung-Welch, MF Lopez, RP Cambria, BL Utterback, WM Skea. Tris-tricine and Tris-borate buffer systems provide better estimates of human mesothelial cell intermediate filament protein molecular weights than the standard Tris-glycine system. Anal Biochem 197:25–33, 1991.

53. H Langen, D Roder, JF Juranville, M Fountoulakis. Effect of protein application mode and acrylamide concentration on the resolution of protein spots separated by two-dimensional gel electrophoresis. Electrophoresis 18:2085–2090, 1997.

54. JA Lott, VA Stephan, KA Pritchard Jr. Evaluation of the Coomassie Brilliant Blue G-250 method for urinary protein. Clin Chem 29:1946–1950, 1983.

55. V Neuhoff, N Arold, D Taube, W Ehrhardt. Improved staining of proteins in polyacrylamide gels including isoelectric focusing gels with clear background at nanogram sensitivity using Coomassie Brilliant Blue G-250 and R-250. Electrophoresis 9:255–262, 1988.

56. CR Merril, D Goldman, ML van Keuren. Silver staining methods for polyacrylamide gel electrophoresis. Methods Enzymol 96:230–239, 1983.

57. C Scheler, S Lamer, Z Pan, XP Li, J Salnikow, P Jungblut. Peptide mass fingerprint sequence coverage from differently stained proteins on two-dimensional electrophoresis patterns by matrix assisted laser desorption/ionization–mass spectrometry (MALDI-MS). Electrophoresis 19:918–927, 1998.

58. F Gharahdaghi, CR Weinberg, DA Meagher, BS Imai, SM Mische. Mass spectrometric identification of proteins from silver-stained polyacrylamide gel: a method for the removal of silver ions to enhance sensitivity. Electrophoresis 20:601–605, 1999.

59. WF Patton, MJ Lim, D Shepro. Protein detection using reversible metal chelate stains. Methods Mol Biol 112:331–339, 1999.

60. L Castellanos-Serra, W Proenza, V Huerta, RL Moritz, RJ Simpson. Proteome analysis of polyacrylamide gel-separated proteins visualized by reversible negative staining using imidazole-zinc salts. Electrophoresis 20:732–737, 1999.

61. TH Steinberg, LJ Jones, RP Haugland, VL Singer. SYPRO Orange and SYPRO Red protein gel stains: one-step fluorescent staining of denaturing gels for detection of nanogram levels of protein. Anal Biochem A 239:223–237, 1996.

62. TH Steinberg, RP Haugland, VL Singer. Applications of SYPRO Orange and SYPRO Red protein gel stains. Anal Biochem 239:238–245, 1996.

63. CD Fultz, FA Witzmann. Locating Western blotted and immunostained proteins within complex two-dimensional patterns. Anal Biochem 251:288–291, 1997.

64. JB Hunter, SM Hunter. Quantification of proteins in the low nanogram range by staining with the colloidal gold stain AuroDye. Anal Biochem 164:430–433, 1987.

65. AJ Link. Autoradiography of 2-D gels. Methods Mol Biol 112:285–290, 1999.

66. KH Lee, MG Harrington. Double-label analysis. Methods Mol Biol 112:291–295, 1999.

67. J Taylor, NL Anderson, AE Scandora Jr, KE Willard, NG Anderson. Design and implementation of a prototype Human Protein Index. Clin Chem 28:861–866, 1982.

68. RD Appel, DF Hochstrasser. Computer analysis of 2-D images. Methods Mol Biol 112:363–381, 1999.

69. R Aebersold, SD Patterson. Current problems and technical solutions in protein biochemistry. In: RH Angeletti, ed. Proteins: Analysis and Design. San Diego: Academic Press, 1998.

70. WN Burnette. "Western blotting": electrophoretic transfer of proteins from sodium dodecyl sulfate—polyacrylamide gels to unmodified nitrocellulose and radiographic detection with antibody and radioiodinated protein A. Anal Biochem 112: 195–203, 1981.

71. D Egger, K Bienz. Protein (Western) blotting. Mol Biotechnol 1:289–305, 1994.
72. A Gatti, X Wang, PJ Robinson. Protein kinase C-alpha is multiply phosphorylated in response to phorbol ester stimulation of PC12 cells. Biochim Biophys Acta 1313: 111–118, 1996.
73. TG Myers, EC Dietz, NL Anderson, EA Khairallah, SD Cohen, SD Nelson. A comparative study of mouse liver proteins arylated by reactive metabolites of acetaminophen and its nonhepatotoxic regioisomer, 3'-hydroxyacetanilide. Chem Res Toxicol 8:403–413, 1995.
74. P Edman, G Begg. A protein sequenator. Eur J Biochem 1:80–91, 1967.
75. M Kamo, A Tsugita. N-terminal amino acid sequencing of 2-DE spots. Methods Mol Biol 112:461–466, 1999.
76. RH Aebersold, J Leavitt, RA Saavedra, LE Hood, SB Kent. Internal amino acid sequence analysis of proteins separated by one- or two-dimensional gel electrophoresis after in situ protease digestion on nitrocellulose. Proc Natl Acad Sci USA 84: 6970–6974, 1987.
77. I Maillet, G Lagniel, M Perrot, H Boucherie, J Labarre. Rapid identification of yeast proteins on two-dimensional gels. J Biol Chem 271:10263–10270, 1996.
78. JX Yan, MR Wilkins, K Ou, AA Gooley, KL Williams, JC Sanchez, O Golaz, C Pasquali, DF Hochstrasser. Large-scale amino-acid analysis for proteome studies. J Chromatogr A 736:291–302, 1996.
79. M Fountoulakis, JF Juranville, P Berndt. Large-scale identification of proteins of *Haemophilus influenzae* by amino acid composition analysis. Electrophoresis 18: 2968–2977, 1997.
80. JX Yan, JC Sanchez, L Tonella, KL Williams, DF Hochstrasser. Studies of quantitative analysis of protein expression in *Sacchromyces cerevisiae*. Electrophoresis 20:738–742, 1999.
81. SD Patterson, R Aebersold. Mass spectrometric approaches for the identification of gel-separated proteins. Electrophoresis 16:1791–1814, 1995.
82. WJ Henzel, TM Billeci, JT Stults, SC Wong, C Grimley, C Watanabe. Identifying proteins from two-dimensional gels by molecular mass searching of peptide fragments in protein sequence databases. Proc Natl Acad Sci USA 90:5011–5015, 1993.
83. P James, M Quadroni, E Carafoli, G Gonnet. Protein identification by mass profile fingerprinting. Biochem Biophys Res Commun 195:58–64, 1993.
84. M Mann, P Hojrup, P Roepstorff. Use of mass spectrometric molecular weight information to identify proteins in sequence databases. Biol Mass Spectrom 22: 338–345, 1993.
85. DJC Pappin, P Hojrup, AJ Bleasby. Rapid identification of proteins by peptide-mass fingerprinting. Curr Biol 3:327–332, 1993.
86. JR Yates III, S Speicher, PR Griffin, T Hunkapiller. Peptide mass maps: a highly informative approach to protein identification. Anal Biochem 214:397–408, 1993.
87. M Quadroni, P James. Proteomics and automation. Electrophoresis 20:664–677, 1999.
88. PL Courchesne, SD Patterson. Identification of proteins by matrix-assisted laser desorption/ionization mass spectrometry using peptide and fragment ion masses. Methods Mol Biol 112:487–511, 1999.

89.   A Shevchenko, M Wilm, O Vorm, M Mann. Mass spectrometric sequencing of
      proteins from silver-stained polyacrylamide gels. Anal Chem; 68:850–858, 1996.
90.   X Jin, Y Chen, DM Lubman, D Misek, SM Hanash. Capillary electrophoresis/
      tandem mass spectrometry for analysis of proteins from two-dimensional sodium
      dodecyl sulfate polyacrylamide gel electrophoresis. Rapid Commun Mass Spec-
      trom 13:2327–2334, 1999.
91.   AL Burlingame, RK Boyd, SJ Gaskell. Mass spectrometry. Anal Chem 70:647R–
      716R, 1998.
92.   JR Yates III. Mass spectrometry and the age of the proteome. J Mass Spectrom
      33:1–19, 1998.
93.   O Vorm, P Roepstorff, M Mann. Improved resolution and very high sensitivity in
      MALDI TOF of matrix surfaces made by fast evaporation. Anal Chem 66:3281–
      3287, 1994.
94.   T Keough, RS Youngquist, MP Lacey. A method for high-sensitivity peptide se-
      quencing using postsource decay matrix-assisted laser desorption ionization mass
      spectrometry. Proc Natl Acad Sci USA 96:7131–7136, 1999.
95.   CW Sutton, CH Wheeler, U Sally, JM Corbett, JS Cottrell, MJ Dunn. The analysis
      of myocardial proteins by infrared and ultraviolet laser desorption mass spectrome-
      try. Electrophoresis 18:424–431, 1997.
96.   C Eckerskorn, K Strupat, D Schleuder, D Hochstrasser, JC Sanchez, F Lottspeich,
      F Hillenkamp. Analysis of proteins by direct-scanning infrared-MALDI mass spec-
      trometry after 2D-PAGE separation and electroblotting. Anal Chem 69:2888–2892,
      1997.
97.   PA Haynes, N Fripp, R Aebersold. Identification of gel-separated proteins by liquid
      chromatography–electrospray tandem mass spectrometry: comparison of methods
      and their limitations. Electrophoresis 19:939–945, 1998.
98.   A Shevchenko, ON Jensen, AV Podtelejnikov, F Sagliocco, M Wilm, O Vorm, P
      Mortensen, A Shevchenko, H Boucherie, M Mann. Linking genome and proteome
      by mass spectrometry: large-scale identification of yeast proteins from two dimen-
      sional gels. Proc Natl Acad Sci USA 93:1440–1445, 1996.
99.   JA Loo, H Muenster. Magnetic sector-ion trap mass spectrometry with electrospray
      ionization for high sensitivity peptide sequencing. Rapid Commun Mass Spectrom
      13:54–60, 1999.
100. SC Henderson, SJ Valentine, AE Counterman, DE Clemmer. ESI/ion trap/ion
      mobility/time-of-flight mass spectrometry for rapid and sensitive analysis of bio-
      molecular mixtures. Anal Chem 71:291–301, 1999.
101. AA Gooley, NH Packer. The importance of protein co- and post-translational modi-
      fication in proteome projects. In: MR Wilkins, KL Williams, RD Appel, DF Hoch-
      strasser, eds. Proteome Research: New Frontiers in Functional Genomics. Berlin:
      Springer-Verlag, 1997, pp 65–91.
102. AJ Link, K Robison, GM Church. Comparing the predicted and observed properties
      of proteins encoded in the genome of *Escherichia coli* K-12. Electrophoresis 18:
      1259–1313, 1997.
103. E Gianazza. Isoelectric focusing as a tool for the investigation of post-translational
      processing and chemical modifications of proteins. J Chromatogr A 705:67–87,
      1995.

104. NL Anderson, DC Copple, RA Bendele, GS Probst, FC Richardson. Covalent protein modifications and gene expression changes in rodent liver following administration of methapyrilene: a study using two-dimensional electrophoresis. Fundam Appl Toxicol 18:570–580, 1992.

105. Y Qiu, LZ Benet, AL Burlingame. Identification of the hepatic protein targets of reactive metabolites of acetaminophen in vivo in mice using two-dimensional gel electrophoresis and mass spectrometry. J Biol Chem 273:17940–17953, 1998.

106. B Kuster, M Mann. Identifying proteins and post-translational modifications by mass spectrometry. Curr Opin Struct Biol 8:393–400, 1998.

107. R Hoffmann, S Metzger, B Spengler, L Otvos. Sequencing of peptides phosphorylated on serines and threonines by post-source decay in matrix-assisted laser desorption/ionization time-of-flight mass spectrometry. J Mass Spectrum 34:1195–1204, 1999.

108. R Apweiler, H Hermjakob, N Sharon. On the frequency of protein glycosylation, as deduced from analysis of the SWISS-PROT database. Biochim Biophys Acta 1473:4–8, 1999.

109. MR Wilkins, E Gasteiger, AA Gooley, BR Herbert, MP Molloy, PA Binz, K Ou, JC Sanchez, A Bairoch, KL Williams, DF Hochstrasser. High-throughput mass spectrometric discovery of protein post-translational modifications. J Mol Biol 289: 645–657, 1999.

110. B Bjellqvist GJ Hughes, C Pasquali, N Paquet, F Ravier, JC Sanchez, S Frutiger, D Hochstrasser. The focusing positions of polypeptides in immobilized pH gradients can be predicted from their amino acid sequences. Electrophoresis 14:1023–1031, 1993.

111. DK Sanghera, T Kristensen, RF Hamman, MI Kamboh. Molecular basis of the apolipoprotein H (beta 2-glycoprotein 1) protein polymorphism. Hum Genet 100: 57–62, 1997.

112. J Palyga, E Gornicka-Michalska, A Kowalski. Genetic polymorphism of histone H1.z in duck erythrocytes. Biochem J 294:859–863, 1993.

113. PF Lemkin. Comparing two-dimensional electrophoretic gel images across the Internet. Electrophoresis 18:461–470, 1997.

114. PF Lemkin, JM Myrick, Y Lakshmanan, MJ Shue, JL Patrick, PV Hornbeck, GC Thornwal, AW Partin. Exploratory data analysis groupware for qualitative and quantitative electrophoretic gel analysis over the Internet-WebGel. Electrophoresis 20:3492–3507, 1999.

115. CR Merril, MP Goldstein, JE Myrick, PF Lemkin. The protein disease database of human body fluids. I. Rationale for the development of this database. Appl Theor Electrophor 5:49–54, 1995.

116. PF Lemkin, GA Orr, MP Goldstein, GJ Creed, JE Myrick, CR Merril. The Protein Disease Database of human body fluids. II. Computer methods and data issues. Appl Theor Electrophor 5:55–72, 1995.

117. NL Anderson, J Taylor, JP Hofmann, R Esquer-Blasco, S Swift, NG Anderson. Simultaneous measurement of hundreds of liver proteins: application in assessment of liver function. Toxicol Pathol 24:72–76, 1996.

118. PK Jensen, L Pasa-Tolic, GA Anderson, JA Horner, MS Lipton, JE Bruce, RD Smith. Probing proteomes using capillary isoelectric focusing-electrospray ioniza-

tion Fourier transform ion cyclotron resonance mass spectrometry. Anal Chem 71: 2076–2084, 1999.

119. W Tong, A Link, JK Eng, JR Yates III. Identification of proteins in complexes by solid-phase microextraction/multistep elution/capillary electrophoresis/tandem mass spectrometry. Anal Chem 71:2270–2278, 1999.

120. AJ Link, J Eng, DM Schieltz, E Carmack, GJ Mize, DR Morris, BM Garvik, JR Yates III. Direct analysis of protein complexes using mass spectrometry. Nat Biotechnol 17:676–682, 1999.

121. SP Gygi, B Rist, SA Gerber, F Turecek, MH Gelb, R Aebersold. Quantitative analysis of complex protein mixtures using isotope-coded affinity tags. Nat Biotechnol 17:994–999, 1999.

122. H Thiellement, N Bahrman, C Damerval, C Plomion, M Rossignol, V Santoni, D de Vienne, M Zivy. Proteomics for genetic and physiological studies in plants. Electrophoresis 20:2013–2026, 1999.

123. D Arnott, KL O'Connell, KL King, JT Stults. An integrated approach to protome analysis: identification of proteins associated with cardiac hypertrophy. Anal Biochem 258:1–18, 1998.

124. M Hubbard. Proteomic analysis of enamel cells from developing rat teeth: big returns from a small tissue. Electrophoresis 19:1891–1900, 1998.

125. PR Jungblut, A Otto, J Favor, M Löwe, EC Müller, M Kastner, K Sperling, J Klose. Identification of mouse crystallins in 2D protein patterns by sequencing and mass spectrometry. Application to cataract mutants. FEBS Lett 435:131–137, 1998.

126. JE Celis, M Ostergaard, NA Jensen, I Gromova, HH Rasmussen, P Gromov. Human and mouse proteomic databases: novel resources in the protein universe. FEBS Lett 430:64–72, 1998.

127. Y Nishizawa, N Komori, J Usukura, KW Jackson, SL Tobin, H Matsumoto. Initiating ocular proteomics for cataloging bovine retinal proteins: microanalytical techniques permit the identification of proteins derived from a novel photoreceptor preparation. Exp Eye Res 69:195–212, 1999.

128. PR Jungblut, U Zimny-Arndt, E Zeindl-Eberhart, J Stulik, K Koupilova, KP Pleissner, A Otto, EC Müller, W Sokolowska-Köhler, G Grabher, G Stöffler. Proteomics in human disease: cancer, heart and infectious diseases. Electrophoresis 20:2100–2110, 1999.

129. ES Robinson, TP Dooley, KL Williams. UV-Induced melanoma cell lines and their potential for proteome analysis: a review. J Exp Zool 282:48–53, 1998.

130. PS Nelson, N Clegg, B Eroglu, V Hawkins, R Bumgarner, T Smith, L Hood. The Prostate Expression Database (PEDB): status and enhancements in 2000. Nucleic Acids Res 28:212–213, 2000.

131. MJ Page, B Amess, RR Townsend, R Parekh, A Herath, L Brusten, MJ Zvelebil, RC Stein, MD Waterfield, SC Davies, MJ O'Hare. Proteomic definition of normal human luminal and myoepithelial breast cells purified from reduction mammoplasties. Proc Natl Acad Sci USA 96:12589–12594, 1999.

132. Y Qiu, LZ Benet, AL Burlingame. Identification of the hepatic protein targets of reactive metabolites of acetaminophen in vivo in mice using two-dimensional gel electrophoresis and mass spectrometry. J Biol Chem 273:17940–17953, 1998.

133. FA Witzmann, MD Bauer, AM Fieno, RA Grant, TW Keough, SE Kornguth, MP

Lacey, FL Siegel, Y Sun, LS Wright, RS Young, ML Witten. Proteomic analysis of simulated occupational jet fuel exposure in the lung. Electrophoresis 20:3659–3669, 1999.

134. MJ Page, B Amess, C Rohlff, C Stubberfield, R Parekh. Proteomics: a major new technology for the drug discovery process. Drug Disc Today 2:55–62, 1999.

135. L Aicher, D Wahl, A Arce, O Grenet, S Steiner. New insights into cyclosporine A nephrotoxicity by proteome analysis. Electrophoresis 19:1998–2003, 1998.

136. S Steiner, L Aicher, J Raymackers, L Meheus, R Esquer-Blasco, L Anderson, A Cordier. Cyclosporine A mediated decrease in the rat renal calcium binding protein calbindin-D 28kDa. Biochem Pharmacol 51:253–258, 1996.

137. L Aicher, G Meier, A Norcross, J Jakubowski, MC Varela, A Cordier, S Steiner. Decrease in kidney calbindin-D as a possible mechanism mediating CsA and FK-506-induced calciuria and tubular mineralization. Biochem Pharmacol 53:723–731, 1997.

138. A Arce, L Aicher, D Wahl, R Esquer-Blasco, NL Anderson, A Cordier, S Steiner. Changes in the liver proteome of female Wistar rats treated with the hypoglycemic agent SDZ PGU 693. Life Sci 63:2243–2250, 1998.

139. NL Anderson, R Esquer-Blasco, JP Hofmann, NG Anderson. A two-dimensional gel database of rat liver proteins useful in gene regulation and drug effects studies. Electrophoresis 12:907–930, 1991.

140. M Quadroni, P James. Proteomics and automation. Electrophoresis 20:664–667, 1999.

141. Binz PA, Muller M, Walther D, Bienvenut WV, Gras R, Hoogland C, Bouchet G, Gasteiger E, Fabbretti R, Gay S, Palagi P, Wilkins MR, Rouge V, Tonella L, Paesano S, Rossellat G, Karmime A, Bairoch A, Sanchez JC, Appel RD, Hochstrasser DF. A molecular scanner to automate proteomic research and to display proteome images. Anal Chem 71:4981–4988, 1999.

142. E Strauss. New ways to probe the molecules of life. Science 282:1406–1407, 1998.

143. V Hatzimanikatis, LH Choe, KH Lee. Proteomics: theoretical and experimental considerations. Biotechnol Prog 15:312–318, 1999.

15

Bioinformatics
WWW Resources

Siu Tang and Daiga Helmeste
University of California, Irvine, Irvine, California

1 INTRODUCTION

Genome research relies heavily on the World Wide Web (WWW or the Web). The genome research community was indeed an early adopter of the Web and computer technology. There are two good reasons for this. Firstly, there are immense amounts of genetic sequence and data generated rapidly and continuously from many areas of the world. Secondly, researchers have a need for early access to this ever changing database. Distributed computing offered by the Internet provides an ideal platform for the retrieval, exchange, and computing of this voluminous, heterogeneous, and constantly evolving genetic information.

Many newcomers to bioinformatics are baffled when they encounter the unfamiliar terminology and methods of computer sciences and the Web. This is particularly true for physicians or pharmacologists without a background in computer science. This chapter provides an overview of the Web resources on bioinformatics and explains commonly encountered concepts and terminology in computer and information technology.

2 WORLD WIDE WEB RESOURCES

The Weizmann GenCard site refers to the number of different data sources and their high degree of heterogeneity in the WWW as an "information labyrinth." Useful Web sites are scattered worldwide. The Internet allows us to transcend the geographic barrier and access these sites. However, the situation is not different from the one you encounter in a library, with your topic of interest scattered among the many books in different areas of the library. While many of the books seem useful and interesting, it is impractical to search through every book in the library. There would be duplication of materials, redundancy, and unnecessary information scattered among the needed data. You would need an efficient tool to retrieve the target information. Modern Internet search engines are like indexing systems in a library, except that a number of them are extremely powerful.

Web information search and retrieval may be carried out in many different ways. The commonest entry point is through many of the commercial portals. These portals generally supply so-called search engines, which are software for identifying information of interest from their own archives or providing links to other portals. To illustrate the magnitude of the literature accumulated on bioinformatic sites on the Web, we input the keyword "bioinformatics" into several popular portals and search engines. At the time of this writing, this search returned a manageable number of 105 sites from Yahoo to a high of 99,840 sites from AltaVista, followed by 32,451 sites from Lycos. As Web resources are not static, the numbers will be different but possibly higher when readers try out their own searches after reading this chapter. Web addresses may also change over time. Some Web content could be outdated as the responsible host failed to remove the obsolete materials. A small number of portals require registration, mostly free. Of the major sites, only the NCSA workbench requires registration to establish your workspace.

One may group bioinformatic sites in many different ways. These sites could be grouped according to the type of organization sponsoring the site (e.g., governmental vs. university vs. commercial), the subject matter emphasized (e.g., proteins vs. nucleotides vs. diseases), or their functional nature (e.g., sequence search vs. structure database search vs. analysis vs. education). Some sites concentrate on special interest topics while others are multipurpose and comprehensive. There are university sites that have become "the site" for a particular topic. There are sites put together by individual professors or departments, which are useful portals. Some of these portals are updated regularly and offer good overviews of the field of bioinformatics.

As mentioned above, WWW bioinformatics sites are essentially a mixed bag with regard to their content and purpose. While there are many ways to classify these hundreds of sites, major sites generally include databases and search engines, accompanying literature, and links to other important sites. Many important sites also represent joint efforts between universities and governments, or are cosponsored by universities and industry. Some of the megasites have become the one-stop center for researchers due to their extensive database collections and tools. The huge NCBI's site, for example, is such a site and will be described in more detail. However, there are other sites run by organizations and laboratories, offering valuable up-to-date original data, maps and protocols, experimental conditions, and phenotypes, which will not appear or only appear in NCBI's Entrez database later. This chapter attempts to serve only as a yellow page for and provide the reader with a bird's eye view of the WWW resources available today. The readers are encouraged to visit these sites themselves, as the Internet is an ever-changing resource. We will not discuss applications or the tools as the other chapters cover these. There are also excellent texts (e.g., *Bioinformatics* by Baxevanis and Ouellette, John Wiley & Sons, 1998; *Guide to Human Genome Computing* by Bishop, Academic Press, 1998) addressing that aspect.

3 MAJOR DATABASE SITES

3.1 International Nucleotide Sequence Database Collaboration

The collaboration consists of three partners: GenBank, built by the National Center for Biotechnology Information (NCBI) at NIH, the DNA Database of Japan (DDBJ) in Mishima, Japan, and the European Bioinformatics Institute (EBI)'s European Molecular Biology Laboratory (EMBL) nucleotide database in Hinxton, England.

The most important source of new data for the collections is direct submissions from scientists worldwide. Most peer-review journals now expect that DNA and amino acid sequences will be submitted to a sequence database before publication. While having their own points of data submission, the three organizations exchange data on a daily basis and make similar databases available to the community.

3.1.1 NCBI Web Site (www.ncbi.nlm.nih.gov)

The NCBI's homepage gives the following description: "Established in 1988 as a national resource for molecular biology information, NCBI creates public databases, conducts research in computational biology, develops software tools for analyzing genome data, and disseminates biomedical information" (Fig. 1). The NCBI pages show clear links to all kinds of important protein and nucleotide databases, literature (PubMed), and search and analysis tools. The NCBI site is probably the most comprehensive bioinformatic site at present.

3.1.1.1 Database. Popular databases include their own GenBank sequence database, OMIM (Online Mendelian Inheritance in Man), MMDB (Mo-

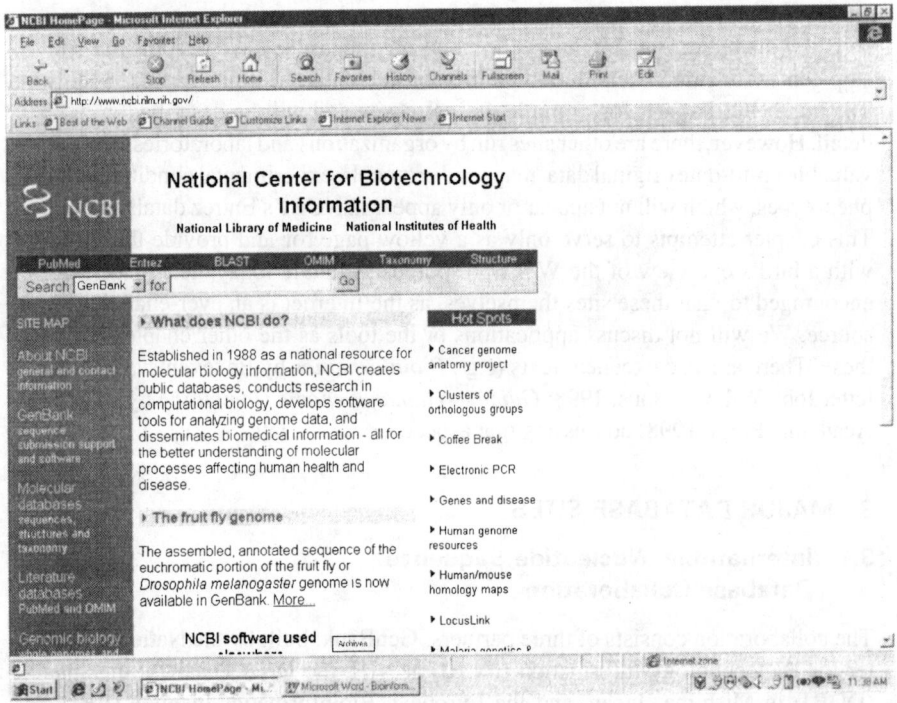

FIGURE 1   NCBI's home page (April 2000).

lecular Modeling Database), UniGene (Unique Human Gene Sequence Collection), dbEST (Database of Expressed Sequence Tags), dbSTS (Database of Sequence Tagged Sites) and SNP (single-nucleotide polymorphism).

To illustrate the magnitude of the growth of the GenBank database, GenBank has published a graph and table showing the statistics from 1982 to 1999. These could be viewed at http://www.ncbi.nlm.nih.gov/Genbank/genbankstats. html. After an essentially flat growth from 1982 to 1990, it took off exponentially from then on. In 1982, the number of base pairs in the collection was 680,338 and the sequences 606. In 1990, the corresponding numbers were 49,179,285 and 39,533. The numbers increased to 2,008,761,784 and 2,837,897 in 1998 and then to 3,841,163,011 and 4,864,570 in 1999.

3.1.1.2   Data Submission.   Data submission is an important function of the GenBank site. There are two ways to submit to GenBank. BankIt is a Web submission tool for simple submissions. Sequin is a stand-alone submission tool for more control over annotating entry, segmented records, or very long entries.

The submission can be sent via e-mail to gb-sub@ncbi.nlm.nih.gov or through FTP. As an alternative, the submission file can be copied to floppy disk and mailed to GenBank Submissions at: GenBank Submissions, National Center for Biotechnology Information, National Library of Medicine, Bldg. 38A, Room 8N-803, Bethesda, MD 20894. It is important to remember that the trend is toward direct Web submission for many database sites.

3.1.1.3 Search. The NCBI's Entrez is a powerful database search engine. This integrated search engine provides a drop-down menu offering the user selections to search for biomedical literature (PubMed), nucleotide and protein sequences, along with 3D protein structures, complete genomes, and population study data sets (PopSet). The textfield next to the drop down menu allows the user to enter text to direct the search (Fig. 2).

3.1.1.4 Links. The NCBI pages offer valuable links to some important databases. For example, the Human Genome Resources site (Fig. 3) is a very

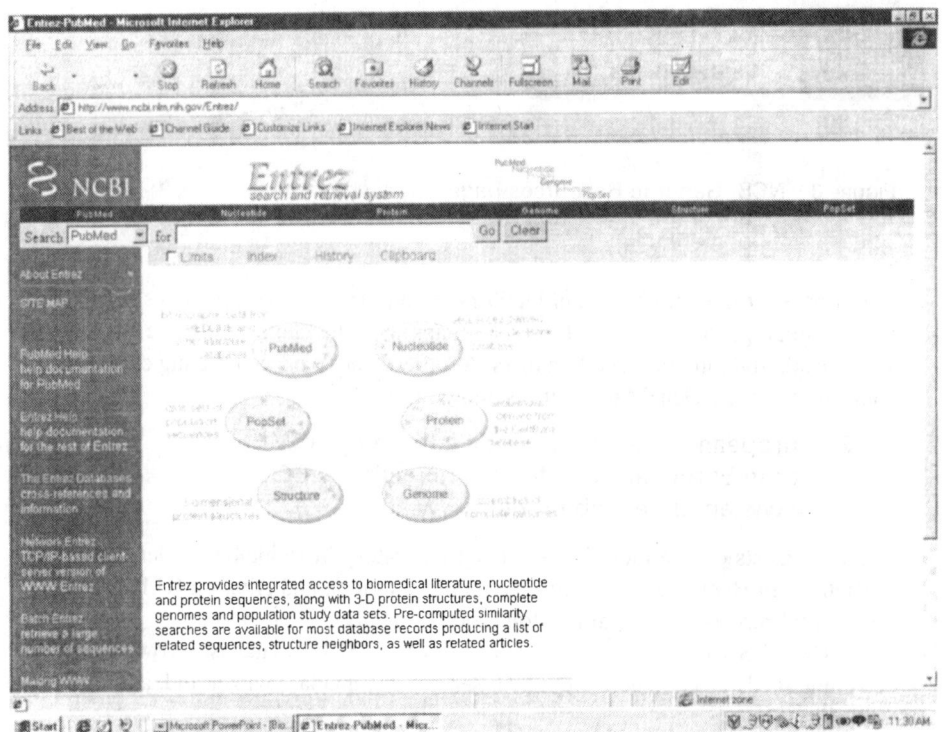

FIGURE 2 Entrez home page.

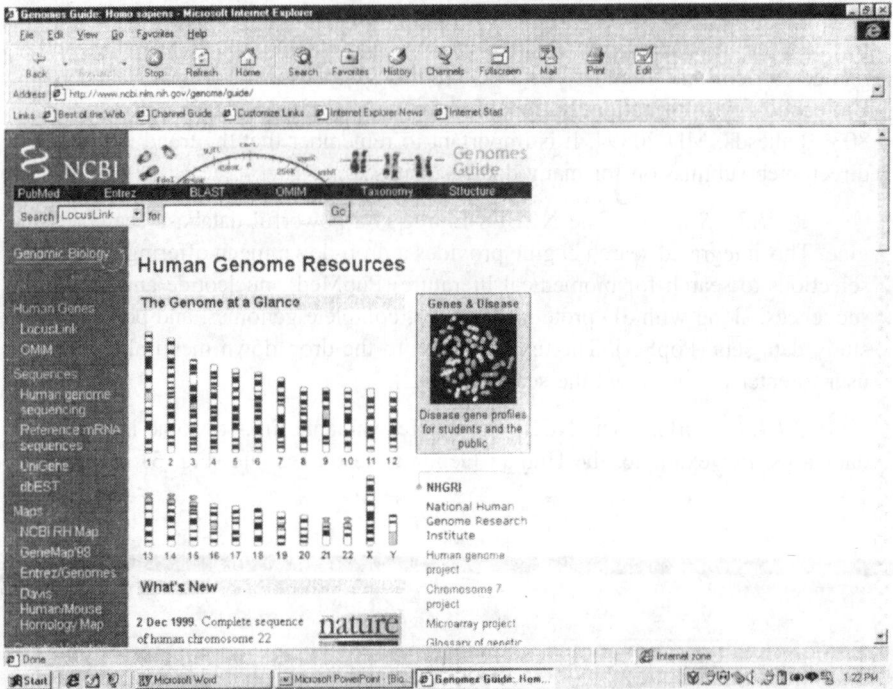

FIGURE 3   NCBI Genome Resources page.

useful page. It links to the GeneMap99 pages and many other resources related to the human genome. It also offers STS maps with the choices of GeneMap99, Whitehead, Stanford, or Généthon links. A representative page depicting chromosome 16 from the GeneMap99 site is shown (Fig. 4).

3.1.2   European Molecular Biology Laboratory (EMBL) at the European Bioinformatics Institute (EBI) (www.embl-heidelberg.de; www.ebi.ac.uk)

EMBL consists of five facilities: the main laboratory in Heidelberg (Germany); outstations in Hamburg (Germany), Grenoble (France), and Hinxton (U.K.); and an external research program in Monterotondo (Italy).

The SRS (Sequence Retrieval System) is EMBL's database browser for searching its database. There are mirror servers in Canada, Switzerland, and Taiwan (Fig. 5).

The EMBL/EBI site also offers many important database links and analytic tools.

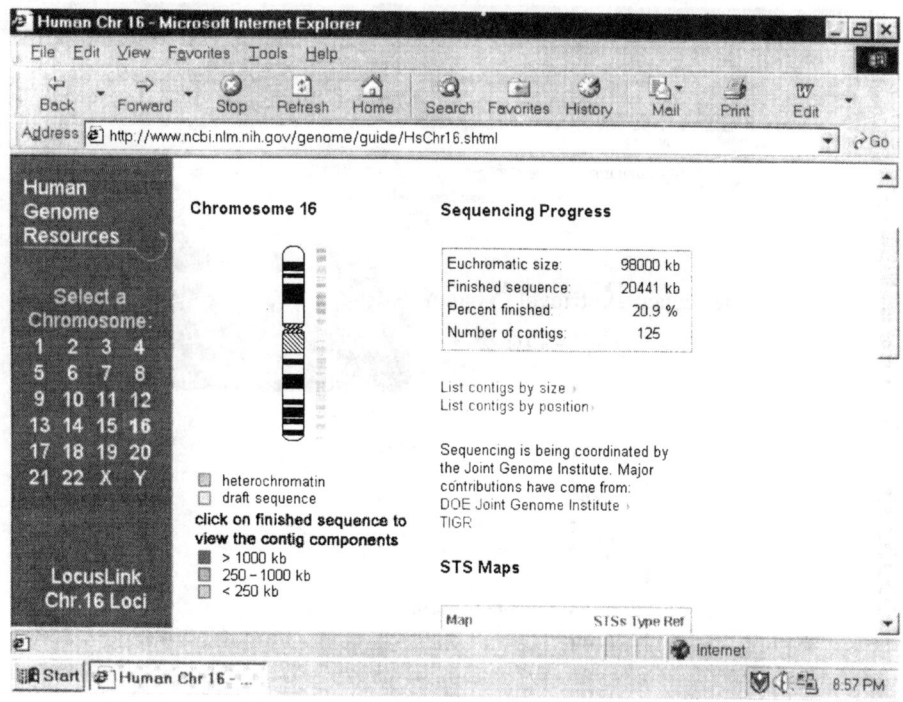

FIGURE 4 An NCBI GeneMap99 page.

3.1.3 Database of Japan (DDBJ) (DNA DataBank of Japan) (www.ddbj.nig.ac.jp)

Similar to the site maintained by their U.S. and European collaborators, this Japanese site offers both submission and database search facilities (Fig. 6).

3.2 Other Database Sites

3.2.1 SWISS-PROT and PROSITE (www.expasy.ch; also accessible through most major sites)

ExPASy stands for Expert Protein Analysis System. The ExPASy Molecular Biology Server is the proteomics server of the Swiss Institute of Bioinformatics (SIB). This server is dedicated to the analysis of protein sequences and structures. The SWISS-PROT Protein Sequence Database is a database of protein sequences derived from translations of DNA sequences from the EMBL Nucleotide Sequence Database, adapted from the Protein Identification Resource (PIR) collec-

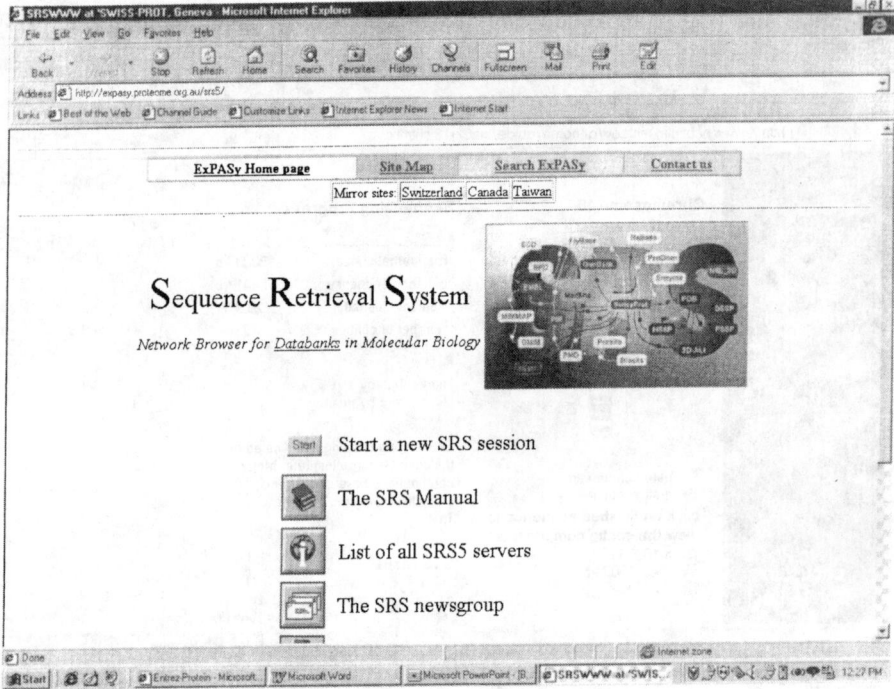

FIGURE 5   The EMBL's database browser page. Note mirror sites in Switzerland, Canada, and Taiwan.

tion, extracted from the literature and directly submitted by researchers. It contains high-quality annotation, is nonredundant, and cross-referenced to several other databases. PROSITE is a database of protein families and domains. It consists of biologically significant sites, patterns, and profiles that help to identify to which known protein family a new sequence belongs.

3.2.2   GDB (Genome Database) (http://www.gdb.org)

The important GDB site presents mapping data and interconnects many important databases from the Human Genome project with search tools (Fig. 7).

3.2.3   Généthon (www.genethon.fr)

The objective of Généthon II is to localize, and then isolate genes. Apart from many useful links, its many projects, and public data, it has a special database for neuromuscular disorders, skin, neurological, and rheumatological diseases (Fig. 8).

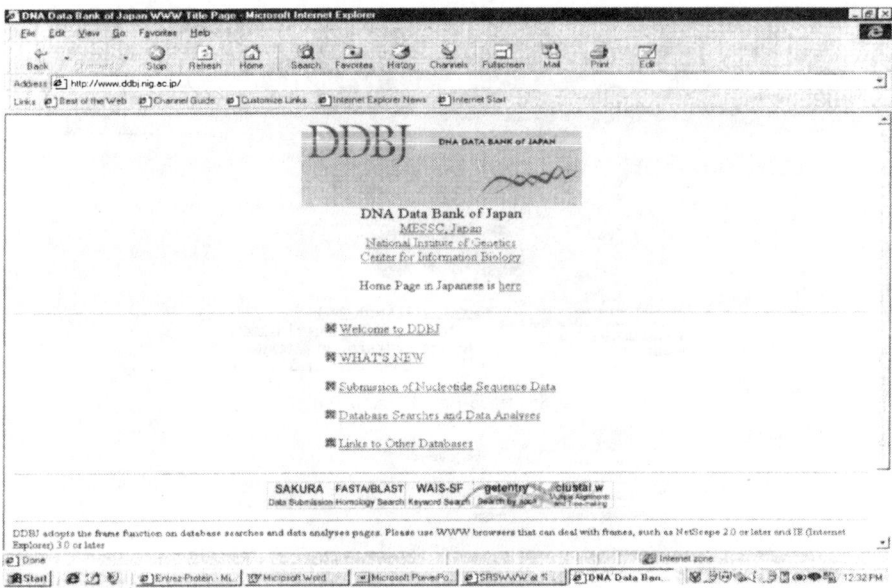

FIGURE 6 The DNA Data Bank of Japan home page.

3.2.4 TIGR (www.tigr.org)

The TIGR databases are a large collection of curated databases containing DNA and protein sequence, gene expression, cellular role, protein family, and taxonomic data for microbes, viral, parasites, plants (such as rice), and humans. Anonymous FTP access to sequence data is provided. Their main page offers vast selections to human, plant, and microbial databases. Gene Indices represent analysis of the transcribed sequences represented in the world's public EST data. Their expressed gene anatomy database links expression data, cellular roles, and alternative splicing information to a curated, nonredundant set of human transcript sequences (Fig. 9).

4 UNIVERSITIES AND INSTITUTES

There are many important sites maintained by universities around the world. Their pages provide rich materials, maps, and tools. For example, chromosome-specific physical maps are available on many of these sites: University of Texas Health Science Center, Emory University, University of Pennsylvania, Columbia University, Yale, the Hospital for Sick Children in Toronto, Stanford, and many other North American and European sites. It is impractical to review the large

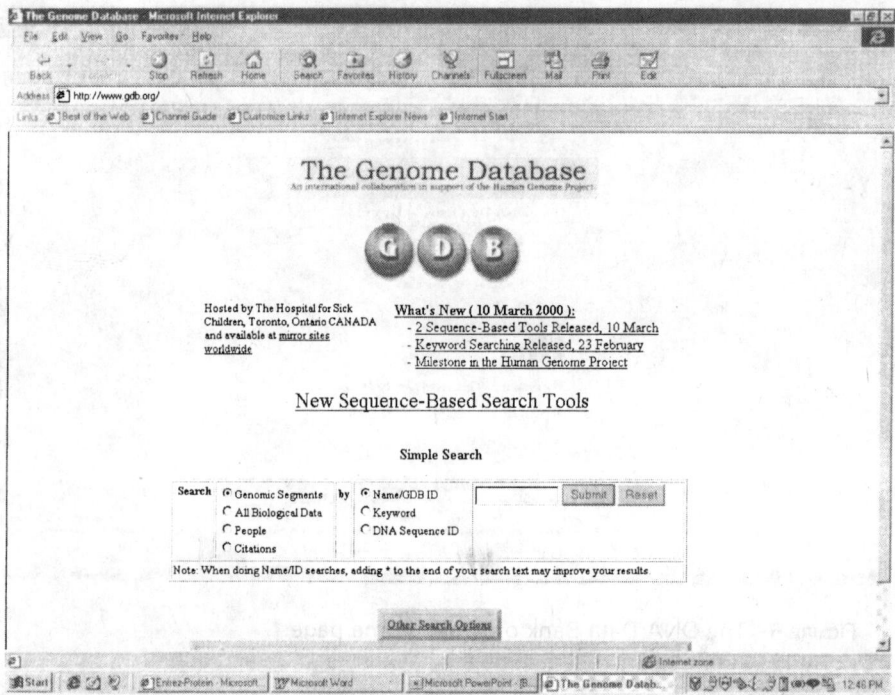

FIGURE 7   The GDB home page, hosted by the Hospital for Sick Children in Toronto. Mirror sites are available worldwide.

number of the university sites. The list below represents just a small fraction of university Web sites frequently mentioned in the literature.

4.1   Weizmann Institute of Science Genome Center (www.bioinfo.weizmann.ac.il/bioinfo.html)

This site offers its own database as well as links to other public databases. It also gives valuable information regarding many of its research projects and education materials.

4.2   Whitehead/MIT Center for Genome Research (www.wi.mit.edu/bio/biology.html)

This site has extensive database collections on human, rat and mouse genetic materials.

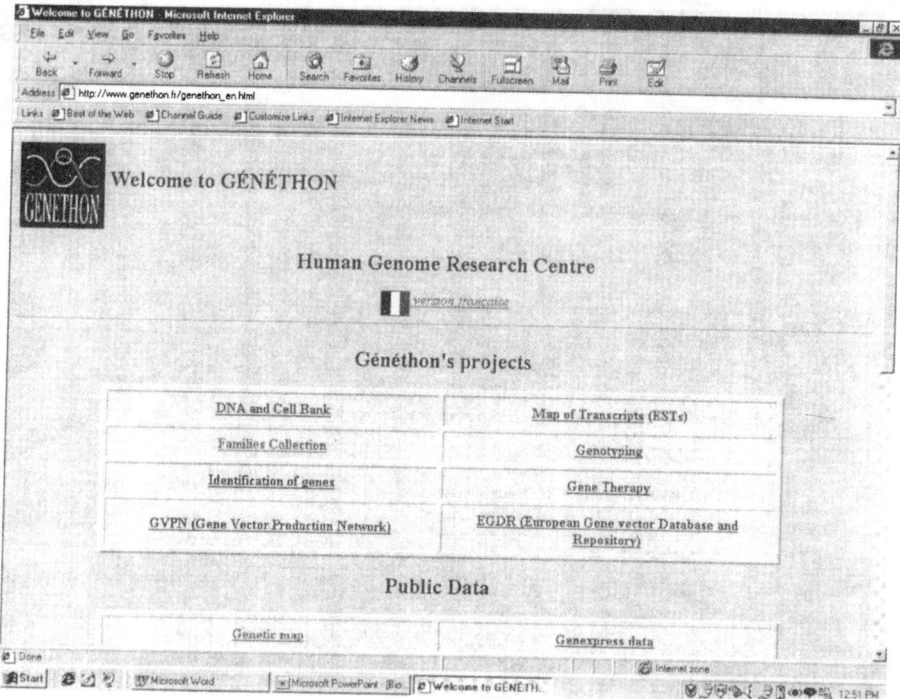

FIGURE 8   The Généthon home page.

4.3   Washington University Genome Sequencing Center (http://genome.wustl.edu/gsc/gschmpg.html)

Home of some large-scale sequencing projects. Human and mouse ESTs and *C. elegans* sequencing are some of the important information on this site.

4.4   Stanford Human Genome Center (http://shgc.stanford.edu)

One of the aims of the Human Genome Project is to build a high resolution radiation hybrid map using sequence-tagged sites (STS) as landmarks. The Stanford Human Genome Center focuses on aligning the radiation hybrids to fit the growing framework of STSs. The complete set of arranged STSs will form a continuous map of the human genome. Maps to a 500-kb (the Stanford G3 panel) resolution has been built using a panel of 83 radiation hybrids and >10,000 STSs, derived using random genomic DNA sequences, previously mapped genetic markers, and expressed sequences.

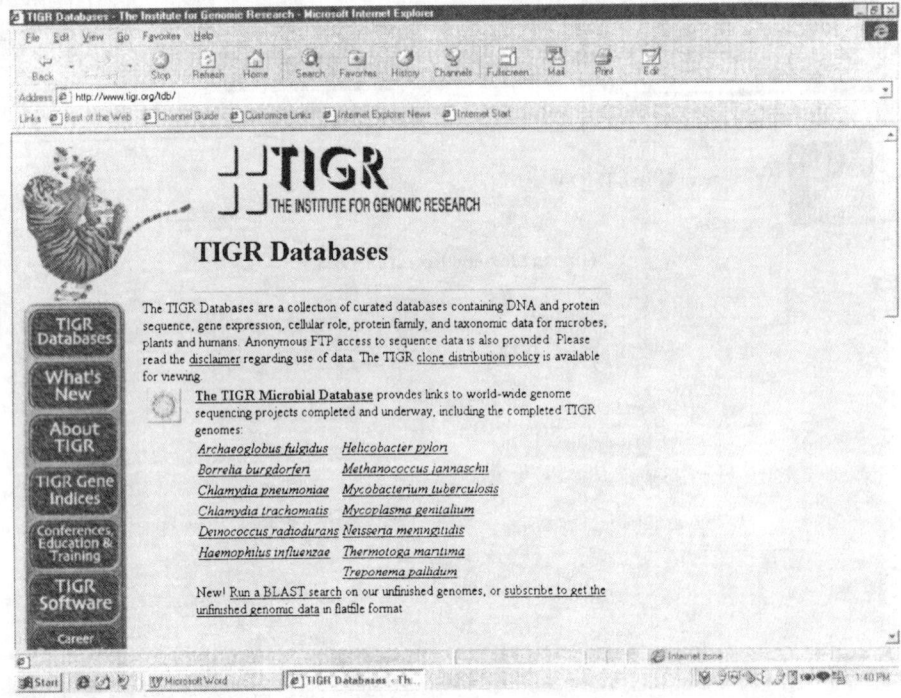

FIGURE 9   The TIGR Databases.

4.5 Cardiff Mutation Database (www.uwcm.ac.uk/uwcm/mg/hgmd0.html)

At the point of writing, the University of Wales Cardiff Human Gene Mutation database (HGMD) contains 21,382 mutations in 996 genes and provides 873 reference cDNA sequences.

4.6 Baylor College of Medicine's MBCR (Molecular Biology Computation Resources) Biological Databases

This Web site contains links for Medline and other molecular genetic searches as well as analytic tools. It is also devoted to the dissemination of biological databases developed by Baylor faculty. This site demonstrates the importance of the university sites, aside from the one-stop megasites, to provide current information and data on genetic research. The databases are in various stages of completion and include databases such as breast cancer gene, small RNA database, mammary transgene interactive database, and the tumor gene database. This database includes oncogenes, proto-oncogenes, tumor supressor genes/antioncogenes, regulators, and substrates.

4.7 GENATLAS (www.citi2.fr/GENATLAS/)

The GENATLAS database compiles the information relevant to the mapping efforts of the Human Genome Project. This information is collected from original articles in the literature or from the proceedings of Human Gene Mapping and Single Chromosome Workshops. GENATLAS/GEN is a repertory of three types of objects: genes, phenotypes, and markers. At present (1999) 9,396 genes are recorded, either individually or as components of a cluster.

4.8 Additional Useful Bioinformatics or Genome Research Sites

Brookhaven Protein Databank (www.rcsb.org/pdb)

George Mason University (www.science.gmu.edu/~michaels/Bioinformatics)

Harvard Genome Research Databases (http://golgi.harvard.edu; http://cgr.harvard.edu)

Hospital for Sick Children (www.gdb.org)

Kyoto University (www.genome.ad.jp/dbget/dbget.links.html)

UK MRC Human Genome Mapping Project Resource Center (www.hgmp.mrc.ac.uk)

5 NONHUMAN DATABASES

Nonhuman databases include those described in the following sections and the Human/Mouse Homology Relationship Page (NCBI) at www.ncbi/nlm.nih.gov/Homology/ (see Fig. 10).

5.1 MGD (Mouse Genome Database) (http://www.jax.org)

A large number of transgenic animals have been produced worldwide for use in both basic and applied research. This is a large mouse genetic mapping repository maintained by the Jackson Laboratory in Bar Harbor, Maine. The Transgenic/Targeted Mutation Database TBASE is an attempt to organize information on transgenic animals and targeted mutations generated and analyzed worldwide.

5.2 SGD (*Saccharomyces* Genome Database) (http://genome-www.standford.edu/Saccharomyces/)

Housed at the Stanford Human Genome Center, the SGD is the entire *Saccharomyces* genome. This important yeast site offers a simple but powerful search engine to search for yeast data. The site also offers a chromosome map, and

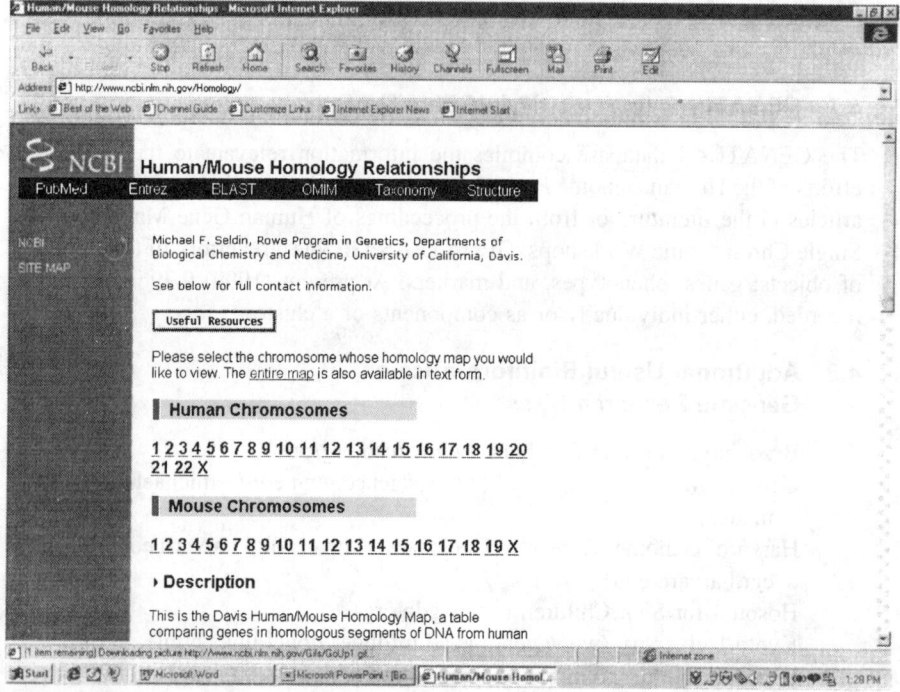

FIGURE 10   The NCBI's Human/Mouse Homology Relationships page.

allows user to download data and to register yeast genes. It provides links to other yeast WWW sites.

6   SOME SPECIFIC DATABASES

Immunogenetics (http://hiv-web.lanl.gov/immuno/index.html; www.ebi. ac.uk/imgt)
G Protein Coupled Receptor (www.sandler.embl-heidelberg.de/7tm)
Glucocorticoid Receptor (http://nrr.georgetown.edu/GRR/GRR.html)
Mitochondrial Genome Database (www.gen.emory.edu/mitomap.html)
Thyroid Hormone Receptors (http://xanadu.mgh.harvard.edu//receptor/ trrfront.html)

7   ONLINE ANALYTIC TOOLS

Many analytic tools are available on-line and they could be accessed through most of the major sites described above. Examples include BLAST (NCSA, SRS,

NCBI), PRIMER (Whitehead/MIT), Whitehead's radiation hybrid mapping service, Baylor's Genefinder for exon prediction (to find the location of potential genes, paste sequence to field, and choose prediction algorithm), and the integrated NCSA's Biology workbench for integrated search and analysis.

7.1 BLAST (Basic Local Alignment Search Tool)

BLAST is a popular set of similarity search programs designed to explore all of the entire available sequence databases regardless of whether the query is protein or DNA sequence based. Sample search algorithms include blastn, to compare sequence to database with parameters for nucleotides, and blastp, to compare sequence to database with parameters for protein sequences. For a better understanding of BLAST you can make use of the NCBI online tutorials which explain the basics of the BLAST algorithm.

7.2 FASTA

This is another tool used to find homologies and is available at the EBI page.

7.3 NCSA Biology WorkBench (http://biology.ncsa.uiuc.edu)

The Biology WorkBench is a Web-based computing environment. It integrates many standard protein and nucleic acid sequence databases, and a wide variety of sequence analysis programs into a single interface. The WorkBench allows users to perform database searches and analyze the results without worrying about the technical aspects of computer file formats, command line options, and flags. WorkBench jobs run on NCSA servers, giving anyone with access to a web browser access to the computational resources of NCSA. Biology WorkBench tutorials are available online.

7.4 Bioinformatic Information Pages (Catalogs, Portal, Index, Links)

Aside from the major sites mentioned above, there are many other useful Web sites maintained by individuals, departments, government, or organizations around the world offering information on bioinformatics. They provide a useful and sometimes extensive menu with links to important databases, search engines, molecular biology, software, tools, education, and conferences. The following are some good examples:

> www.sdsc.edu/ResTools/biotools/biotools4.html
> www.cmgm.stanford.edu/~plf58/page4.html
> http://info.er.usgs.gov/network/science/biology/index.html (US Geological Survey)

www.public.iastate.edu/~pedro/research_tools.html
www.genome.ad.jp/dbget/dbget.links.html (Japan)
www.infobiogen.fr/services/dbcat (Catalogs of databases, France)
http://biochem.kaist.ac.kr/bioinformatics.html
http://www2.nchc.gov.tw/~c00chh00/bioinfo.html (Taiwan)
www.yk.rim.or.jp/~aisoai/index.html (Japan)
http://biobase.dk/cgi-bin/celis (Denmark)

8   EDUCATION SITES IN BIOINFORMATICS

As this field continues to expand, so do the courses offering education in bioinformatics. The number of courses offered has grown exponentially over the past 2–3 years. As discussed by Altman (A Curriculum for Bioinformatics: The Time Is Ripe, Bioinformatics 14:549–550, 1998; see http://www-smi.stanford.edu/pubs/SMI_Reports/SMI-98-0744.pdf), there are two basic models for instruction. In the first model, students with either a biology or computer science background, enter the program to train in computational biology. Depending on the program, one can emerge as a "computer scientist who specializes in biology" or a "biologist who specializes in computer science." This allows individuals with either background to enter into a given program and emerge with a relatively even level of expertise in both biology and computer science, or a special emphasis in one. In the second model, students enter into the bioinformatics/computational biology program without a background in either biology or computer science. This may be at the undergraduate (see University of Waterloo, undergraduate degree in bioinformatics, http://www.cs.uwaterloo.ca/undergrad/current/BioInfo.html/) or graduate school training levels. To make training programs complete, topics should optimally include biology, computer science, statistics, and bioinformatics. Altman (cited above) recommends addition of an ethics component as well.

In many of these programs, the molecular biology training includes genetics and biochemistry as they relate to protein structure and function. These would include an analysis of the characteristics of gene regulatory regions, coding and noncoding sequences in a gene, and typical characteristics of functional domains in proteins. Specific bioinformatics topics include computational methods in molecular biology. Types of analyses that the students learn include finding genes and gene control regions in a sequence, phylogenetic trees, alignment of sequences, secondary and tertiary structure predictions, and finding features and domains in proteins. In some of these programs, prerequisites may include programming skills (Perl, C++, Unix) and math (matrix mathematics, linear algebra, calculus). (For example, the Stanford Center for Professional Development Clinical and Bio Informatics Short Course prerequisites (http://scpd.stanford.edu/smiseries/racmb.html) or the University of Southern California Professional Master of Science in Computational Molecular Biology requirements (http://www-hto.

usc.edu/compbiomasters/admission.html) for typical course prerequisites and instructional topics.) Students entering a program without a computer science background need courses in programming and data structures/algorithms among others. Statistics courses would be expected to include probability theory, experimental statistical design and analysis, and stochastic processes (Altman, 1998). With the appropriate prerequisites/courses under his/her belt, the student is ready to tackle topics such as optimization, dynamic programming algorithms for alignment of biological sequences, cluster analysis, neural networks, and Bayesian inference.

As of the time of writing of this chapter (spring 2000), a number of educational institutions have started to offer degree-based programs in addition to short courses. Both web-based and traditional classroom style courses are available to choose from. As mentioned above, a professional master of science in computational molecular biology is given by the University of Southern California (http://www.hto.usc.edu/compbiomasters/admission.html). In addition, distance learning options (with or without a degree) are increasingly available. These include the Virtual School of Natural Sciences at the University of Bielefeld, Germany (http://www.techfak.uni-bielefeld.de/bcd/welcome.html); courses on distant homologies, motifs, patterns and profiles at the International Centre for Genetic Engineering and Biotechnology, Trieste, Italy (http://www.icgeb.trieste.it/net/courseware/Title.htm); biocomputing and bioinformatics at the University of Manchester, England (http://mbisg4.sbc.man.ac.uk:8900/index.html); the Virtual school of molecular sciences at the University of Nottingham, England (http://www.vsms.nottingham.ac.uk/vsms/biotools/index.html); bioinformatics at the Universite de Paris, France (http://www.citi2fr/bio2/biocours/intro.html); and the Stanford Clinical and Bio Informatics short course series online (http://scpd.stanford.edu/smiseries/racmb.html).

Computational biology/bioinformatics programs are now offered at over 50 institutions worldwide, including the W.M. Keck Center for Computational Biology (Pennsylvania and Texas), the Department of Molecular Biotechnology (University of Washington, Seattle), Waterloo University (Ontario, Canada), Stanford University (California), MIT (Massachusetts), the Pasteur Institute (France), Oxford University (England), the Weizmann Institute of Science (Israel), and many others. Virtually every continent has bioinformatic courses available. To attempt a "complete" inventory of such courses/programs would be hopeless since they are expanding and changing every day. The reader is instead referred to the Web-based lists of courses that have been compiled by organizations such as the International Society for Computational Biology, as shown below.

List of bioinformatics/computational biology courses and degree programs compiled by the International Society for Computational Biology (http://www.iscb.org/univ.html)

List of bioinformatics courses compiled at Rockefeller University (http://linkage.rockefeller.edu/wli/bioinfocourse.html)

List of bioinformatics courses compiled at the University of Bielefeld (http://www.techfak.uni-bielefeld.de/bcd/Curric/syllabi.html)

List of bioinformatics courses compiled at the University of Texas (http://biotech.icmb.utexas.edu/pages/bioinform/biprograms us.html)

9 COMMON COMPUTER AND INFORMATION TECHNOLOGY TOOLS AND TERMINOLOGY

9.1 Bandwidth

The measure of telecommunication link capacity. The broader the bandwidth, the more information can be transmitted within a time unit. The industry is looking toward low-cost broad bandwidth connections. University offices and laboratories generally have fast connections via T1 lines. For many families, the final connection to the computer via phone lines is generally the limiting factor for fast information transmission. Cable and DSL connection are changing the scenario for some homes. New apartment buildings in some countries now have built-in fiber-optic connections offering broad bandwidth Internet connections.

9.2 Bioinformatics

The use of computer tools for the acquisition, management, and analysis of biological information, incorporating elements of molecular biology, computational biology, and database computing. The Internet and WWW resources play an important part in bioinformatics.

9.3 Browsers

Browsers are software tools designed for browsing Internet and WWW information. Popular browsers include Internet Explorer and Netscape; both are free and downloadable from the Web. Browsers carry with them different features or capabilities. As many Web sites now require advanced features that are only found in the later editions of the browsers, it is advisable to update the browser periodically. Some HTML codes and Java applets are also not supported by some browsers.

9.4 CGI(Common Gateway Interface)

CGI is a protocol, not a language. It is the common way browsers communicate with Web servers.

9.5 CGI Scripts

These are scripts written in some form of languages (usually but not necessary Perl) for server communication.

9.6 Client

The user's computer visiting a server hosting the information is referred to as the client.

9.7 Compilers

A computer does not read human language. Programming languages (codes) are invented by humans to instruct the computer to carry out jobs. A compiler translates codes of a computer programming language into machine language before execution. Some computer languages, such as C and C++, need to be compiled before execution. Some are directly interpreted without compiling. Java is a compiled and interpreted language while Perl is an interpreted language.

9.8 Computer Operation System

Operation system (OS) is the system that runs the computer and determines its capabilities. The common OSs include Microsoft's Windows and Windows NT, Apple's OS, and the UNIX/LINUS operation system. As UNIX is designed for multiuser multitasking, many bioinformatic databases run on UNIX platforms.

9.9 Computer Programming Languages

Computer languages are instructions or codes written according to language specification of the language to direct the computer to perform certain tasks. Common modern programming languages include C, C++, and Java. Perl in particular is the common computer languages for bioinformatic applications. Scripting languages such as Java Scripts are not traditionally referred to as programming languages. They are generally smaller and perform smaller, specific functions.

9.10 HTML

HTML stands for Hypertext Markup Language. It is the native language of the Web. HTML is like a text/typing instruction set; documents written in HTML are interpretable by browsers. Web pages written in HTML when browsed through browsers will take their final form as the pages seen on screen. Hypertext, a form of electronic cross-reference, also makes information interactive and links Web documents. The reader may jump from topic to topic unhindered by geography. Browsers do not support all HTML codes the same way, and some browsers do not support certain HTML codes.

9.11 Internet Connections

There are many choices for establishing an Internet connection. Depending on your geographic location and budget, connections varying from slow to fast, with increasing bandwidth: Telephone lines → ISDN/DSL → cable → T1 → T3 → fiber optics. Wireless connections are by satellites and other wireless transmission technology. Portable phones in some countries are now Internet capable.

9.12 Java Applets and Applications

Java applets are small programs written in Java codes developed by SUN Microsystems, which could be deployed over the Internet to the users' computers and viewed within an HTML page. Java applications are formal computer programs written in Java codes but are standalone programs not requiring a browser to run.

9.13 Perl

Perl is an acronym for Practical Extraction and Reporting Language. It is an interpreted language developed by Larry Wall in 1986. It consists of various UNIX tools, shell scripting, C, and occasional OOP features. Perl is a powerful text (string, arrays, lists) and pattern manipulation tool. It is cross-platform and portable. These attributes make it a suitable language for data manipulation and genetic research. There are many uses for WWW interactivity (processing forms, guestbooks, counting visits), and Perl has been generally accepted as the standard for writing CGI scripts and Web server maintenance. Some Perl terminology encountered in bioinformatics includes scalars ($, a piece of data, constant or variable), arrays (@, collection of scalars), and hashes (%, collection of scalar in pairs).

9.14 Server

Servers are simply computers handling requests for information.

9.15 Site, Web Page, Home Page

Web pages are pages residing on servers around the world and are accessible through the Internet. Site is a collection of pages, indexed by its Internet address. Home page is the central or first page of the collection of pages of a site. Web page is a single page of the file to display on the screen.

9.16 TCP/IP

This is the telecommunications protocol for the Internet independent of the connecting computer's platform or OS.

16

Applied Bioinformatics

David L. Hyndman
Hitachi Chemical Research Center, Irvine, California

Masato Mitsuhashi
Hitachi Chemical Research Center and University of California, Irvine,
Irvine, California

1 INTRODUCTION

Bioinformatics is the use of computers for the storage or analysis of biological information. With the explosive growth of the Internet, the low cost of fast personal computers, and the enormous amounts of genetic sequence information that have become available, bioinformatics has probably touched everyone who does biological research. From the most humble use, such as simply retrieving a gene sequence from GenBank, to the most complex, such as data mining, successful research in biology will depend on the ability to use computer technology.

From the earliest uses of computers, most applications primarily took advantage of the calculating speed of computers to make tasks possible that could not otherwise be practically done. With many bioinformatics functions this is the underlying power. In recent years, however, several other aspects of computer technology have become useful in bioinformatics. Not the least of these is the ability of computers to communicate and transfer information, as exemplified by the Internet. Another useful function is the ability to make three-dimensional (3D) representations of chemical structures for the analysis of molecular function. Finally, what may eventually become the most powerful aspect of computer technology is the development of computers that can make decisions of the type hitherto made only by human beings. Generally referred to as artificial intelligence, these technologies may one day do much of the work that currently must be done by scientists.

In this chapter we summarize the basic concepts and applications of bioinformatics. We discuss the various forms of biological information and many types of software for analysis and manipulation of this information. We discuss particular software products for many bioinformatics applications and where to find these programs. So, with a general understanding of the available resources and possibilities of bioinformatics, biological scientists will more effectively be able to utilize these technologies.

2 TYPES OF BIOLOGICAL INFORMATION

Biological information can come in many forms. Some of these forms are easily stored and manipulated by computers, such as genetic sequence data. Other forms of information, however, are not as easily analyzed or manipulated by computers. These include biochemical pathway knowledge and experimental results from the scientific literature. Until now, these latter types of information have not been incorporated into any practical software, although there are current efforts to do exactly that.

2.1 Sequence Data

Sequence data are data which can be stored as a linear two-dimensional (2D) sequence. This is primarily limited to DNA/RNA sequence and protein sequence data.

2.2 GenBank and Other Public Sequence Databases

GenBank is the database administered by NCBI (the National Center for Biotechnology Information) that contains all publicly available DNA and RNA sequences. Protein sequences are included as derivatives of the DNA or RNA sequences. EMBL, the European Molecular Biology Laboratory, and DDBJ, the DNA Database of Japan, are similar public databases. These three centers accept submissions of sequences and exchange data daily so that the same sequence data is available from all three. The discussion of genetic sequence databases here will primarily focus on GenBank.

2.3 GenBank Divisions

The sequences in GenBank are put into one of 16 divisions. Originally all the divisions were made along taxonomic lines, such as primates or bacteria, but now several other divisions have been added which are defined by the experimental means in which the sequences have been determined. The taxonomic divisions contain sequences that are of high quality and generally have some annotation with regard to function. The other divisions contain sequences that often contain errors, and so researchers should not depend on the accuracy of those sequences. A list of the divisions are shown in Table 1.

The largest GenBank division is the Expressed Sequence Tag database (dbEST). dbEST contains data from "single-pass" cDNA sequences from a number of organisms. At the time of writing, there are 2,903,395 sequences with 1,114,300,950 base pairs of sequence in this category.

dbSTS sequences are Sequence Tagged Sites, which are short genomic landmark sequences used for mapping the genome.

The Genome Survey Sequences database (dbGSS) is similar to dbEST except that the sequences are genomic in origin. These may be, but are not limited to, cosmid/BAC/YAC end sequences, exon-trapped genomic sequences, or Alu sequences.

TABLE 1 GenBank Divisions

Division	Entries	Bases	Description
PRI	103,447	538,441,557	Primate sequence entries
ROD	48,993	71,658,191	Rodent sequence entries
MAM	20,142	18,365,645	Other mammalian sequence entries
VRT	30,591	29,290,899	Other vertebrate sequence entries
INV	48,880	171,282,436	Invertebrate sequence entries
PLN	138,410	50,175,564	Plant sequence entries (including fungi and algae)
BCT	64,198	153,577,633	Bacterial sequence entries
VRL	74,084	66,195,702	Viral sequence entries
PHG	1,458	3,509,472	Phage sequence entries
PAT	134,494	41,728,002	Patent sequence entries
SYN	3,425	8,076,054	Synthetic and chimeric sequence entries
UNA	491	371,508	Unannotated sequence entries
EST	2,903,395	1,114,300,950	EST (expressed sequence tag) sequence entries
GSS	1,008,904	518,917,227	GSS (genome survey sequence) sequence entries
HTG	3,573	433,486,687	HTGS (high throughput genomic sequencing) sequence entries
STS	83,056	29,543,013	STS (sequence tagged site) sequence entries

The High-Throughput Genomic Sequences database (dbHTS) contains sequences generated by high-throughput sequencing projects.

2.4 Sequence File Formats

Each GenBank sequence entry contains a contiguous sequence of DNA or RNA. There are three generally used formats for displaying DNA or RNA sequence data. One common format is the GenBank Flat File Format (GBFF), as shown in Table 2, and is used by GenBank as well as the DNA Database of Japan. The EMBL flat file format, used by EMBL, is shown in Table 3. Another common format is the FASTA format, shown in Table 4.

2.5 Parts of a GenBank File Format Entry

The GBFF can be separated into three parts. The Header gives information about the entry as a whole. The Features section describes parts of the sequence that have a particular function or property, and the Sequence section gives the actual sequence itself.

2.5.1 Header

The first item of information for the entry is the LOCUS. This is a unique identifier for the sequence entry. Originally this was designed to indicate the name of the organism and the gene, but because of many redundant entries for the same genes, the LOCUS is often meaningless. The length of the sequence in base pairs is shown after the LOCUS on the first line. The next piece of information is the type of molecule sequenced. This is usually DNA or RNA, but sometimes mRNA, tRNA, rRNA, or uRNA. After that is the GenBank division, as discussed above, and finally the date of the submission.

The second line contains the sequence definition, which usually is the gene name or gene product name. Some sequences may contain the descriptions "complete cds" or "partial cds," but these annotations have not been used consistently.

The third line contains the accession number. The accession number is the same among the three major gene sequence depositories and is the most reliable way to identify a sequence.

Other header information includes the organism from which the sequence was derived and the journals in which it was published.

2.5.2 Features

The Features section indicates portions of the sequence which contain some property. Features include nucleic acid regions of functionality, such as promoters; the region coding for protein (CDS); and amino acid sequence regions with func-

TABLE 2 Example of a GenBank Flat File Format (GBFF) Record

LOCUS   HUMCFTR10   203 bp   DNA   PRI   01-NOV-1994
DEFINITION   Human cystic fibrosis transmembrane conductance regulator
   (CFTR) gene, exon 10.
ACCESSION   M55034
NID   g180298
VERSION   M55034.1   GI:180298
KEYWORDS   cystic fibrosis; transmembrane conductance regulator.
SOURCE   Human DNA.
   ORGANISM   Homo sapiens
      Eukaryota; Metazoa; Chordata; Craniata; Vertebrata; Mammalia;
      Eutheria; Primates; Catarrhini; Hominidae; Homo.
REFERENCE   1 (bases 1 to 203)
   AUTHORS   Kerem, B.-S., Zielenski, J., Markiewicz, D., Bozon, D., Gazit,
      E., Yahav, J., Kennedy, D., Riordan, J.R., Collins, F.S., Rommens,
      J.M. and Tsui, L.-C.
   TITLE   Identification of mutations in regions corresponding to the two
      putative nucleotide (ATP)-binding folds of the cystic fibrosis gene
   JOURNAL   Proc. Natl. Acad. Sci. U.S.A. 87 (21), 8447–8451 (1990)
   MEDLINE   91046014
FEATURES   Location/Qualifiers
      source   1..203
            /organism = "Homo sapiens"
            /db_xref = "taxon: 9606"
            /map = "7q31–q32"
      exon   8..199
            /gene = "CFTR"
            /note = "G00-120-584; putative"
            / number = 10
      gene   8..199
            /gene = "CFTR"
      mutation   130..131
            /gene = "CFTR"
            /note = "G00-120-584; putative"
            /replace = "tatca"
BASE COUNT   66 a   34 c   43 g   60 t
ORIGIN   Chromosome 7q31–q32.
        1 tttccagact tcacttctaa tgatgattat gggagaactg gagccttcag agggtaaaat
       61 taagcacagt ggaagaattt cattctgttc tcagttttcc tggattatgc ctggcaccat
      121 taaagaaaat atctttggtg tttcctatga tgaatataga tacagaagcg tcatcaaagc
      181 atgccaacta gaagaggtaa gaa
//

TABLE 3 Example of an EMBL Formatted Record

ID HSCFTR10 standard; DNA; HUM; 203 BP.
XX
AC M55034;
XX
SV M55034.1
XX
DT 16-JAN-1991 (Rel. 26, Created)
DT 02-JUL-1999 (Rel. 60, Last updated, Version 4)
XX
DE Human cystic fibrosis transmembrane conductance regulator (CFTR)
DE gene, exon 10.
XX
KW cystic fibrosis; transmembrane conductance regulator.
XX
OS Homo sapiens (human)
OC Eukaryota; Metazoa; Chordata; Craniata; Vertebrata; Mammalia;
    Eutheria;
OC Primates; Catarrhini; Hominidae; Homo.
XX
RN (1)
RP 1-203
RX MEDLINE; 91046014.
RA Kerem B.-S., Zielenski J., Markiewicz D., Bozon D., Gazit E., Yahav J.,
RA Kennedy D., Riordan J.R., Collins F.S., Rommens J.M., Tsui L.-C.;
RT "Identification of mutations in regions corresponding to the two
    putative
RT nucleotide (ATP)-binding folds of the cystic fibrosis gene";
RL Proc. Natl. Acad. Sci. U.S.A. 87(21):8447-8451 (1990).
XX
DR GDB; 120584; CFTR.
XX
FH Key   Location/Qualifiers
FH
FT source   1..203
FT   /db_xref = "taxon:9606"
FT   /organism = "Homo sapiens"
FT   /map = "7q31-q32"
FT exon   8..199
FT   /note = "G00-120-584; putative"
FT   /number = 10
FT   /gene = "CFTR"
FT gene   8..199
FT   /gene = "CFTR"

TABLE 3 Continued

```
FT   mutation      130..131
FT              /note = "G00-120-584; putative"
FT              /replace = "tatca"
FT              /gene = "CFTR"
XX
SQ   Sequence 203 BP; 66 A; 34 C; 43 G; 60 T; 0 other;
     tttccagact tcacttctaa tgatgattat gggagaactg gagccttcag agggtaaaat   60
     taagcacagt ggaagaattt cattctgttc tcagttttcc tggattatgc ctggcaccat   120
     taaagaaaat atctttggtg tttcctatga tgaatataga tacagaagcg tcatcaaagc   180
     atgccaacta gaagaggtaa gaa                       203
//
```

---

tional features, such as a signal peptide. A complete list of features are shown in Table 5.

2.5.3 Sequence

After the Features section, the Sequence itself follows the line with the word ORIGIN. The Sequence contains the standard IUPAC characters for nucleotides. Note that u (for uracil) is never used, but rather t (for thymidine), even when the Sequence is an RNA sequence. The standard characters are listed in Table 6.

2.6 Unigene Databases

Due to the redundancy found in several of the databases, NCBI has created Unigene databases for human, mouse, and rat gene sequences. In these databases, all sequences are clustered such that all sequences for the same gene are in the same cluster. The Unigene databases will contain sequences from dbEST, dbHTG, dbGSS, and dbSTS in addition to the annotated sequences from the Primate and Rodent divisions. A unique sequence database is available that contains the most reliable sequence from each cluster. The Unigene databases can be accessed on the Internet at following Web site (http://www.ncbi.nlm.nih.gov/Unigene).

2.7 Complete Genomes

Some complete genomes have been sequenced and are available for download from GenBank. At the time of writing, available complete genomes include yeast, 18 bacteria, and several viruses. The available complete genomes can be downloaded over the Internet from ftp://ncbi.nlm.nih.gov/genbank/genomes. Also

TABLE 4 Example of a FASTA Formatted Record

>gi | 180298 | gb | M55034.1 | HUMCFTR10 Human cystic fibrosis transmembrane conductance regulator (CFTR)
gene, exon 10
TTTCCAGACTTCACTTCTAATGATGATTATGGGAGAACTGGAGCCTTCAGAGGGTAAAATTAAGCACAGT
GGAAGAATTTCATTCTGTTCTCAGTTTCCTGGATTATGCCTGGCACCATTAAGAAGAAATATCTTTGGTG
TTTCCTATGATGAATATAGATACAGAAGCGTCATCAAGCATGCCAACTAGAGAGGTAAGAA

available are partial genomes of *C. elegans*, *Drosophila*, mice, rats, and humans.

2.8 Single-Nucleotide Polymorphism Database

The Single-Nucleotide Polymorphism database (dbSNP) began in September 1999 as a central repository of data for single-nucleotide variations as well as short deletion and insertion polymorphisms. At the time of writing, the database contains 21,134 entries. The database can be searched in various ways or can be used for a BLAST search. In addition to the sequence, dbSNP also contains information for assaying for the given allele and the use of a given SNP with individuals and populations. The Web site for dbSNP is www.ncbi.nlm.nih.gov/SNP.

3 RETRIEVING SEQUENCES

The starting point for searching GenBank on the Internet is the NCBI World Wide Web site at www.ncbi.nlm.nih.gov/GenBank/GenBankSearch.html. From this site, you can access the Entrez retrieval system, the ftp server, and information regarding the e-mail server system.

3.1 Entrez

Entrez is a system for retrieving GenBank sequence data via the world wide web. Entrez provides a web interface for finding GenBank entries using various types of search criteria such as Accession number, keyword, organism, author, etc. The Entrez web site is www.ncbi.nlm.nih.gov/Entrez/nucleotide.html.

Entrez also has a batch search function in which the user may do many searches, or a single search with many matches, and download the results sequences to a file on a local computer hard drive. For example, batch searches can save all sequences for a given organism. The web page for the Entrez batch search is at www.ncbi.nlm.nih.gov/Entrez/batch.html.

3.2 Ftp Server

The GenBank flat files can be downloaded from the ftp server at ftp://ncbi.nlm.nih.gov/genbank. All of the various GenBank divisions are divided into individual files, or multiple files when the size of the data exceeds 250 megabytes. The files are given the *.Z file extension, which means that they are compressed, and can be decompressed with the WinZip program or some other decompression utility.

3.3 E-mail Server

An easy way to retrieve many different sequences is through the GenBank e-mail server. Queries can be sent to NCBI via e-mail and the results will be sent

TABLE 5   Feature Key Words in GenBank Flat File Records

allele	Related strain contains alternative gene form
attenuator	Sequence related to transcription termination
C_region	Span of the C immunological feature
CAAT_signal	'CAAT box' in eukaryotic promoters
CDS	Sequence coding for amino acids in protein (includes stop codon)
conflict	Independent sequence determinations differ
D-loop	Displacement loop
D_segment	Span of the D immunological feature
enhancer	Cis-acting enhancer of promoter function
exon	Region that codes for part of spliced mRNA
gene	Region that defines a functional gene, possibly including upstream (promotor, enhancer, etc) and downstream control elements, and for which a name has been assigned.
GC_signal	'GC box' in eukaryotic promoters
iDNA	Intervening DNA eliminated by recombination
intron	Transcribed region excised by mRNA splicing
J_region	Span of the J Immunological feature
LTR	Long terminal repeat
mat_peptide	Mature peptide coding region (does not include stop codon)
misc_binding	Miscellaneous binding site
misc_difference	Miscellaneous difference feature
misc_feature	Region of biological significance that cannot be described by any other feature
misc_recomb	Miscellaneous recombination feature
misc_RNA	Miscellaneous transcript feature not defined by other RNA keys
misc_signal	Miscellaneous signal
misc_structure	Miscellaneous DNA or RNA structure
modified_base	The indicated base is a modified nucleotide
mRNA	Messenger RNA
mutation	A mutation alters the sequence here
N_region	Span of the N immunological feature
old_sequence	Presented sequence revises a previous version
polyA_signal	Signal for cleavage & polyadenylation
polyA_site	Site at which polyadenine is added to mRNA
precursor_RNA	Any RNA species that is not yet the mature RNA product
prim_transcript	Primary (unprocessed) transcript
primer	Primer binding region used with PCR
primer_bind	Non-covalent primer binding site

TABLE 5   Continued

promoter	A region involved in transcription initiation
protein_bind	Non-covalent protein binding site on DNA or RNA
RBS	Ribosome binding site
rep_origin	Replication origin for duplex DNA
repeat_region	Sequence containing repeated subsequences
repeat_unit	One repeated unit of a repeat_region
rRNA	Ribosomal RNA
S_region	Span of the S immunological feature
satellite	Satellite repeated sequence
scRNA	Small cytoplasmic RNA
sig_peptide	Signal peptide coding region
snRNA	Small nuclear RNA
source	Biological source of the sequence data represented by a GenBank record. Mandatory feature, one or more per record.
	For organisms that have been incorporated within the NCBI taxonomy database, an associated /db_xref = "taxon:NNNN" qualifier will be present (where NNNNN is the numeric identifier assigned to the organism within the taxon database).
stem_loop	Hair-pin loop structure in DNA or RNA
STS	Sequence Tagged Site; operationally unique sequence that identifies the combination of primer spans used in a PCR assay
TATA_signal	'TATA box' in eukaryotic promoters
terminator	Sequence causing transcription termination
transit_peptide	Transit peptide coding region
transposon	Transposable element (TN)
tRNA	Transfer RNA
unsure	Authors are unsure about the sequence in this region
V_region	Span of the V immunological feature
variation	A related population contains stable mutation
-(hyphen)	Placeholder
-10_signal	'Pribnow box' in prokaryotic promoters
-35_signal	'-35 box' in prokaryotic promoters
3'clip	3'-most region of a precursor transcript removed in processing
3'UTR	3' untranslated region (trailer)
5'clip	5'-most region of a precursor transcript removed in processing
5'UTR	5' untranslated region (leader)

TABLE 6 IUPAC Codes

Character	Meaning
A	adenosine
C	cytidine
G	guanine
T	thymidine/uracil
R	G or A (purine)
Y	T or C (pyrimidine)
K	G or T (keto)
W	A or T (weak)
M	A or C (amino)
S	G or C (strong)
D	G, A, or T
B	G, T, or C
H	A, C, or T
V	G, C, or A
N	A, G, C, or T (any)

back to the user's e-mail address. This can be done for sequence retrieval as well as BLAST searches. For instructions on sending queries, refer to the Web page www.ncbi.nlm.nih.gov/GenBank/GenBankEmail.html.

3.4 Other Database Web Sites

EMBL can be accessed from www.ebi.ac.uk/embl/index.html, and DDBJ can be access from www.ddbj.nig.ac.jp.

4 OTHER TYPES OF BIOLOGICAL INFORMATION

4.1 Swiss-Prot

SWISS-PROT is a curated protein sequence database which has been maintained by the Swiss Institute of Bioinformatics and is available through subscription from Geneva Bioinformatics (www.genebio.com). The SWISS-PROT database is well annotated with respect to functions of proteins, domains, structures, and any posttranslational modifications. SWISS-PROT has tried to merge redundant data that may be found in other databases to reduce redundancy in the database.

4.2 3D Structural Data

PDB is a Protein Data Bank that contains 3-dimensional macromolecular structure data primarily determined by X-ray crystallography and NMR. PDB is organized by the Research Collaboratory for Structural Bioinformatics (RCSB). In addition to protein structures, RNA, DNA and other 3D structures are also stored in the database. The database can be searched and structures and sequences can be retrieved. The Web site is www.rcsb.org/pdb.

MMDB is the Molecular Modeling Database and is maintained by the NCBI structure group. MMDB contains macromolecular 3D structures, as well as tools for visualization and comparative analysis. The database contains experimentally determined biopolymer structures obtained from the Protein Data Bank (PDB). MMDB can be accessed on the Web at www.ncbi.nlm.nih.gov/Structure/MMDB/mmdb.shtml.

4.3 3D Structure Software

Cn3D, NCBI's software for viewing 3D structures can be downloaded from NCBI's Web site and used to view structures from MMDB. Other software for viewing 3D structures are MAGE and RasMol. Structure files in all three formats are available for downloading from MMDB.

VAST 3D Comparison Software can find 3D structures that are similar to a given query structure. For all structures in MMDB, this analysis has already been done and neighbors (i.e., similar structures) have been identified. For newly determined 3D structures that are not already in the MMDB database, the VAST search service can be used to identify neighbors.

4.4 Taxonomy Database

The Taxonomy database is accessible from the NCBI web page at www.ncbi.nlm.nih.gov/Taxonomy/tax.html. This database contains a tree with every species for which at least one nucleic acid or protein sequence has been submitted.

4.5 TRANSFAC Database

The Transcription Factor Database (TRANSFAC) is a database of eukaryotic cis-acting regulatory DNA elements and trans-acting factors [1]. TRANSFAC contains entries for the DNA sequence of the sites themselves, for the transcription factors, and for the genes in which they are found. It can be accessed through www.cbi.pku.edu.cn/TRANSFAC.

4.6 HOVERGEN

HOVERGEN [2] is a database of homologous vertebrate genes. HOVERGEN allows a user to easily select sets of homologous genes from a given set of vertebrate species. This is particularly useful for comparative sequence analysis, phylogeny, and molecular evolution studies. HOVERGEN can be downloaded, but the software to view it can currently only run on a UNIX X-WINDOWS system. However, some of the functions can be accessed from the web page at pbil.univ lyon1.fr/databases/hovergen.html.

4.7 Online Mendelian Inheritance in Man

The Online Mendelian Inheritance in Man (OMIM) is a catalog of human genes and genetic disorders authored and edited by Dr. Victor A. McKusick and his colleagues at Johns Hopkins and elsewhere. The database is accessible at NCBI's Web site (www.ncbi.nlm.nih.gov/omim) and contains textual information, pictures and reference information.

4.8 Medline

PubMed, the publicly accessible Web version of Medline is available through the NCBI web site at www.ncbi.nlm.nih.gov/PubMed.

5 BIOINFORMATICS SOFTWARE

The storage and retrieval of biological information are valuable functions for the biologist. It is, however, the software that is used to analyze the data that is the most valuable aspect of bioinformatics. The strategies and methods used within computer software to complete specific tasks are referred to as algorithms. The development of algorithms for solving biological problems is referred to as computational biology. It is from the area of computational biology that the job of the biologist will be greatly enhanced and changed in years to come.

5.1 Homology Analysis

Homology is the characteristic of a group of genes that are descended from a common ancestor. Through a pairwise comparison of two DNA or amino acid sequences, the homology analysis is meant to determine whether the sequences are homologous and, if so, how closely related they are.

An alignment is a matching of a position of one sequence with a position of another sequence. An optimal alignment is that alignment in which the greatest similarities are found. A given alignment can be assigned a homology score, which is a measure of the degree of similarity. A simple system for calculating a homology score would be a match/mismatch scheme in which every match is given the same value and every mismatch, or every gap, is given the same penalty. In analyzing the similarity of two proteins, however, a substitution matrix is generally used in which specific amino acid substitutions are assigned specific penalty values [3,4]. Because certain amino acid substitutions are well tolerated, a

	A	B	C	D	E	F	G	H	I	K	L	M	N	P	Q	R	S	T	V	W	Y	Z
A	2	0	-2	0	0	-4	1	-1	-1	-1	-2	-1	0	1	0	-2	1	1	0	-6	-3	0
B	0	2	-4	3	2	-5	0	1	-2	1	-3	-2	2	-1	1	-1	0	0	-2	-5	-3	2
C	-2	-4	12	-5	-5	-4	-3	-3	-2	-5	-6	-5	-4	-3	-5	-4	0	-2	-2	-8	0	-5
D	0	3	-5	4	3	-6	1	1	-2	0	-4	-3	2	-1	2	-1	0	0	-2	-7	-4	3
E	0	2	-5	3	4	-5	0	1	-2	0	-3	-2	1	-1	2	-1	0	0	-2	-7	-4	3
F	-4	-5	-4	-6	-5	9	-5	-2	1	-5	2	0	-4	-5	-5	-4	-3	-3	-1	0	7	-5
G	1	0	-3	1	0	-5	5	-2	-3	-2	-4	-3	0	-1	-1	-3	1	0	-1	-7	-5	-1
H	-1	1	-3	1	1	-2	-2	6	-2	0	-2	-2	2	0	3	2	-1	-1	-2	-3	0	2
I	-1	-2	-2	-2	-2	1	-3	-2	5	-2	2	2	-2	-2	-2	-2	-1	0	4	-5	-1	-2
K	-1	1	-5	0	0	-5	-2	0	-2	5	-3	0	1	-1	1	3	0	0	-2	-3	-4	0
L	-2	-3	-6	-4	-3	2	-4	-2	2	-3	6	4	-3	-3	-2	-3	-3	-2	2	-2	-1	-3
M	-1	-2	-5	-3	-2	0	-3	-2	2	0	4	6	-2	-2	-1	0	-2	-1	2	-4	-2	-2
N	0	2	-4	2	1	-4	0	2	-2	1	-3	-2	2	-1	1	0	1	0	-2	-4	-2	1
P	1	-1	-3	-1	-1	-5	-1	0	-2	-1	-3	-2	-1	6	0	0	1	0	-1	-6	-5	0
Q	0	1	-5	2	2	-5	-1	3	-2	1	-2	-1	1	0	4	1	-1	-1	-2	-5	-4	3
R	-2	-1	-4	-1	-1	-4	-3	2	-2	3	-3	0	0	0	1	6	0	-1	-2	2	-4	0
S	1	0	0	0	0	-3	1	-1	-1	0	-3	-2	1	1	-1	0	2	1	-1	-2	-3	0
T	1	0	-2	0	0	-3	0	-1	0	0	-2	-1	0	0	-1	-1	1	3	0	-5	-3	-1
V	0	-2	-2	-2	-2	-1	-1	-2	4	-2	2	2	-2	-1	-2	-2	-1	0	4	-6	-2	-2
W	-6	-5	-8	-7	-7	0	-7	-3	-5	-3	-2	-4	-4	-6	-5	2	-2	-5	-6	17	0	-6
Y	-3	-3	0	-4	-4	7	-5	0	-1	-4	-1	-2	-2	-5	-4	-4	-3	-3	-2	0	10	-4
Z	0	2	-5	3	3	-5	-1	2	-2	0	-3	-2	1	0	3	0	0	-1	-2	-6	-4	3

FIGURE 1   The PAM250 score matrix.

substitution matrix gives a more functionally significant scoring of homology. An example of a substitution matrix is shown in Figure 1.

The first widely used algorithm for homology analysis was the Needleman-Wunsch algorithm [5]. This algorithm used a programming technique referred to as dynamic programming to find the best global alignment between two sequences. Needleman-Wunsch allowed for the use of a substitution matrix to generate a homology score.

A very important alteration of the Needleman-Wunsch algorithm came with the Smith-Waterman algorithm [6]. Smith-Waterman was a modification of the Needleman-Wunsch algorithm that found the best local alignments, as opposed to the best global alignments. A local alignment is a local region of similarity that does not necessarily include all positions of the sequences. An optimal local alignment is one in which the score does not improve by either increasing or decreasing the extent of the alignment.

5.2 Similarity Searches

The work horse of bioinformatics is the similarity search, which can identify homologous genes within a genomic database. This is useful when a researcher has sequenced a new gene and wants insight into possible functions of the gene.

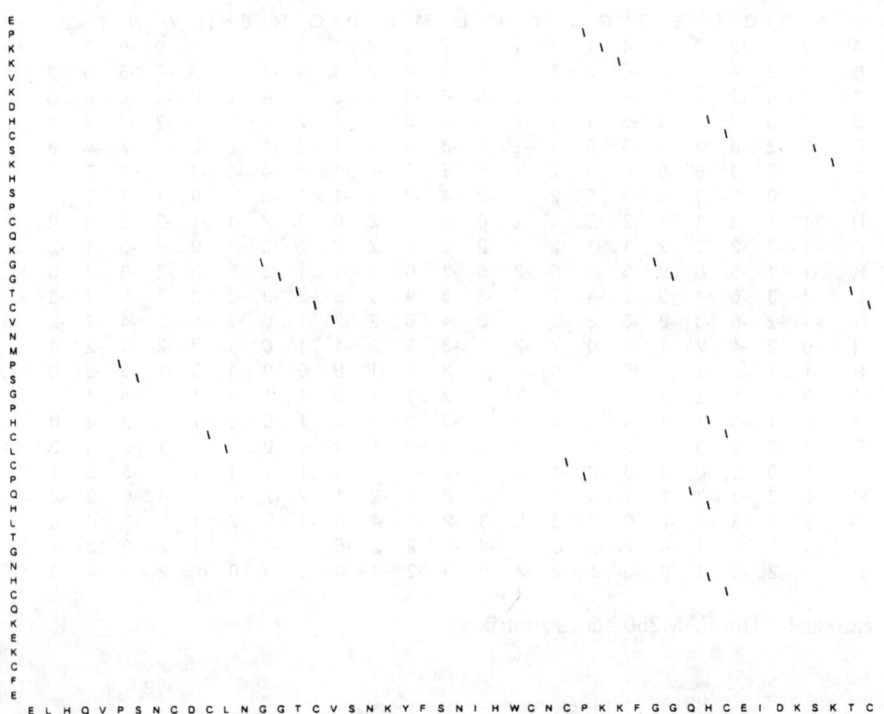

FIGURE 2 FASTA dot matrix comparison of human plasminogen activator and human urokinase plasminogen activator.

Because the Smith-Waterman algorithm is very computationally intensive, it would be prohibitively time-consuming to do such a search against the thousands or millions of sequences found in current genomic databases. So, more streamlined, heuristic methods had to be developed.

The first of these algorithms was FASTA, written by William Pearson and David Lipman [7]. With FASTA, you set a given length for which to find matching areas. This is called the k-tup. Then, a matrix is generated, as shown in Figure 2, in which areas of consecutive k-tup matches are shown. The best combination of nonoverlapping matches are combined and a preliminary score is determined. When good candidates are found, the Smith-Waterman algorithm is then applied to generate the optimal alignment and the homology score is calculated.

The next major algorithm for similarity searching after FASTA was the BLAST algorithm (Basic Local Alignment Search Tool) [8]. The original BLAST, though significantly faster than FASTA, was unable to find alignments that contained gaps (which FASTA can). In 1997, however, BLAST 2.0 became

TABLE 7 Types of Blast

Search type	Query type	Query translation	Comparison sequences	Comparison translation
blastp	Amino acid sequence	no	Proteins	no
blastn	Nucleotide sequence	no	Nucleotide sequences	no
blastx	Nucleotide sequence	yes	Proteins	no
tblastn	Amino acid sequence	no	Nucleotide sequences	yes
tblastx	Nucleotide sequence	yes	Nucleotide sequences	yes

available. BLAST 2.0 is claimed to be three times as fast as the original BLAST and now has the ability to find alignments with gaps.

One more additional BLAST function is PSI BLAST. This uses sequences from a first BLAST search to refine the search parameters for subsequent searches. This can allow the identification of more distantly related sequences that may not have been identified with regular BLAST.

5.3 Using BLAST

BLAST can be used on the NCBI web site to search all GenBank sequences. The web site is www.ncbi.nlm.nh.gov/BLAST. The user inputs either actual sequence or an accession number and selects the search database and the type of BLAST search (see below).

5.3.1 Types of BLAST

There are five different types of BLAST searches that can be done, and they are listed in Table 7. The first distinction is whether the query sequence is an amino acid sequence (blastp and tblastn) or a nucleotide sequence (blastn, blastx, or tblastx). If the query is a nucleotide sequence, the distinction must be made whether to use the nucleotide query sequence "as is" for comparison (blastn), or if the query sequence should be translated. Because translation can occur in three different frames on either of the two strands, six possible amino acid sequences are generated. The next distinction of the programs is with respect to the database. If an untranslated nucleotide sequence is used for the query (blastn), then the only possibility is to use the untranslated nucleotide database for the search. For the other cases in which the query is an amino acid sequence or is translated into amino acid sequence, the query can be either a protein sequence database (blastp, or blastx) or the six possible translations of the nucleotides sequences (tblastn or tblastx).

5.3.2 Genetic Code Selection

Advanced BLAST options allow the user to select the Genetic Codes that will be used for the translation of the query sequence (for blastx or tblastx.)

5.3.3 Matrix Selection

Several different substitution matrices can be used for weighting the different matches. As discussed earlier, a substitution matrix incorporates rules for the penalties assigned for different types of substitutions. Possible matrices are the following:

> PAM30
> PAM70
> BLOSSUM80
> BLOSSUM62
> BLOSSUM45

The difference between using the different matrices for a BLAST search is that some matrices are more suited for identifying closely related sequences while others are better for identifying more divergent sequences. For the PAM matrices, higher PAM values will identify sequences with greater divergence [9]. For the BLOSSUM matrices, higher BLOSSUM values are better for identifying more closely related sequences [4].

5.4 Hybridization Simulation

An analogous but unique use of genetic sequence data is in the identification of hybridizable sequences to a given candidate oligonucleotide probe. This algorithm, referred to as Hybridization Simulation [10], applies a thermodynamic hybridization model to calculate melting temperature or free energy of hybridization, rather than a substitution model as used by homology analysis programs. The HYBsimulator software, which incorporates the Hybridization Simulation algorithm, enables users to screen a list of candidate oligonucleotide sequences (probes or primers) against a GenBank database to determine where and to what degree these oligonucleotides will hybridize to nonspecific sequences. The software has been widely used to design specific probes, primers, and antisense oligonucleotides.

5.5 Multiple Sequence Alignment

Sometimes a researcher will have a group of related sequences and will wish to align the sequences together. This process can help to deduce a function of a new gene or to develop a hierachy or phylogenetic tree of the sequences to see which ones are more closely related. This is done by using a multiple sequence alignment (MSA) program.

5.5.1 CLUSTAL W

CLUSTAL W [11] is one of the most widely used multiple sequence alignment programs and is freely available on the World Wide Web (www2.ebi.ac.uk/clus talw). The algorithm starts by doing a pairwise alignment of all of the sequences against each other. The degree of divergence, or distance, is calculated for each pair. The distances between the different sequences are then used to create a phylogenetic tree. The tree is used to do pairwise alignments of the most closely related sequences. Then new sequences are added one at a time to expand the alignment.

5.5.2 MultAlin

MultAlin is another MSA algorithm based on building a phylogenetic tree from the results of pairwise alignments. It uses an iterative process of rebuilding the phylogenetic tree as sequences are added to the alignment. Results will differ from those of CLUSTAL W, though there is no consensus as to which algorithm is more accurate. MultAlin can be used on the Web at www.toulouse.inra.fr/multalin.html.

6 ANALYSIS OF A NEW SEQUENCE

When a new DNA or RNA sequence is determined, the biologist will look to bioinformatics to learn as much as possible about the sequence. If the sequence is genomic DNA, the researcher would like to identify the promoter sites or transcription factor-binding sites, the regions that would be transcribed into mRNA, and where the intron-exon splice sites are located. If the sequence is mRNA, the researcher would like to identify the open reading frame that encodes the protein. Having determined the amino acid sequence of a protein, the researcher may like to know if any closely related sequences are known or if there are any structural features or motifs that will give an indication of the function of the protein.

6.1 Database Searching

As mentioned earlier, the most commonly used technique for learning about new sequences is a database similarity search. If closely related sequences are identified, knowledge about these related sequences may provide insight into the function of the new sequence. A direct nucleotide similarity search of dbEST can also provide information. Since dbEST sequences are all derived from expressed mRNA, if the new sequence is found in dbEST, there will be information regarding the tissues or conditions in which the gene is expressed. Furthermore, if the new sequence is a genomic DNA sequence, intron-exon splice junctions might be identified.

6.2 Gene Prediction Programs

There are several programs for the identification of promoter regions, intron-exon splice sites, and transcriptional stop sites of new genomic DNA sequences. Algorithms vary from simply using codon usage tables and examining codon bias to identifying homology to known sequence motifs to artificial intelligence techniques such as Hidden Markov Models or neural networks.

GRAIL [12] is a well-known program for identifying the genes in naked DNA sequence. GRAIL can be used through a web page at avalon.epm.ornl.gov/ Grail-bin/EmptyGrailForm. GRAIL can also be used via an email server. For information on using the GRAIL email server, refer to the following Internet site: ftp://arthur.epm.ornl.gov/pub/xgrail/Manual.grail-genquest.July94.

GENSCAN [13] is another program for Gene Prediction that is available through a Web interface at http://bioweb.pasteur.fr/seqanal/interfaces/genscan-simple.html.

Promoter Scan [14], at the Web site bimas.dcrt.nih.gov/molbio/proscan, will predict promoter regions based on scoring homologies with putative eukaryotic Pol II promoter sequences.

NetGene2 [15] World Wide Web server is a service that produces neural network predictions of splice sites in human, *C. elegans* and *A. thaliana* DNA. It can be accessed at www.cbs.dtu.dk/services/NetGene2.

6.3 Identification of the Open Reading Frame of mRNA Sequences

Several programs are available for identifying the correct open reading frame of an mRNA sequence. For eukaryotic mRNA sequences, the correct ORF can usually be identified by using Kozak's rules [16]. For prokaryotes, the problem lies in reliably localizing the ribosome binding site. A number of programs are available for this purpose [17].

6.4 Identification of Protein Sequence Features

When an amino acid sequence of a protein has been determined, a researcher can use bioinformatics tools to try to gain some understanding as to the structure and function of the protein.

6.5 Amino Acid Composition

Some programs exist which use the amino acid composition of the protein to identify other proteins that may be in the same family. It has been documented that amino acid composition across species boundaries is well conserved [18] and that by considering amino acid composition, investigators can detect weak similarities between proteins whose sequence identity falls below 25% [19].

AACompldent and AACompSim are two programs that can be accessed through ExPASy (Expert Protein Analysis System). They both find similar proteins by using amino acid composition to search a database. They can be accessed through ExPASy's web site at www.expasy.ch.

PROPSEARCH is another program for finding similar proteins in a database based on amino acid composition [19]. PROPSEARCH can be accessed from a Web site at www.embl-heidelberg.de/prs.html.

6.6 Identifying Physical Properties of a Protein from Its Sequence

The isoelectric point and molecular weight of a protein can be calculated based on an input sequence by a program called Compute pl/MW. Compute pl/MW is available from the ExPASy Web site at www.expasy.ch.

6.7 Protease Cleavage Products

PeptideMass, also available from the ExPASy web site at www.expasy.ch/toos/peptide-mass.html, will calculate the fragments that will result from the digestion of an input protein sequence by a user-selected protease.

6.8 Hydrophobicity

Several programs, including GREASE, can provide a graph of the hydrophobicity of the protein based on the amino acid sequence [20]. GREASE can be used on the Web at fasta.bioch.Virginia.edu/fasta/grease.htm.

6.9 Protein Secondary Structure Prediction

Using a neural network algorithm, nnpredict can predict whether a given residue will be part of an alpha helix, a beta strand, or neither. The program can be accessed through the Web at www.cmpharm.ucsf.edu/~nomi/nnpredict.html.

PredictProtein is a program that does several searches for homologous proteins and motifs and then predicts secondary structure, transmembrane helix do-

mains, and protein globularity. It can be accessed on the Web at www.embl
heidelberg.de/predictprotein.

6.10 Identification of Specialized Structures

The TMpred program makes predictions of transmembrane domains. TMpred
uses a database of transmembrane proteins called TMbase [21] to predict the
presence of a transmembrane domain in a protein sequence. The TMpred web
interface can be accessed at www.isrec.isb-sib.ch/ftp-server/tmpred/www/
TMPRED_form.html.

    SignalP is a program that will detect a signal peptide and its cleavage site.
A signal peptides is a portion of the amino acid sequence which targets the protein
to a particular membrane or organelle. SignalP, developed by the Center of Biological Sequence Analysis at the Technical University of Denmark, uses a neural
network-based algorithm and a database of prokaryotic and eukaryotic sequences
that have known signal sequences. SignalP can be accessed through its Web
interface at www.cbs.dtu.dk/services/SignalP.

6.11 RNA Secondary Structure Prediction

Many research areas can make use of secondary structure information of an RNA
molecule. Such information can be useful in identifying good sites for probes or
antisense oligonucleotides by selecting sites that are not blocked by the secondary
structure of the RNA molecule. The algorithms make use of nearest neighbor
parameters for RNA duplex formation. RNA secondary structure can be predicted
with the mfold program developed by Michael Zuker [22,23]. Mfold can be accessed on the Web at mfold2.wustl.edu/~mfold/ma/form1.cgi.

7 DATA MINING

Data mining is the use of algorithms to analyze large amounts of data and find
patterns, relationships, or correlations that are not readily visible. Data mining
techniques have been applied to several areas of biology. One of the most challenging and possibly valuable areas is in the analysis of expression profile data.

7.1 Gene Expression Data Analysis

The advent of several technologies for the expression profiling of many mRNA
levels at several time points, under various conditions, or with different cell types
has begun to generate huge amounts of data. There have also been some developments in expression profiling on the protein level.

    The analysis of this data will ultimately become extremely valuable. The
amount of data alone suggests the amount of valuable insights that may be learned

from it. Such large amounts of data provide new challenges for software developers to develop algorithms that can handle this data efficiently and correctly. There are currently several products that are available for analysis of this data. However, many questions remain unanswered as to the best way to analyze the data and future developments should prove quite useful.

7.2   Clustering of Genes with Similar Expression Profiles

Typical expression profiles will have several time points, or conditions, and will follow hundreds of different genes. This results in thousands of data points. One common strategy for mining these data is to cluster the genes by their expression profiles. Genes that respond in similar ways to a given condition may have something in common, and so it is valuable to be able to cluster genes in this way. There are several computational methods for clustering data points that have been in common use for some time, but it is not clear if these should be applied directly to expression profiles. Recent developments in this area have shown promise, and this question may be successfully resolved soon [24].

7.3   Mining for DNA Sequence Motifs in Clustered Genes

One of the rationales behind clustering genes is to find common expression control elements. Analyzing the sequences of genes whose expression profiles cluster together may reveal transcriptional control elements for yet unknown transcription factors. Because of the complexity of biological systems in which many genes will be turned on and off by various different transcription factors, this problem will not be solved by a simple sequence analysis approach. There have recently been some interesting developments in this area using Artificial Intelligence techniques [25].

8   OTHER APPLICATIONS OF BIOINFORMATICS

8.1   Oligonucleotide Probe, Primer, or Antisense Design Software

There have been several software products for designing oligonucleotides for various purposes. Oligo, Primer Premier, and RightPrimer are specifically developed for design of PCR or sequencing primers. HYBsimulator is more general in its ability to design oligonucleotides for all purposes, including antisense. The types of analyses done by software to design oligonucleotides generally are calculations of Tm, G/C content, and hairpin structure formation of candidate oligonucleotides. HYBsimulator has some very useful functions for designing multiplex probe cocktails and, as mentioned above, can do a Hybridization Simulation analysis with a database to design the most specific oligonucleotides.

8.2   Using Gene Expression Data to Identify Drug Candidates

Researchers are often trying to identify a drug that will elicit a specific physiological effect. Gene expression profiling can be used to identify candidate compounds. Some physiological responses, such as apoptosis (programmed cell death), can be elicited by various types of treatments. These treatments also cause specific gene expression changes in the cell. If a drug that can elicit a similar effect is desired, drug candidates can be identified which provoke a similar gene expression profile.

8.3   Cheminformatics for Combinatorial Chemistry Drug Screening

A common strategy for pharmaceutical companies to find compounds that have some desired effect is to screen many thousands of compounds and identify those that have the desired effect. This type of brute-force screening strategy requires enormous resources and can take many years to identify new drugs. Some companies have tried another approach by using structural chemistry models to classify compounds into groups which are predicted to have similar types of active groups. A representative candidate of each group is screened for the desired effect in the system. When compounds that have the desired effect are identified, other members of the same family are then screened to find those with the most efficacy.

One example of a program that enables this sort of analysis is the FlexX program. This program can use protein structural information and can predict how well a given compound will serve as a ligand for the protein. Information about FlexX can be found at www.tripos.com.

8.4   Concordance Analysis Using a Relational Database with Homology Results

One strategy for developing antibacterial agents is to identify genes that are essential to a set of bacteria but are not present in humans. These genes can provide targets for antibacterial agents. One technique for identifying such genes is to perform a homology analysis between every combination of genes in all known organisms. The results of these analyses can then be stored in a relational database. A relational database allows quick selection of genes that have significant homology among a specified list of bacteria while not having significant homology to any animal genes. Compounds which inhibit these gene products would theoretically kill the bacteria but not affect an animal [26].

One application of this strategy is referred to as SEEBUGS (Software for the Examination, Exploration, and Broad Understanding of Genome Sequences). SEEBUGS is available from Congenomics and can be accessed free of charge at http://www.congen.com.

8.5 Knowledge Bases

Several efforts have been underway to develop databases that contain not only sequence data but actual knowledge regarding the biological systems and pathways. Because this knowledge exists in the literature in a form that is not easy for a computer to parse, the entry of this information must be done by scientists reading the literature. Obviously, this is a daunting task and at this time there are no available products that have adequately solved this problem.

9 WHAT THE FUTURE HOLDS FOR BIOINFORMATICS

The ultimate goal of bioinformatics at this point is to put all of these tools at our fingertips in an easy to use, integrated way. Several companies have been working on systems that will attempt to accomplish this by integrating databases, homology, and search functions with knowledge bases, literature databases and expression profile data. Whether or not this will be accomplished soon is hard to say, but it is apparent that the work of the biologist will become more and more dependent on information technology as time goes on.

REFERENCES

1. T Heinemeyer, E Wingender, I Reuter, H Hermjakob, AE Kel, OV Kel, EV Ignatieva, EA Ananko, OA Podkolodnaya, FA Kolpakov, NL Podkolodny, NA Kolchanov. Databases on transcriptional regulation: TRANSFAC, TRRD, and COMPEL. Nucleic Acids Res 26:364–370, 1998.
2. L Duret, D Mouchiroud, M Gouy, HOVERGEN, a database of homologous vertebrate genes. Nucleic Acids Res 22:2360–2365, 1994.
3. MO Dayhoff, RM Schwarz, BC Orcutt. A model of evolutionary change in proteins. In: MO Dayhoff, ed. Atlas of Protein Sequence and Structure. Washingon, DC: National Biomedical Research Foundation, 1978, pp 345–352.
4. S Henikoff, JG Henikoff. Amino acid substitution matrices from protein blocks. Proc Natl Acad Sci USA 89:10915–10919, 1992.
5. SB Needleman, C Wunsch. A general method applicable to the search for similarities in the amino acid sequence of two proteins. J Mol Biol 48:443–453, 1970.
6. TF Smith, MS Waterman. Identification of common molecular subsequences. J Mol Biol 147:195–197, 1981.
7. WR Pearson, DJ Lipman. Improved tools for biological sequence comparison. Proc Natl Acad Sci USA 85:2444–2448, 1988.
8. SF Altschul, W Gish, W Miller, EW Myers, DJ Lipman. Basic local alignment search tool. J Mol Biol 215:403–410, 1990.
9. SF Altschul. Amino acid substitution matrices from an information theoretic perspective. J Mol Biol 219:555–565, 1991.
10. D Hyndman, A Cooper, S Pruzinsky, D Coad, M Mitsuhashi. Software to determine optimal oligonucleotide sequences based on hybridization simultion data. Biotechniques 20(6):1090–1094, 1096–97, 1996.

11. DG Higgins, JD Thompson, TJ Bibson. Using CLUSTAL for multiple sequence alignments. Methods Enzymol 266:383–402, 1996.

12. Y Xu, JR Einstein, RJ Mural, M Shah, EC Uberbacher. An improved system for exon recognition and gene modeling in human DNA sequences. In: R Altman, D Brutlag, P Karp, R Lathrop, D Searls, eds. Proceedings of the Second International Conference on Intelligent Systems for Molecular Biology. Menlo Park, CA: AAAI Press, 1994, pp 376–383.

13. C Burge, S Karlin. Prediction of complete gene structures in human genomic DNA. J Mol Biol 268:78–94, 1997.

14. DS Prestridge. Predicting Pol II Promoter Sequences Using Transcription Factor Binding Sites. J Mol Biol 249:923–932, 1995.

15. SM Hebsgaard, PG Korning, N Tolstrup, J Engelbrecht, P Rouze, S Brunak. Splice site prediction in *Arabidopsis thaliana* pre-mRNA by combining local and global sequence information. Nucleic Acids Res 24(17):3439–3452, 1996.

16. M Kozak. Interpreting cDNA sequence: some insights from studies on translation. Mamm Genome 7:563–574, 1996.

17. MS Gelfand. Prediction of function in DNA sequence analysis. J Comput Biol 2: 87–115, 1995.

18. SJ Cordwell, MR Wilkins, A Cerpa-Poljak, AA Gooley, M Duncan, KL Williams, I Humphery-Smith. Cross-species identification of proteins separated by two-dimensional electrophoresis using matrix-assisted laser desorption ionization/time-of-flight mass spectrometry and amino acid composition. Electrophoresis 16:438–443, 1995.

19. UI Hobohm, CA Sander. A sequence property approach to searching protein databases. J Mol Biol 251:390–399, 1995.

20. J Kyte, RF Doolittle. A simple method for displaying the hydropathic character of a protein. J Mol Biol 157:105–132, 1982.

21. K Hofmann, W Stoffel. Tmbase: A database of membrane-spanning protein segments. Biol Chem Hoppe-Seyler 347:166, 1993.

22. M Zuker, DH Mathews, DH Turner. Algorithms and thermodynamics for RNA secondary structure prediction: a practical guide. In: J Barciszewski, C Clark, eds. RNA Biochemistry and Biotechnology, NATO ASI Series Kluwer Academic Publishers, Norwell, MA, 1999.

23. DH Mathews, J Sabina, M Zuker, DH Turner. Expanded sequence dependence of thermodynamic parameters provides robust prediction of RNA secondary structure. J Mol Biol 288:911–940, 1999.

24. UI Alon, N Barkai, DA Notterman, K Gish, S Ybarra, D Mack, AJ Levine. Broad patterns of gene expression revealed by clustering analysis of tumor and normal colon tissues probed by oligonucleotide arrays. Proc Natl Acad Sci USA 96(12): 6745–6750, 1999.

25. L Pickert, I Reuter, F Klawonn, E Wingender. Transcription regulatory region analysis and detection and fuzzy clustering. Bioinformatics 14(3):244–251, 1998.

26. R Bruccoleri, TJ Dougherty, DB Davison. Concordance analysis of microbial genomes. Nucleic Acids Res 26(19):4482–4486, 1998.

17

Mapping of Disease Loci

Glenys Thomson
University of California, Berkeley, Berkeley, California

1 INTRODUCTION

The genetic and physical maps, and technologies for gene identification that have already emerged from the Human Genome Project (HGP) have had a tremendous impact on the research community's ability to discover the genes that underlie human genetic variation [1,2]. Recent successes in the genetic mapping of Mendelian traits and diseases have been remarkable. However, progress has been exceedingly slow in elucidating the genetic components of complex diseases and traits such as cardiovascular diseases, asthma, diabetes, rheumatoid arthritis, obesity, alcoholism, and schizophrenia. Complex diseases involve multiple genes, environmental effects, and their interactions. Rather than being due to specific and relatively rare mutations, complex diseases and traits may result principally from genetic variation that is relatively common in the general population. Examples include apolipoprotein E gene (APOE) variation and age of onset of Alzheimer's disease, the angiotensin-converting enzyme gene (ACE) and myocardial infarction, the chemokine receptor CCR5 gene (CMKBR5) and the risk of infection in those exposed to HIV, and the many diseases for which immune response genes of the HLA region have been implicated.

In the following, the shorthand of only talking about Mendelian or complex diseases, with the understanding that the statements also apply to nondisease traits is used throughout. Diseases caused by a single major gene or biochemical pathway defect are referred to as Mendelian, or single-gene traits. Complicating factors such as incomplete penetrance—not all genetically predisposed individuals manifest the disease, as in polydactyly, and variable age of onset effects, as in Huntington's disease—are often present. However, the basic single-gene nature of the inheritance pattern is often evident, with Mendelian segregation patterns according to recessive, dominant, or sex chromosome X-linked inheritance [see 2 for review].

A Mendelian disease can have complex clinical effects; e.g., sickle cell anemia affects many organ systems. Even with the same allelic mutation, as in individuals with sickle cell anemia, there may be considerable variation in disease severity, due to modifier genes. The majority of Mendelian traits also show allele and/or locus heterogeneity. Different alleles at one gene may give rise to disease, e.g., cystic fibrosis, which can result in variation in the disease expression. Different genes may also be responsible for disease in different families, e.g., the BRCA1 and BRCA2 genes and early-onset familial breast cancer.

In contrast to Mendelian diseases, complex (or multifactorial) diseases are generally more common, and result from the interaction of multiple genes and environmental factors. Studies of rates of occurrence of disease in twins and other family members compared to population level rates are used to demonstrate the role of genetic and environmental factors in complex diseases [see 3 for review].

Genetically, complex diseases may exhibit the following properties: incomplete penetrance—not all susceptible individuals are affected; the involvement of several disease-predisposing loci—some of which may have a major effect, but many of which may have a relatively minor effect; interaction effects between these loci and with environmental factors; and heterogeneity—so that different loci and/or alleles cause disease in different groups. As a result it is difficult with complex diseases to localize disease genes, ascertain the number and relationship of disease loci involved, understand modes of inheritance and interaction effects, determine the molecular basis of disease, and understand the mechanism(s) by which these genetic changes give rise to disease, including all genetic and environmental factors and their interactions.

For many complex diseases the fact that a large number of genes, many with relatively small effects, are involved drastically complicates efforts to identify genetic regions involved in the disease process, and makes replication of results difficult. Additionally, each complex disease can present its own set of unique problems and statistical issues in the localization of disease genes and definition of disease predisposing factors, including a low or high disease prevalence, late-onset diseases for which parental data may be difficult to obtain, and infectious diseases where family studies are difficult and issues of exposure confound the analyses.

The distinction in terminology between Mendelian and complex traits is not meant to imply that complex diseases do not follow in general the rules of Mendelian inheritance, but merely that a simple pattern of inheritance is not obvious. While the boundary between these two categories is not precisely defined, a large number of diseases clearly fall into each category. It is important to also remember that although we often use the shorthand notation of disease gene, or disease-causing gene, we are talking about variation at genes involved in normal human health and development, specific variations of which may lead to a disease state [4].

Sir Archibald Garrod's brilliant studies in 1908 of the genetics and biochemical pathways involved in "inborn errors of metabolism" laid the conceptual foundation for all later studies in human genetics [2]. The single-gene Mendelian nature of a large number of traits and diseases was subsequently identified. Gene mapping in humans before the 1970s was, however, essentially limited to the X chromosome, based on the specific pattern of inheritance. Future progress in biochemical genetics and gene mapping awaited advances in molecular biology.

2 MAPPING STRATEGIES, DNA POLYMORPHISMS, AND POPULATION PARAMETERS

2.1 Mapping Genes Involved in Disease

There are three main approaches to mapping the genetic variants involved in a disease: functional cloning, the candidate gene strategy, and positional cloning [2]. In functional cloning, identification of the underlying protein defect leads to localization of the responsible gene (disease—function—gene—map). Sickle cell anemia was the first human disease to be successfully understood at the molecular level and isolation of the mutant molecule led to the localization of the β-globin gene on chromosome 11. Functional cloning is, however, only useful in a subset of Mendelian traits where the biological basis is known, and in very few complex traits.

In the candidate gene approach, genes with a known or proposed function with the potential to influence the disease phenotype are investigated for a direct role in disease [2]. The most successful application of the candidate gene approach to mapping complex diseases in humans has been with the HLA region on chromosome 6p21, the major histocompatibility complex of humans. Genes in the HLA region have been implicated in the etiology of >100 diseases [5]. These include: complex autoimmune diseases such as type 1 diabetes (until recently called insulin-dependent diabetes mellitus—IDDM), rheumatoid arthritis, and multiple sclerosis; cancers, e.g., Hodgkin's disease; infectious diseases such as malaria, tuberculosis, and AIDS; and also other diseases such as narcolepsy.

Positional cloning is used when the biochemical nature of a disease is unknown. Marker genes not related to disease physiology and genomewide screens are then the starting point for mapping the genetic components of the disease. The aim is first to identify the genetic region within which a disease-predisposing gene lies and, once this is found, to localize the gene and determine its functional and biological role in the disease (disease—map—gene—function). Most markers used nowadays are DNA based.

Landmarks in positional cloning have included genetic linkage of Huntington's disease in 1983 to an RFLP (restriction fragment length polymorphism) marker (see Sect. 2.2 below) on chromosome 4 (the gene was cloned in 1993) and the cloning of the cystic fibrosis gene on chromosome 7 in 1989. By 1990, when the Human Genome Project (HGP) began, a handful of additional successes had accrued. In 1994, the early-onset familial breast/ovarian cancer (BRCA1) gene was cloned, and the early-onset familial breast cancer (BRCA2) gene in 1995. By 1997 close to 100 Mendelian disease loci had been identified by positional cloning [1,2].

A complementary array of approaches is available to uncover the different genetic facets of both Mendelian and complex traits and diseases [6]. Two complementary analytic methods—linkage analyses and association (linkage disequilibrium) mapping (see Sects. 3 and 4 below)—are used to detect the specific genetic regions and genes involved in the disease process. These approaches can be applied without prior knowledge of the biological basis of the disease using genomewide studies, together with the candidate gene approach and comparative analyses using animal models of disease.

2.2 DNA Polymorphisms

Markers such as protein and blood group loci were initially used in the analysis of genetic traits; however, they were limited in utility due to low variation. Early in the 1980s these markers began to be replaced with DNA polymorphisms, initially RFLPs which are detected by the ability of a segment of DNA to be cut, or to not be cut, by a specific restriction enzyme.

Microsatellites have rapidly replaced RFLP markers in studies to map disease predisposing genes since they occur frequently and randomly across the human genome, have high levels of variation, are easy to type, and can be amplified using the polymerase chain reaction (PCR) methodology and hence only a small amount of template DNA is required. Single-nucleotide polymorphisms (SNPs) are the most recent type of genetic marker to be considered. They are the most common type of human DNA genetic variation, occurring on average 1 per 1000 base pairs [7]. SNPs are mostly biallelic and less informative than microsatellites; however, they are more frequent and mutationally more stable than microsatellites, and more amenable to automation and DNA chip technology.

The completion of the HGP in the near future, yielding the complete sequence of the 3000 million bases (Mb) of the human genome is eagerly awaited. While this accomplishment will greatly aid studies of Mendelian and complex diseases, it will not provide an immediate solution to their genetics, especially for complex diseases. We must first address the daunting prospect of documenting the genetic variation of human genomes at the population level within and across ethnic groups. Only then, correlating this extensive genetic variation with disease, can we uncover the complete genetics of complex diseases and traits, and determine the environmental factors impacting on each disease [4].

2.3 Linkage Disequilibrium

Before discussing linkage and association mapping it is important to distinguish between two concepts: physical linkage and linkage disequilibrium. The description of genetic variation at the population level begins with consideration of allelic variation at a single genetic locus. The next step is to consider genetic variation at two or more loci simultaneously, including nonrandom associations. The nonrandom association of alleles at different genetic loci is termed linkage disequilibrium; random association is described as linkage equilibrium. The pairwise linkage disequilibrium parameter, usually denoted D, is the difference between the observed frequency of a two-locus gametic (chromosome) type—usually referred to as a haplotype, and the frequency expected on the basis of random association of alleles in gametes, i.e., $D = f(AB) - f(A)f(B)$, where $f(.)$ denotes the frequency of a gamete (haplotype) or allele.

There is a relationship between D and the recombination fraction θ between two loci: the value of D decreases by a fraction $(1 - \theta)$ each generation under random mating and a neutral model. Thus the more loosely two loci are linked, the faster the decay of linkage disequilibrium. It is possible, although relatively rare, for loci that are unlinked to be in significant linkage disequilibrium, and for loci that are physically very closely linked to be in linkage equilibrium. However, in general, linkage disequilibrium is usually only seen between very closely linked loci and is rare otherwise. General-population-level observations are that there is an overall proportionality between linkage disequilibrium and the inverse of the recombination distance [8]. This rule, however, breaks down in very closely linked regions [8–10].

Linkage disequilibrium can occur in populations as a consequence of a number of factors [see 11 for review]: mutation—when a new mutant arises, it occurs in one individual and is in linkage disequilibrium with all polymorphic loci in the population; selection—either acting directly on the two loci, or transient linkage disequilibrium can also be created with neutral loci via a hitchhiking event with a selected locus [12]; migration or admixture—generation of linkage disequilibrium by these forces requires that the allelic frequencies of both loci in the two populations be different, and this difference must be substantial to generate very much linkage disequilibrium; and random genetic drift—while the expected value of pairwise linkage disequilibrium due to drift over many generations is zero, the variance is large for closely linked loci in small populations.

The amount of linkage disequilibrium observed in a population is also affected by a number of factors: recombination—significant linkage disequilibrium may be maintained for a long time between very closely linked loci; selection— if the selection is sufficiently strong compared to the recombination rate linkage disequilibrium can be maintained at an equilibrium state, and will occur transiently with a hitchhiking event; nonrandom mating—high levels of inbreeding and self-fertilization in plants can retard the rate of approach to linkage equilibrium; and population demographics—a small founder population or a bottleneck in the recent past can cause significant linkage disequilibrium due to genetic drift for closely linked loci, and while less linkage disequilibrium will be generated by genetic drift in a rapidly growing population [13], any linkage disequilibrium present before or during the early phase of the expansion will persist.

Selection is expected to produce linkage disequilibrium nonrandomly across the genome, whereas all the other factors should act randomly over the genome. In study of the CEPH families, linkage disequilibrium was found to be nonrandomly distributed throughout the genome [8]. Some regions, such as HLA, showed strong evidence of selection and significant linkage disequilibrium which spanned 3 cM or more, and an additional 10 genetic regions showed linkage disequilibrium equal to or greater than in the HLA region.

Population and evolutionary aspects of a genetic region are highly relevant to the study of Mendelian and complex diseases. These relate to our ability to localize and identify disease-predisposing variants, and to our understanding of the mechanisms by which some disease-predisposing genes can become relatively common in a population.

3 LINKAGE MAPPING

3.1 Linkage Analyses

Linkage analyses test for cosegregation of a marker and disease phenotype within a pedigree (implicating physical linkage between the marker gene and a gene involved in the disease process, and such loci are then said to be "linked") [14–16]. Linkage analyses do not require linkage disequilibrium between the marker and disease loci. Different marker alleles may segregate with disease in each pedigree.

Linkage analyses can be performed using single-marker locus variation, and any kind of inherited difference can potentially be a genetic marker. For genomewide linkage analyses, testing for cosegregation with disease of about 300–400 highly polymorphic markers, usually microsatellites, distributed approximately evenly over the genome (average spacing between markers is then on the order of 10cM, i.e., 10% recombination) is the usual practice. The increasing availability of more markers across the genome, combined with multipoint analyses using a number of closely linked markers, such as microsatellites and SNPs, hence increasing the informativeness with respect to cosegregation, will increase the power of linkage studies.

When large multigeneration pedigrees are available, linkage analysis is a powerful technique for localizing disease genes and has been successfully applied to a number of monogenic traits, e.g., Huntington's disease and the familial breast cancer genes BRCA1 and BRCA2. With diabetes, it has been used to map MODY (maturity-onset diabetes of the young) genes. The occurrence of multiple alleles at one genetic locus involved in disease, as in cystic fibrosis, does not affect the power of linkage analyses. However, if different Mendelian genes are involved in disease in different families as in MODY, power can be reduced if all the families are analyzed together.

For complex diseases, the involvement of many genes and the strong influence of environmental factors mean that large multigeneration pedigrees are rarely, or never, seen. Linkage analysis of nuclear families with both parents and two children affected with the disease, although less powerful, is therefore more commonly used to map complex traits [4,17,18]. Consider an affected sib pair family (Fig. 1), and assume for simplicity we can distinguish all four parental chromosomes in the genetic region under study. Deviation from the Mendelian random expectations of 25%, 50%, and 25%, that the affected sibs will on average share 2, 1, and 0 parental chromosomes in common that are identical by descent (ibd) implicates a disease-predisposing gene in the region.

3.2 Linkage Studies in Complex Diseases

Linkage of the HLA region to type 1 diabetes was demonstrated initially with 15 affected sib pairs [19] (Table 1a). This linkage, termed IDDM1, has been confirmed in many studies (Table 1b), with a mean ibd sharing of parental alleles for HLA of 72% [20–23]. For some other HLA-associated diseases, e.g., multiple sclerosis and rheumatoid arthritis, the initial number of affected sib pairs required to show evidence of linkage has been larger—at least 50 and sometimes around 100 [24,25].

The existence of non-HLA genes in many of the HLA-associated diseases was established from theoretical considerations involving population prevalence, risks to relatives, and HLA ibd values in affected sib pairs [26–28]. Type 1

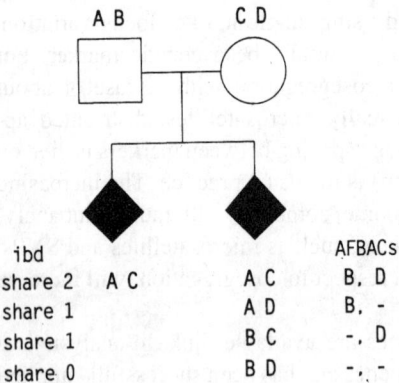

			AFBACs
ibd			
share 2	A C	A C	B, D
share 1		A D	B, -
share 1		B C	-, D
share 0		B D	-, -

FIGURE 1 Affected sib pair families. A nuclear family pedigree is shown with the father (square) and mother (circle) in the first row and the two affected children of either sex (shaded diamonds) in the 2nd row. Assume for simplicity we can distinguish all four parental alleles, denoted A, B, C, and D, in the genetic region under study, with the parental alleles ordered such that A and C are transmitted from the father and mother respectively to the first affected child [17,18]. Four possible configurations among the two offspring with respect to the alleles inherited from the parents are possible: they can share both parental alleles (AC); they can share an allele from the father (A) but differ in the alleles received from the mother (C and D); they can share an allele from the mother (C) but differ in the alleles received from the father (A and B); or they can share no parental alleles in common. These four configurations are equally likely if there is no influence of the genetic region under consideration on the disease. The parental alleles that are never transmitted to the affected sib pair in each family type are used as a control population in association studies using nuclear family data, the so-called AFBAC (affected family based control) sample (see Sect. 4.2). (From Refs. 17, 18.)

diabetes shows an increased risk in siblings over population prevalence (λ_s) of 15 in Caucasian populations [28], of which HLA contributes 3.4: approximately 45% of the type 1 diabetes genetic component under a multiplicative model [29].

Given the relative ease with which linkage was demonstrated for many HLA-associated diseases, it seemed a logical progression to use genomewide linkage scans on affected sib pair families to investigate all complex diseases. Such studies of many complex disorders are in progress: to map the non-HLA genes in a number of diseases such as type 1 diabetes, multiple sclerosis, rheumatoid arthritis, celiac disease, and Crohn's disease; and for many other complex diseases, for example type 2 diabetes, hypertension, coronary artery disease, alcoholism, and schizophrenia.

TABLE 1 HLA and IDDM Affected Sib Pair Values

a. Cudworth and Woodrow 1975 [19]			
ibd sharing	2	1	0
Observed	10	4	1	Total 15
Observed %	67%	27%	6%
$\chi_2^2 = 14.07$, $P < .001$, mean ibd sharing = 0.805			
b. Payami et al. 1985, 538 families [20]			
ibd sharing	2	1	0
Observed	373	283	55	Total 711
Observed %	52%	40%	8%
$\chi_2^2 = 314.03$, $P < 10^{-5}$, mean ibd sharing = 0.724			

Type 1 diabetes was the first complex disease for which genomewide linkage scans in affected sib pairs was carried out [30–32]. Many other studies using genomewide scans to detect non-HLA type 1 diabetes genes have followed since these papers [reviewed in 21]. Apart from HLA, no evidence of a major gene effect has been found. Using ~500 affected sib pairs, linkages for the chromosomal regions IDDM4 (11q13), IDDM5 (6q25), and IDDM8 (6q27) were confirmed [33] using the criteria of Lander and Kruglyak [34]. The mean ibd sharing values in these cases were much closer to the 50% expected randomly than seen with IDDM1: 0.58, 0.58, and 0.60, respectively for IDDM4, IDDM5, and IDDM8. IDDM6 (18q12-21), IDDM10 (10p11-q11), and IDDM12 (2q33) have more recently been considered confirmed, using a combination of affected sib pair and association/linkage tests [21,35–37]. Over seven additional chromosomal regions have shown evidence of linkage to type 1 diabetes in one or more studies [reviewed in 21–23].

3.3 Observations from Genomewide Linkage Scans in Complex Diseases

A common feature of all complex disease studies has been difficulty in both detecting and replicating linkages, with considerable heterogeneity seen between data sets both within and between populations and ethnic groups. The possible involvement in disease of relatively common alleles of a large number of loci, each with a relatively small effect overall, requiring study of many hundreds, and usually thousands, of affected sib pairs to establish linkage, can explain this phenomenon [22,38,39]. The additional possible involvement in some cases of complex disease of relatively rare variants further confounds our abilities to detect all genes involved in the disease process.

Two recent second-generation type 1 diabetes genome scans continue to illustrate the heterogeneity seen in linkage studies in complex diseases [22,23]. Even more surprising, little or no support was found for most reported type 1 diabetes loci in one of these studies [23] even with a very large sample size. The use of stratification analyses based on known IDDM loci such as in the HLA region (IDDM1) may have contributed to more examples of evidence of IDDM loci in the second study [22] (see Sect. 7.2).

Despite initial anxieties with genomewide linkage scans that we would be flooded with false positives [34], this has not been the case. An excess of false linkages has never been a problem with complex diseases. Instead, we are scrambling to find any evidence of disease-predisposing genes. In an insightful review of the many factors that need to be considered in the design of genomewide scans and interpretation of linkage results, Rao [40] pointed out that application of stringent criteria drastically reduces power, and leads to many disease genes remaining undetected [also see 41, 42]. Rao's recommendation was that "we tolerate/accept, on average, one false positive per individual scan." The issue is to have a reasonable balance between false positives and false negatives, while understanding that false negatives are the more serious concern [40,43,44].

4 ASSOCIATION (LINKAGE DISEQUILIBRIUM) MAPPING

4.1 Association Analyses in Case/Control Data

Association studies compare marker frequencies in unrelated cases and controls, and test for the co-occurrence of a marker and disease at the population level; a significant association with disease may implicate a candidate gene in the etiology of a disease. Alternatively, an association can be due to linkage disequilibrium of a marker allele(s) with the disease-predisposing gene, and this will usually imply close physical linkage of the marker and disease-predisposing gene (see Sect. 2.3 above) [6], reflecting the historical origin of a mutation on a specific chromosome with a characteristic set of variation. In association studies it is essential that the patient and control groups be ethnically matched [11,45]. If they are not, a spurious association of an unlinked marker with disease can result from population stratification, i.e., if there is a mixture of two groups in the patient and control samples with different frequencies of the marker allele and the disease.

The success of association (linkage disequilibrium) studies to fine-map Mendelian traits following initial localization of chromosomal regions by linkage analysis is well documented in many different populations [9]. In these studies linkage disequilibrium extended on average >500 kb (0.5% recombination). There are exceptions to the use of association data in localizing disease genes; the breast cancer gene BRCA1 could not be localized using linkage disequilibrium mapping, as different mutations were implicated in each family.

Association mapping may in many cases be more efficient than linkage analyses in detecting genetic regions involved in disease [39]. IDDM2—the minisatellite VNTR (variable number of tandem repeats) 5′ to the insulin gene [46], which is easily detected by association, is difficult to detect by linkage analysis [47]. The well-established and strong HLA association with multiple sclerosis is not picked up in all genome linkage scans [48]. As with linkage studies, haplotype level analyses can be more powerful than single-locus analyses [49,50].

At least 12,000 highly polymorphic, evenly spaced markers, giving an average distance between markers of 0.25 cM (250 kb), is required for an initial disease genomic association scan. Association scans are thus over an order of magnitude higher than the 300 to 400 markers at 10 cM typically used for linkage genome scans. The use of pooled samples of DNA for the study of RFLP [51], microsatellite [52–54], and SNP variation [55], as well as the current development of DNA chip technology for the study of SNPs [78], has opened the way for future routine and extensive use of association mapping in the study of complex diseases. Genomewide association scans in complex diseases are starting to be used, currently with DNA pooling and microsatellites. Methods for correction with microsatellites of stutter artifact and preferential amplification have been demonstrated [53]. Note, however, that a pooled DNA genomic association screen can be carried out without using these correction factors; no bias is introduced as patient and control samples are similarly affected under the null hypothesis of no marker association with disease.

Many researchers feel that the number of false positives that will result from genomewide association scans make them unmanageable. A preliminary discussion of power and a multistage strategy to reduce false positives in genomewide association studies is outlined [53]. As with linkage studies [40,44], power should be high in an initial association scan, to reduce missing associations (false negatives), and sample sizes of 500–1000 are recommended [53,56]. Long and Langley [56] have demonstrated that greater power is achieved in association genome scans by increasing the sample size than by increasing the number of markers.

The potential power of association studies to detect disease genes depends on several unknown parameters, and cannot be determined accurately, especially given that common genetic variants may often be involved in complex diseases [57–60]. For example, the nature of mutations involved in the disease process will influence the power of association studies to detect disease genes [57]. Also, the power of genome association scans will vary across the genome, due to variation in linkage disequilibrium values [8], as well as between populations. The full development of SNPs will eventually permit routine typing for variation in every human gene and its regulatory region, the ultimate association study [7,61,62].

Association mapping is appropriate for monogenic and complex diseases, and may always be preferable to linkage analyses for late-onset diseases where it is difficult to obtain nuclear families, rare diseases for which multiplex pedigrees may not be available—e.g., type 1 diabetes and multiple sclerosis in China—and infectious diseases. Study design can incorporate disease heterogeneity and interaction effects between loci (also see Sect. 7.2).

4.2 Association Analyses in Nuclear-Family-Based Data

The use of nuclear-family data in association studies was initially developed to avoid possible ethnic mismatching between patients and randomly ascertained controls [63]. The parental marker alleles not transmitted to an affected child, or never transmitted to an affected sib pair, form the so-called AFBAC population [17,18] (see Fig. 1). In a random mating population, when there is a marker association with disease, the AFBAC population provides an unbiased estimate of the overall population (control) marker alleles when the recombination fraction between the marker and disease genes is sufficiently small that it can be taken as zero ($\theta = 0$), and differences between patient and AFBAC frequencies can be tested, for example, by a contingency table analysis for heterogeneity.

Of more importance, however, is the fact that concerns about population stratification effects creating associations between unlinked loci are completely removed with family-based data. Testing for a 50% transmission ratio from parents heterozygous for a marker allele (the TDT—transmission disequilibrium test) detects significant differences with marker alleles that are in both linkage disequilibrium and linked to the disease predisposing gene [64–66]. This is because a compound null hypothesis is always being tested which involves a term which is zero if the marker and disease are unlinked, and a term which is zero if there is no linkage disequilibrium at the population level. Thus, associations at the population level of unlinked marker loci with disease caused by population stratification, migration, or admixture are eliminated, and significant effects are only seen for marker loci linked and in linkage disequilibrium with the disease loci. Further, results across populations can be combined using the TDT statistic, although it is important to keep in mind that power could be reduced if the same association(s) is not seen in all populations.

The recent emphasis on use of only family-based association/linkage tests has ignored the readily available resource of case/control data [45], where sampling and then study of many thousands of samples are feasible with new techniques. Provided the patient and control groups are carefully matched for ethnicity, population stratification effects creating spurious associations are eliminated. The large collections of multiplex families now available for linkage

TABLE 2 HLA-Associated Diseases*

HLA	Patients	Controls
Ankylosing spondylitis		
B27	90%	9%
Type 1 diabetes		
DR3	52%	23%
DR4	74%	24%
DR3 or DR4	93%	43%
Multiple sclerosis		
DR2	86%	33%
Rheumatoid arthritis		
DR4	81%	33%
Narcolepsy		
DR2	>95%	33%

* For each disease, the frequency of the associated HLA allele is given in patients and controls. The letter designation denotes the HLA gene, while the number is assigned to a specific allele at the gene. For ease of reading, the data shown are older serological level HLA typing, rather than more recent molecular typing. (From Ref. 5.)

studies in many complex diseases are obviously also a valuable resource for association screens [53,67].

4.3 Association Studies in Complex Diseases

Association mapping has been the main approach in implicating genes of the HLA region in disease etiology (Table 2). Association studies in the early 1970s distinguished type 1 (HLA-associated) from type 2 (not HLA-associated) diabetes. In some cases the classical HLA class I or class II genes have been implicated as directly involved in disease, e.g., ankylosing spondylitis (class I), and type 1 diabetes, rheumatoid arthritis, celiac disease, and narcolepsy (class II). In other cases, the association with classical HLA genes was due to linkage disequilibrium, as with hemochromatosis. Association mapping has also been involved in mapping non-HLA genes. In a small subset of type 2 diabetes cases association studies have identified the role of candidate genes in disease, e.g., the insulin gene, insulin receptor gene, glukokinase gene, and genes in the mitochondrial genome [see 68 for references].

The potential of association studies as the optimal strategy for follow-up of regions showing preliminary evidence of linkage for complex diseases has been demonstrated [22] and awaits full utilization. As with linkage studies, heterogeneity in association results for complex diseases is also seen between studies, especially between populations, and is expected [22,36,56]. In their simulation study, Long and Langley [56] concluded that association studies have a low repeatability unless sample sizes are on the order of 500 individuals.

4.4 Genomewide Association Studies

Escamilla et al. [69], in a study of bipolar mood disorder in an isolated population from Costa Rica, using microsatellite markers spaced at ~6 cM intervals across chromosome 18, concluded that linkage disequilibrium methods will be useful in this case in a larger sample. There is debate with regard to the best type of population to use for association mapping. Lander and Schork [6] state that the ideal population will be isolated, have a narrow population base, and be sampled not too many generations from the time during which a disease-causing mutation has occurred. The Finnish and Costa Rican populations are considered ideal, since they are relatively homogeneous and show linkage disequilibrium over a wider recombination distance than other populations. However, linkage disequilibrium is routinely seen for closely linked loci and around disease genes in all populations. With sufficiently closely linked markers, including haplotype-level analyses [49,50], association mapping should be a powerful and informative approach in many, and possibly most, populations [45].

5   ANIMAL MODELS OF DISEASE

When a particular genetic region is implicated in an animal model of disease, both linkage and association studies can focus on the corresponding syntenic chromosomal region in humans [21,22,70], or study of the specific gene if one has been identified. Demonstration of the involvement of the HLA region in type 1 diabetes led to study, and demonstration of a role of, the corresponding major histocompatibility regions (MHCs) in the diabetic mouse and rat. Genomewide quantitative trait locus (QTL) linkage analyses in the mouse have identified genetic regions and genes involved in several multifactorial traits and diseases, leading to the identification of human homologs, for example, in hypertension [see 6]. The ability with animal and plant studies to control crosses and in most cases to also study large numbers of offspring makes them very powerful.

Animal models of human disease can also be informative for physiological studies of genetic and environmental factors, and can be used to test novel therapeutics [6]. For both Mendelian and complex diseases, genes that modify disease severity can also be investigated in animal models by studying animal strains that are severely or mildly affected by the same gene defect, combined with knock-out and knock-in models.

6 DETERMINING THE GENETIC COMPONENTS INVOLVED IN DISEASE

Initial study of the HLA component to type 1 diabetes gave results compatible with a simple recessive model (with incomplete penetrance) [20,71]. Only later did the extensive heterogeneity of the HLA component to type 1 diabetes emerge. Genetic heterogeneity was definitively established by the demonstration that the HLA class II DR3 and DR4 serological associations at the DRB1 locus showed increased risk for DR3/DR4 heterozygotes [72]. In a joint collaborative study of Caucasian type 1 diabetes patients and controls, Thomson et al. [73] confirmed further heterogeneity by study of relative predispositional effects [74]: after removal of the DR3 and DR4 effects (~93% of patients have one or two copies of DR3 and/or DR4 compared to 43% of controls), DR2 was shown to be protective, followed by predisposing effects of DR1 and DR8. Cross-ethnic studies have now confirmed that the three closely linked class II genes—DRB1, DQA1, and DQB1—all contribute directly to type 1 diabetes [see 75 for references]. A hierarchy of very susceptible, through intermediate, to very protective HLA type 1 diabetes allele, haplotype, and genotype effects are seen, which no current molecular model fully explains [75].

Determining the precise HLA components of disease is difficult for the following primary reasons: multiple genetic factors are involved; the HLA genes are in strong linkage disequilibrium; HLA region loci have many polymorphic residues; common HLA alleles may be involved in disease; and interaction effects among HLA, and/or non-HLA, disease loci may be important. These characteristics make necessary a multistrategy approach, in which complementary methods are used. These include analysis of data from various ethnically or geographically defined groups, as differences in HLA polymorphism and disease prevalence across groups can point toward the precise genetic factors that are important in disease. The methods that have been applied to HLA data to identify the actual disease predisposing factors, and to determine all disease factors in the region, and the difficulties encountered, apply equally to non-HLA regions.

While linkage disequilibrium is our ally in detecting genetic regions involved in disease, it confounds attempts to identify the actual gene in the region involved in disease and to identify additional genes in the region contributing to disease. The so-called haplotype method to identify disease-predisposing alleles and amino acids in a genetic region is a stratification analysis to take account of the effects of linkage disequilibrium [73,75,76]. If all alleles, or amino acid sites, directly involved in disease in a genetic region have been identified, and haplotypes (chromosome combinations) containing all these sites are considered, the relative frequencies of alleles and amino acid sites on these haplotypes not involved in disease should be the same in patients and controls. The absolute frequencies of these haplotypes will differ between patients and controls, but the ratio of variants at sites not involved in disease will not differ between patients and controls, provided all alleles or amino acids involved in disease have been identified and all these sites are included in the haplotypes considered. Obviously, the haplotype method cannot distinguish between sites which are very highly correlated in a population, however ethnic comparisons can help identify the predisposing factors. The method however can unequivocally determine if all disease predisposing amino acid sites in linkage disequilibrium in a genetic region have *not* been identified.

The original application of the haplotype method was to allele frequency data [73]. Direct roles of only HLA DR3 and DR4 serological types in type 1 diabetes were excluded, since HLA B locus variation on these haplotypes was different in patients and controls. At the amino acid level, a combination of sites at DRB1, DQA1, and DQB1 was shown to be highly correlated with the DR-DQ contribution to type 1 diabetes and to correlate with disease incidence [75].

The role of genes additional to HLA DR-DQ in type 1 diabetes was first demonstrated using affected sib pairs with parents homozygous for the DR3 haplotype [77]. HLA class I B locus data was used to distinguish between the 2 DR3 haplotypes of the homozygous parent. Under the null hypothesis that no HLA region variation additional to that defined by the DR3 haplotype is involved in type 1 diabetes, the affected sib pairs should share the two parental DR3 haplotypes equally frequently. Significant deviation from 50% sharing was observed. Since the DR3 haplotypes examined in this study could be assumed to be homogeneous for their DR-DQ alleles at the molecular level (DRB1*0301 DQA1*0501 DQB1*0201), this test implicated other HLA region loci in type 1 diabetes.

Using the haplotype method, linkage disequilibrium patterns, matching of case/control data for specific DR-DQ combinations, and TDT analysis of heterozygote microsatellite data from parents homozygous for the DR-DQ genes, the role of additional HLA region genes in type 1 diabetes has been clearly demonstrated in a number of additional studies. These include other HLA peptide-presenting molecules, such as DPB1*0301 [78,79], as well as microsatellite associations implicating other regions containing genes involved in the disease process [80,81].

7   THE FUTURE

7.1   Overview

With completion of the HGP, the functional and positional cloning of Mendelian traits and diseases will become fairly routine [2]. Considerable work, however, still lies ahead even with Mendelian diseases: to document worldwide variation in mutations, identify the effects of modifier genes on heterogeneity with respect to age of onset and severity, obtain accurate measurements of the penetrance values of different allelic mutations, study the effects of environmental factors on disease expression, and develop appropriate therapies.

For genetically complex human diseases and traits the HGP will not provide an immediate solution to their genetics, although the ability to identify candidate genes de novo and in a region identified by positional cloning will greatly reduce the time required to home in on the actual genes involved in complex diseases. A concomitant outcome of the HGP will be an increase in the characterization of human gene expression patterns, which will greatly aid our studies of the disease process [82].

A multistrategy approach to the mapping of complex diseases and traits is still appropriate: no single method is sufficient or optimal. Genomewide linkage studies are now routine, although still expensive and time-consuming. Despite extensive efforts by many groups, progress in the mapping of complex diseases has been exceedingly slow; only a few genes and some genetic regions involved in complex diseases have been identified. The general picture is one of difficulty in locating disease genes and replication of reported linkages.

The practical application of association studies in Mendelian and complex diseases in fine-mapping of genetic regions identified by linkage analyses has been demonstrated for many, but not all, disease-predisposing loci. Also, while association mapping can narrow down a genetic region implicated via a linkage study, complete sequencing of this region, which may be many Mb long, is still an arduous task. Genomewide association studies are now feasible with pooled DNA samples and are starting to be used. As with linkage studies, the overall power of association genome scans to detect disease genes is unknown. Power for both linkage and association studies depends on a number of unknown parameters and will vary across the genome, and also between populations and ethnic groups. The increasing availability of more markers across the genome, combined with multipoint analyses using closely linked markers [49,83] will increase the power of linkage and association studies, including the follow-up of regions potentially involved in disease.

When animal models accurately reflect the human disease, these will increasingly be informative. All life forms share many molecular features of gene structure, inheritance, and expression, and protein synthesis and function. Given our increasing understanding of the unifying biological aspects of all life forms, including gene expression, protein synthesis, and protein function, animal models can be used to identify key genes that influence human multifactorial traits.

Identification of the actual genetic variants involved in disease is not a trivial task for complex diseases. Cross-ethnic studies can aid in this venture, as patterns of linkage disequilibrium may differ. Animal models also provide valuable information from study of knock-out and knock-in mice.

Increasing technological advances in molecular biology, such as the development of SNPs combined with DNA chip technology, and biocomputing will allow screening and analysis of large sample sizes, with predicted future rates of data output which are astronomical. The full development of SNPs will eventually permit routine typing for variation in every human gene, and their regulatory regions, the ultimate association study [7,58,61,62]. However, attention must also be given to aspects of genetic epidemiology and population genetics in study design. The issue of disease heterogeneity, including diagnostic criteria, will be of increasing importance.

7.2 Disease Heterogeneity

Rao [40] emphasized that power should be high in an initial linkage genomewide scan, to reduce missing linkages (false negatives). The same argument applies to genomewide association scans [56]. Further, all studies of complex diseases should now be seen as exploratory data analyses, without correction for multiple comparisons, or as confirmational studies, as appropriate.

In the context of genomewide significance levels and false positives, the issue is also raised of whether conditional linkage analyses, stratified by linkage results from established loci such as the confirmed IDDM loci, should be carried out on all genome scan data [22], or whether conditional analyses should be performed only after linkage is established for a specific region [23,83]. Given the intrinsic heterogeneous nature of complex disease genetics, stratification analyses with respect to all aspects of disease definition and population heterogeneity should increase our chances of finding the genes involved in disease. Even though type 1 error will be increased [43,83], stratification approaches have proven their worth as an aid in identifying linkages [21,22]. The reduction in sample size resulting from stratification by genetic and environmental factors means that very large sample sizes are needed.

The use of a number of different disease phenotype definitions in linkage studies is similarly debated. Success stories based on study of a range of disease definitions [50], subsets of the disease phenotype [84], sex effects [85], and age-of-onset effects [86–88] support these approaches. The existence of interaction effects between genes involved in complex diseases, as well as parental effects reportedly modifying the transmission and expression of some genes further complicates studies [21]. To investigate the possibility of interaction effects between disease loci, linkage evidence at one or more regions can be incorporated into analyses of other positions [89]. Standard application of multilocus methods of linkage analysis which are under development should also provide more power [83].

7.3 Sample Sizes, Study Designs

Exceedingly large sample sizes of case/control, simplex, and multiplex family-based data, as well as multigeneration pedigrees when available, are needed for our continuing studies of complex diseases. Obtaining a balance between the information content and the ease of obtaining the different types of data points to requiring very large sample sizes of each. Sample sizes in the thousands are required to allow detection and confirmation of linkages, association genomic level as well as fine mapping, stratification analyses based on various disease phenotypes, including complications, age of onset, genetic, and epidemiological parameters, as well as analyses to determine if the true predisposing factors, and all factors in a genetic region, have been identified.

It was previously argued that detailed study of environmental factors on disease would best be studied once the genetic basis of the disease was established. In this way genetically predisposed individuals could be identified and the impact of environmental factors more clearly identified. However, given the difficulty in identifying the genetic components of complex diseases, it now seems appropriate that we concentrate on environmental factors in conjunction with genetic studies, as the effect of environmental factors on many complex diseases is quite strong.

The recent emphasis on use of only family-based TDT association/linkage tests has ignored the readily available resource of case/control data [45], where sampling and then study of many thousands of samples are feasible with new techniques. Provided the patient and control groups are carefully matched for ethnicity, population stratification effects creating spurious associations are eliminated. The large collections of multiplex families now available for linkage studies in many complex diseases are obviously also a valuable resource for association screens. Further, they allow for study of combined linkage and association results [90,91]. This can yield strong evidence for linkage when the affected sib pairs are analyzed based on the presence or not of the associated allele in the proband, e.g., with IDDM2, where the overall evidence of linkage is very weak [92]. Further, the direct role of a putative disease predisposing gene can be tested [91], and interactive effects of candidate genes studied [92].

Our studies must also include many different populations, including extensive ethnic variation, and not be restricted to relatively homogeneous populations. Only with this approach can we identify all the genes involved, in all populations, in predisposition to and protection from disease, including their interaction effects and their influence on response to environmental factors. The genes involved in multigeneration pedigrees may often be different from those in affected sib pair and/or "sporadic" cases of disease, so both types of pedigrees must be studied.

National and international cooperative efforts for sharing data are mandatory to achieve the large sample sizes required and allow meta-analyses of data [93,94], which can be very powerful. Study of genetic effects common to multiple diseases will also increasingly be of considerable interest [94,95]. The most efficient scheme for completing a pooled association screen is for a large collaborative study of several diseases with division of microsatellites among laboratories [53].

Further study of population level data is also obligatory [57,96–98], including development of methods to understand the evolutionary history of a region [8,57,99]. Only then can the power of different linkage and association methods be completely assessed and the processes understood by which disease-predisposing variants become established, and often frequent, in populations.

REFERENCES

1. FS Collins, MS Guyer, A Charkravarti. Variations on a theme: cataloging human DNA sequence variation. Science 278:1580–1581, 1997.
2. TD Gelehrter, FS Collins, D Ginsberg. Principles of Medical Genetics. Baltimore: Williams and Wilkins, 1998.
3. MC King, GM Lee, NB Spinner, G Thomson, MR Wrensch. Genetic epidemiology. Annu Rev Public Health 5:1–52, 1984.
4. G Thomson, MS Esposito. The genetics of complex diseases: an overview. Trends Genet 15:M17–M20, 1999.
5. E Thorsby. Invited anniversary review: HLA associated diseases. Hum Immunol 53: 1–11, 1997.
6. ES Lander, NJ Schork. Genetic dissection of complex traits. Science 265:2037–2048, 1994.
7. FS Collins, LD Brooks, A Chakravarti. A DNA polymorphism discovery resource for research on human genetic variation. Genome Res 8:1229–1231, 1998.
8. GA Huttley, MW Smith, M Carrington, SJ O'Brien. A scan for linkage disequilibrium across the human genome. Genetics 152:1711–1722, 1999.
9. LB Jorde, WS Watkins, M Carlson, J Groden, H Albertsen, A Thliveris, M Leppert. Linkage disequilibrium predicts physical distance in the adenomatous polyposis coli region. Am J Hum Genet 54:884–898, 1994.
10. W Klitz, JC Stephens, M Grote, M Carrington. Discordant patterns of linkage disequilibrium of the peptide-transporter loci within the HLA class II region. Am J Hum Genet 57:1436–1444, 1995.
11. PW Hedrick. Genetics of Populations. Boston: Science Books International, 1983.
12. G Thomson. The effect of a selected locus on linked neutral loci. Genetics 85:753–788, 1977.
13. M Slatkin. Linkage disequilibrium in growing and stable populations. Genetics 137: 331–336, 1994.
14. J Ott. Analysis of Human Genetic Linkage, 3rd ed. Baltimore: John Hopkins University Press, 1999.
15. RC Elston. Linkage and association. Genet Epidemiol 15:565–576, 1998.
16. RC Elston. Methods of linkage analysis—and the assumptions underlying them. Am J Hum Genet 63:931–934, 1998.
17. G Thomson. Mapping disease genes: family-based association studies. Am J Hum Genet 57:487–498, 1995.
18. G Thomson. Analysis of complex human genetic traits: an ordered-notation method and new tests for mode of inheritance. Am J Hum Genet 57:474–486, 1995.
19. AG Cudworth, JC Woodrow. Evidence for HL-A-linked genes in "juvenile" diabetes mellitus. Br Med J 3:133–135, 1975.

20. H Payami, G Thomson, U Motro, EJ Louis, E Hudes. The affected sib method. IV. Sib trios. Ann Hum Genet 49:303–314, 1985.

21. A Pugliese. Unraveling the genetics of insulin-dependent type 1A diabetes: the search must go on. Diabetes Rev 7:39–54, 1999.

22. CA Mein, L Esposito, MG Dunn, GC Johnson, AE Timms, JV Goy, AN Smith, L Sebag-Montefiore, ME Merriman, AJ Wilson, LE Pritchard, F Cucca, AH Barnett, SC Bain, JA Todd. A search for type 1 diabetes susceptibility genes in families from the United Kingdom. Nat Genet 19:297–300, 1998.

23. P Concannon, KJ Gogolin-Ewens, DA Hinds, B Wapelhorst, VA Morrison, B Stirling, M Mitra, J Farmer, SR Williams, NJ Cox, GI Bell, N Risch, RS Spielman. A second-generation screen of the human genome for susceptibility to insulin-dependent diabetes mellitus. Nat Genet 19:292–296, 1998.

24. H Payami, EJ Louis, W Klitz, SK Lo, G Thomson. Family and population analysis of multiple sclerosis. Genet Epidemiol Suppl 1:381–386, 1986.

25. H Payami, G Thomson, MA Khan, DM Grennan, P Sanders, P Dyer, C Dostal. Genetics of rheumatoid arthritis. Tissue Antigens 27:57–63, 1986.

26. G Thomson. A two locus model for juvenile diabetes. Ann Hum Genet 43:383–398, 1980.

27. JI Rotter, EM Landaw. Measuring the genetic contribution of a single locus to a multilocus disease. Clin Genet 26:529–542, 1984.

28. N Risch. Assessing the role of HLA-linked and unlinked determinants of disease. Am J Hum Genet 40:1–14, 1987.

29. J Noble, AM Valdes, M Cook, W Klitz, G Thomson, H Erlich. The role of HLA class II genes in insulin-dependent diabetes mellitus (IDDM): molecular analysis of 180 Caucasian, multiplex families. Am J Hum Genet 59:1134–1148, 1996.

30. JL Davies, Y Kawaguchi, ST Bennett, JB Copeman, HJ Cordell, LE Pritchard, PW Reed, SC Gough, SC Jenkins, SM Palmer, KM Balfour, BR Rowe, M Farrall, AH Barnett, SC Bain, JA Todd. A genome-wide search for human type 1 diabetes susceptibility genes. Nature 371:130–136, 1994.

31. L Hashimoto, C Habita, JP Beressi, M Delepine, C Besse, A Cambon-Thomsen, I Deschamps, JI Rotter, S Djoulah, MR James, P Froguel, J Weissenbach, GM Lathrop, C Julier. Genetic mapping of a susceptibility locus for insulin-dependent diabetes mellitus on chromosome 11q. Nature 371:161–164, 1994.

32. LL Field, R Tobias, T Magnus. A locus on chromosome 15q26 (IDDM3) produces susceptibility to insulin-dependent diabetes mellitus. Nat Genet 8:189–194, 1994.

33. DF Luo, R Buzzetti, JI Rotter, NK Maclaren, LJ Raffel, L Nistico, C Giovannini, P Pozzilli, G Thomson, JX She. Confirmation of three susceptibility genes to insulin-dependent diabetes mellitus: IDDM4, IDDM5 and IDDM8. Hum Mol Genet 5:693–698, 1996.

34. E Lander, L Kruglyak. Genetic dissection of complex traits: guidelines for interpreting and reporting linkage results. Nat Genet 11:241–247, 1995.

35. P Reed, F Cucca, S Jenkins, M Merriman, A Wilson, P McKinney, E Bosi, G Joner, K Ronningen, E Thorsby, D Undlien, T Merriman, A Barnett, S Bain, J Todd. Evidence for a type 1 diabetes susceptibility locus (IDDM10) on human chromosome 10p11-q11. Hum Mol Genet 6:1011–1016, 1997.

36. T Merriman, R Twells, M Merriman, I Eaves, R Cox, F Cucca, P McKinney, J Shield, D Baum, E Bosi, P Pozzilli, L Nistico, R Buzzetti, G Joner, K Ronningen,

E Thorsby, D Undlien, F Pociot, J Nerup, S Bain, A Barnett, J Todd. Evidence by allelic association-dependent methods for a type 1 diabetes polygene (IDDM6) on chromosome 18q21. Hum Mol Genet 6:1003–1010, 1997.

37. L Esposito, NJ Hill, LE Pritchard, F Cucca, C Muxworthy, ME Merriman, A Wilson, C Julier, M Delepine, J Tuomilehto, E Tuomilehto-Wolf, C Ionesco-Tirgoviste, L Nistico, R Buzzetti, P Pozzilli, M Ferrari, E Bosi, F Pociot, J Nerup, SC Bain, JA Todd. Genetic analysis of chromosome 2 in type 1 diabetes: analysis of putative loci IDDM7, IDDM12, and IDDM13 and candidate genes NRAMP1 and IA-2 and the interleukin-1 gene cluster. IMDIAB group. Diabetes 47:1797–1799, 1998.

38. BK Suarez, CL Hampe, P van Eerdewegh. Problems of replicating linkage claims in psychiatry. In: ES Gershon, CR Cloninger, eds. Genetic Approaches to Mental Disorders. Washington, DC: American Psychiatry Press, 1994, pp 23–46.

39. N Risch, K Merikangas. The future of genetic studies of complex human diseases. Science 273:1516–1517, 1996.

40. DC Rao. CAT scans, PET scans, and genomic scans. Genet Epidemiol 15:1–18, 1998.

41. JS Witte, RC Elston, NJ Schork. Genetic dissection of complex traits. Nat Genet 12:355–356, 1996.

42. D Curtis. Genetic dissection of complex traits. Nat Genet 12:356–358, 1996.

43. AA Todorov, DC Rao. Trade-off between false positives and false negatives in the linkage analysis of complex traits. Genet Epidemiol 14:453–464, 1997.

44. DC Rao, C Gu. False positives and false negatives in genomic scans. In: DC Rao, MA Province, eds. Genetic Dissection of Complex Traits: Challenges for the Next Millennium. San Diego: Academic Press, 2000.

45. NE Morton, A Collins. Tests and estimates of allelic association in complex inheritance. Proc Natl Acad Sci USA 95:11389–11393, 1998.

46. ST Bennett, AM Lucassen, SC Gough, EE Powell, DE Undlien, LE Pritchard, ME Merriman, Y Kawaguchi, MJ Dronsfield, F Pociot, J Nerup, N Bouzekri, A Cambon-Thomsen, KS Ronningen, AH Barnett, SC Bain, JA Todd. Susceptibility to human type 1 diabetes at IDDM2 is determined by tandem repeat variation at the insulin gene minisatellite locus. Nat Genet 9:284–292, 1995.

47. RS Spielman, MP Baur, F Clerget-Darpoux. Genetic analysis of IDDM: summary of GAW 5 IDDM results. Genet Epidemiol 6:43–58, 1989.

48. S Sawcer, PN Goodfellow, A Compston. The genetic analysis of multiple sclerosis. Trends Genet 13:234–239, 1997.

49. LF Barcellos, G Thomson, M Carrington, J Schafer, AB Begovich, P Lin, XH Xu, BQ Min, D Marti, W Klitz. Chromosome 19 single-locus and multilocus haplotype associations with multiple sclerosis. Evidence of a new susceptibility locus in Caucasian and Chinese patients. JAMA 278:1256–1261, 1997.

50. AM Valdes, SK McWeeney, G Thomson. Evidence for linkage and association to alcohol dependence on chromosome 19. Genet Epidemiol 17(suppl 1):S367–S372, 1999.

51. N Arnheim, C Strange, H Erlich, G Thomson. Use of pooled DNA samples to detect linkage disequilibrium of polymorphic restriction fragments and human disease: studies of the HLA class II loci. Proc Natl Acad Sci USA 82:6970–6974, 1985.

52. P Pacek, A Sajantila, AC Syvanen. Determination of allele frequencies at loci with

length polymorphism by quantitative analysis of DNA amplified from pooled samples. PCR Methods Appl 2:313–317, 1993.

53. LF Barcellos, W Klitz, LL Field, R Tobias, AM Bowcock, R Wilson, MP Nelson, J Nagatomi, G Thomson. Association mapping of disease loci, by use of a pooled DNA genomic screen. Am J Hum Genet 61:734–747, 1997.

54. SH Shaw, MM Carrasquillo, C Kashuk, EG Puffenberger, A Chakravarti. Allele frequency distributions in pooled DNA samples: applications to mapping complex disease genes. Genome Res 8:111–123, 1998.

55. S Germer, MJ Holland, R Higuchi. High-throughput SNP allele-frequency determination in pooled DNA samples by kinetic PCR. Genome Res 10:258–266, 2000.

56. AD Long, CH Langley. The power of association studies to detect the contribution of candidate genetic loci to variation in complex traits. Genome Res 9:720–731, 1999.

57. AG Clark, KM Weiss, DA Nickerson, SL Taylor, A Buchanan, J Stengard, V Salomaa, E Vartiainen, M Perola, E Boerwinkle, CF Sing. Haplotype structure and population genetic inferences from nucleotide-sequence variation in human lipoprotein lipase. Am J Hum Genet 63:595–612, 1998.

58. DA Nickerson, SL Taylor, KM Weiss, AG Clark, RG Hutchinson, J Stengard, V Salomaa, E Vartiainen, E Boerwinkle, CF Sing. DNA sequence diversity in a 9.7-kb region of the human lipoprotein lipase gene. Nat Genet 19:233–240, 1998.

59. L Kruglyak. Prospects for whole-genome linkage disequilibrium mapping of common disease genes. Nat Genet 22:139–144, 1999.

60. C Lonjou, A Collins, NE Morton. Allelic association between marker loci. Proc Natl Acad Sci USA 96:1621–1626, 1999.

61. M Cargill, D Altshuler, J Ireland, P Sklar, K Ardlie, N Patil, CR Lane, EP Lim, N Kalayanaraman, J Nemesh, L Ziaugra, L Friedland, A Rolfe, J Warrington, R Lipshutz, GQ Daley, ES Lander. Characterization of single-nucleotide polymorphisms in coding regions of human genes. Nat Genet 22:231–238, 1999.

62. MK Halushka, JB Fan, K Bentley, L Hsie, N Shen, A Weder, R Cooper, R Lipshutz, A Chakravarti. Patterns of single-nucleotide polymorphisms in candidate genes for blood-pressure homeostasis. Nat Genet 22:239–247, 1999.

63. CT Falk, P Rubinstein. Haplotype relative risks: an easy reliable way to construct a proper control sample for risk calculations. Annf Hum Genet 51:227–233, 1987.

64. RS Spielman, RE McGinnis, WJ Ewens. Transmission test for linkage disequilibrium: the insulin gene region and insulin-dependent diabetes mellitus (IDDM). Am J Hum Genet 52:506–516, 1993.

65. SA Monks, NL Kaplan, BS Weir. A comparative study of sibship tests of linkage and/or association. Am J Hum Genet 63:1507–1516, 1998.

66. ER Martin, NL Kaplan, BS Weir. Tests for linkage and association in nuclear families. Am J Hum Genet 61:439–448, 1997.

67. N Risch, J Teng. The relative power of family-based and case-control designs for linkage disequilibrium studies of complex human diseases I. DNA pooling. Genome Res 8:1273–1288, 1998.

68. G Thomson. Strategies involved in mapping diabetes genes: an overview. Diabetes Reviews 5:106–115, 1997.

69. MA Escamilla, LA McInnes, M Spesny, VI Reus, SK Service, N Shimayoshi, DJ

Tyler, S Silva, J Molina, A Gallegos, L Meza, ML Cruz, S Batki, S Vinogradov, T Neylan, JB Nguyen, E Fournier, C Araya, SH Barondes, P Leon, LA Sandkuijl, NB Freimer. Assessing the feasibility of linkage disequilibrium methods for mapping complex traits: an initial screen for bipolar disorder loci on chromosome 18. Am J Hum Genet 64:1670–1678, 1999.

70. G Morahan, D Huang, BD Tait, PG Colman, LC Harrison. Markers on distal chromosome 2q linked to insulin-dependent diabetes mellitus. Science 272:1811–1813, 1996.

71. G Thomson, WF Bodmer. The genetics of HLA and disease associations. In: FB Christiansen, T Fenchel, O Barndorff-Nielson, eds. Measuring Selection in Natural Populations. Heidleberg: Springer-Verlag, 1977, pp 545–564.

72. A Svejgaard, P Platz, LP Ryder. Insulin-dependent diabetes mellitus. In: PI Terasaki, ed. Histocompatibility 1980. Los Angeles: University of California Press, 1980, pp 638–656.

73. G Thomson, WP Robinson, MK Kuhner, S Joe, MJ MacDonald, JL Gottschall, J Barbosa, SS Rich, J Bertrams, MP Baur, J Partanen, B Tait, E Schober, WR Mayr, J Ludvigsson, B Lindblom, NR Farid, C Thompson, I Deschamps. Genetic heterogeneity, modes of inheritance and risk estimates for a joint study of Caucasians with insulin dependent diabetes mellitus. Am J Hum Genet 43:799–816, 1988.

74. H Payami, S Joe, NR Farid, V Stenszky, SH Chan, PPB Yeo, JS Chan, G Thomson. Relative predispositional effects (RPE's) of marker alleles with disease: HLA-DR alleles and Graves disease. Am J Hum Genet 45:541–546, 1989.

75. AM Valdes, S McWeeney, G Thomson. HLA class II DR/DQ amino acids and insulin-dependent diabetes mellitus: application of the haplotype method. Am J Hum Genet 60:717–728, 1997.

76. AM Valdes, G Thomson. Detecting disease-predisposing variants: the haplotype method. Am J Hum Genet 60:703–716, 1997.

77. WP Robinson, G Thomson, SS Rich, J Barbosa. The homozygous parent affected sib pair method for detecting disease predisposing variants: application to insulin dependent mellitus. Genet Epidemiol 10:273–288, 1993.

78. HA Erlich, JI Rotter, JD Chang, SJ Shaw, LJ Raffel, W Klitz, TL Bugawan, A Zeidler. Association of HLA-DPB1*0301 with IDDM in Mexican-Americans. Diabetes 45:610–614, 1996.

79. JA Noble, AM Valdes, G Thomson, HA Erlich. The HLA class II locus DPB1 can influence susceptibility to type 1 diabetes. Diabetes 49:121–125, 2000.

80. PH Moghaddam, P deKnijf, BO Roep, B VanderAuwera, A Naipal, F Gorus, F Schuit, MJ Giphart. Genetic structure of IDDM1: Two separate regions in the major histocompatibility complex contribute to susceptibility or protection. Diabetes 47: 263–269, 1998.

81. B Lie, J Todd, F Pociot, J Nerup, H Akselsen, G Joner, K Dahl-Jorgensen, K Ronningen, E Thorsby, D Undlien. The predisposition to type 1 diabetes linked to the HLA complex (IDDM1) includes at least one non-class II gene. Am J Hum Genet 64:793–800, 1999.

82. PO Brown, L Hartwell. Genomics and human disease-variations on variation. Nat Genet 18:91–93, 1998.

83. A Lernmark, J Ott. Sometimes it's hot, sometimes it's not. Nat Genet 19:213–214, 1998.

84. M Gibbs, JL Stanford, RA McIndoe, GP Jarvik, S Kolb, EL Goode, L Chakrabarti, EF Schuster, VA Buckley, EL Miller, S Brandzel, S Li, L Hood, EA Ostrander. Evidence for a rare prostate cancer-susceptibility locus at chromosome 1p36. Am J Hum Genet 64:776–787, 1999.

85. AD Paterson, A Petronis. Sex of affected sibpairs and genetic linkage to type 1 diabetes. Am J Med Genet 84:15–19, 1999.

86. EW Day, SC Heath, EM Wijsman. Multipoint oligogenic analysis of age-at-onset data with applications to Alzheimer disease pedigrees. Am J Hum Genet 64:839–851, 1999.

87. AM Valdes, G Thomson, HA Erlich, JA Noble. Association between IDDM age of onset and HLA among sib pairs. Diabetes 48:1658–1661, 1999.

88. H Li, L Hsu. Effects of age at onset on the power of the affected sib pair and transmission/disequilibrium tests. Ann Hum Genet 64:239–254, 2000.

89. NJ Cox, M Frigge, DL Nicolae, P Concannon, CL Hanis, GI Bell, A Kong. Loci on chromosomes 2 (NIDDM1) and 15 interact to increase susceptibility to diabetes in Mexican americans. Nat Genet 21:213–215, 1999.

90. F Clerget-Darpoux, MC Babron, B Prum, GM Lathrop, I Deschamps, J Hors. A new method to test genetic models in HLA associated diseases: the MASC method. Ann Hum Genet 52:247–258, 1988.

91. F Clerget-Darpoux, MC Babron, I Deschamps, J Hors. Complementation and maternal effect in insulin-dependent diabetes. Am J Hum Genet 49:42–48, 1991.

92. MH Dizier, MC Babron, F Clerget-Darpoux. Interactive effect of two candidate genes in a disease: extension of the marker-association-segregation χ^2 method. Am J Hum Genet 55:1042–1049, 1994.

93. C Gu, M Province, A Todorov, DC Rao. Meta-analysis methodology for combining non-parametric sibpair linkage results: genetic homogeneity and identical markers. Genet Epidemiol 15:609–626, 1998.

94. LH Wise, JS Lanchbury, CM Lewis. Meta-analysis of genome searches. Ann Hum Genet 63:263–272, 1999.

95. KG Becker, RM Simon, JE Bailey-Wilson, B Freidlin, WE Biddison, HF McFarland, JM Trent. Clustering of non-major histocompatibility complex susceptibility candidate loci in human autoimmune diseases. Proc Natl Acad Sci USA 95:9979–9984, 1998.

96. SA Tishkoff, E Dietzsch, W Speed, AJ Pakstis, JR Kidd, K Cheung, B Bonne-Tamir, AS Santachiara-Benerecetti, P Moral, M Krings. Global patterns of linkage disequilibrium at the CD4 locus and modern human origins. Science 271:1380–1387, 1996.

97. NJ Schork, LR Cardon, X Xu. The future of genetic epidemiology. Trends Genet 14:266–272, 1998.

98. SK Service, DW Lang, NB Freimer, LA Sandkuijl. Linkage-disequilibrium mapping of disease genes by reconstruction of ancestral haplotypes in founder populations. Am J Hum Genet 64:1728–1738, 1999.

99. M Grote, W Klitz, G Thomson. Constrained disequilibrium values and hitchhiking in a three-locus system. Genetics 150:1295–1307, 1998.

18

Positional Cloning and Disease Gene Identification

Mark S. Silverberg
University of Toronto and Mount Sinai Hospital, Toronto, Ontario, Canada

Andrew P. Boright
University of Toronto and Hospital for Sick Children, Toronto,
Ontario, Canada

Katherine A. Siminovitch
University of Toronto and Mount Sinai Hospital, Toronto, Ontario, Canada

1   INTRODUCTION

The advent of modern recombinant DNA technology has provided an unprecedented opportunity to study and understand the molecular pathophysiology of
disease. It is now widely believed that the majority of human diseases arise as
a result of the interplay between environmental factors and genetic background.
The interactions between these genes and environmental exposures plays an essential role in not only disease predisposition, but also in modulating disease
prognosis and other phenotypic characteristics (Fig. 1). Until now, the elucidation
of these complex interactions underlying common disorders has remained ob-
scure. This situation, however, is rapidly changing as the Human Genome Project

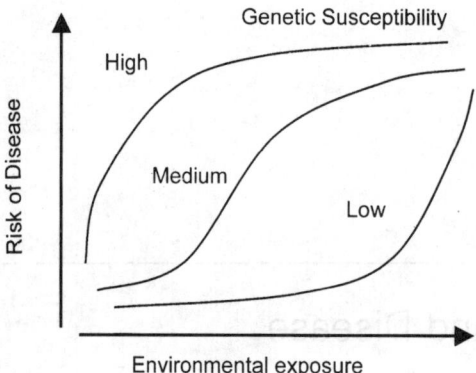

FIGURE 1 In most human diseases, there exists a complex interaction between inherited genetic susceptibility and exposure to environmental factors which, together, determine the risk of acquiring disease.

nears completion and the full genome complement, comprising 80,000–100,000 or so genes is fully elucidated [1]. The major challenge of medical science in this new millennium is to exploit this genetic information so as to delineate the sets of genes responsible for specific illnesses and subsequently unravel the processes by which these genetic determinants influence disease pathophysiology [2]. Such knowledge will lead to the elucidation of molecular markers that can be used to predict disease predisposition, prognosis and drug responsiveness and thus provide the framework for pharmacogenomics to develop and achieve its exciting potential.

In view of the extraordinary potential for disease gene identification to improve health care delivery, an enormous component of human genetics research has been directed at technologies which accelerate the gene discovery process. For many single-gene diseases, knowledge of the pathophysiology has been sufficient to allow for direct screening of newly cloned genes as possible disease gene candidates. This "candidate" gene approach, which builds upon understanding of the disease pathophysiology and a given gene/protein function, has, for example, been used to characterize the molecular basis for phenylketonuria, β-thalassemia, and many other single-gene disorders [3–7].

For the majority of human disease, however, information on etiopathogenesis is insufficient to render candidate gene testing feasible. This situation is true for most single-gene diseases and for virtually all of the common, complex genetic disorders. The problem is compounded in complex genetic disease by many other issues such as lack of knowledge of mode of inheritance, incomplete penetrance, and genetic and allelic heterogeneity [8]. In addition, until relatively re-

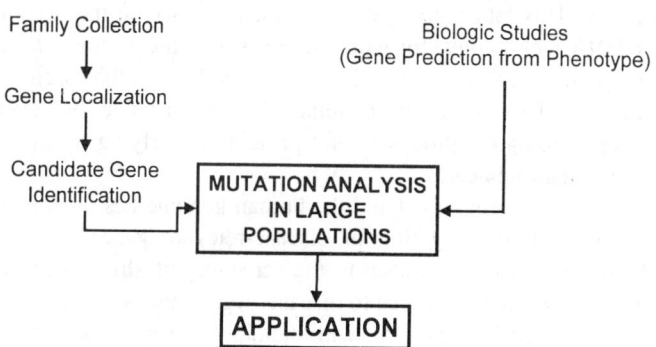

POSITIONAL CLONING   **CANDIDATE GENE APPROACH**

Family Collection

Gene Localization

Candidate Gene Identification

Biologic Studies
(Gene Prediction from Phenotype)

MUTATION ANALYSIS IN LARGE POPULATIONS

APPLICATION

FIGURE 2 Both positional cloning and candidate gene analysis may be used for disease gene discovery. However, these two approaches converge at the point where mutation testing of a candidate gene is required. Once discovered, a disease-causing mutation may then be utilized to develop novel diagnostic tests and therapeutic interventions.

cently, most of the genome had remained uncharacterized. For these reasons, much of the research on disease gene identification has been predicated on an alternate approach, referred to as positional cloning, in which genes are isolated despite lack of information on disease pathophysiology or mode of inheritance [9]. This approach involves discovery of disease genes based on their chromosomal localization, a strategy that has represented a major breakthrough in human genetics. While the initial steps invoked in positional cloning and candidate gene analysis are distinct, positional cloning ultimately involves the identification of a set of candidate genes and as such the methodologies converge (Fig. 2). Accordingly, this chapter incorporates a review of each of these approaches and their value in discovery of disease susceptibility genes.

2 CANDIDATE GENE APPROACHES

In circumstances where disease pathophysiology is well understood, the genes and proteins underlying disease susceptibility are, to a varying degree, predictable. The relevance of such "candidate" genes to a specific disease can be directly established by demonstrating the disease to be associated with allelic variants of the gene(s) in question. Such candidate gene analysis involves investigations of fully characterized genes encoding putative disease-relevant products. Alternatively, the candidate gene analysis may require the isolation of a gene corresponding to a "candidate" disease-related protein, for example using oligo-nucleotide-based probes or antibodies to screen cDNA or cDNA expression libraries, respectively. This latter strategy was frequently used in the early days of recombinant DNA technology, for example, to isolate the Factor VIII gene involved in hemophilia A [3] and the globin genes involved in thalassemia and sickle cell anemia [7]. This approach has relatively limited value, however, as the specific pathophysiological processes and proteins underlying the majority of human disease remain unclear.

As gene cloning has progressed and the human genome has been increasingly well characterized, investigation of disease-relevant genes has largely shifted from the direct cloning approach to the screening of already-identified, novel genes for their potential relevance to disease. Again, this analysis involves some degree of "educated" guesswork, with candidates being selected on the premise of some relevance to disease etiology. This approach is well-illustrated by the example of Marfan's syndrome where the underlying genetic defect was identified by the recognition that a newly cloned gene encoded a protein, fibrillin, which showed functional properties of possible relevance to defects found in Marfan's patients [10,11]. Genes encoding the human leukocyte antigens (HLA) have also been considered and investigated as candidate susceptibility genes for a broad spectrum of diseases, and in particular, autoimmune and other immunological disorders such as asthma, inflammatory bowel disease, multiple sclerosis, type 1 diabetes mellitus, and psoriasis [12]. As the complement of human genes becomes fully elucidated, opportunities for disease gene identification by candidate gene analysis are rapidly increasing, and this approach is now widely used to screen for disease-relevant genes.

The increasing feasibility of candidate gene-based disease gene identification has engendered enormous interest in genetic association studies, in which the relevance of a given gene to a disease phenotype is examined by comparing the frequencies of specific allelic variants of the gene of interest in affected individuals and matched controls (Fig. 3) [13,14]. These case-control studies involve analysis of putative susceptibility (positively associated) or resistance (negatively associated) alleles. This methodology has many advantages over traditional linkage analysis for disease gene discovery, with the association approach, for example, not requiring family collection. The association method also involves analysis of gene variants (polymorphisms) which may not only exhibit linkage disequilibrium with the gene defect of interest but which may actually represent the disease-relevant defect per se [13]. A key consideration, however, in case-control genetic association studies is the ethnic constitution of the case versus control group; ethnic divergence among these groups can represent a major source of spurious results in view of the potential for significant differences in allele frequencies among different ethnic populations. This problem, that is, population admixture, together with inadequate sample sizes, incomplete or inaccurate dis-

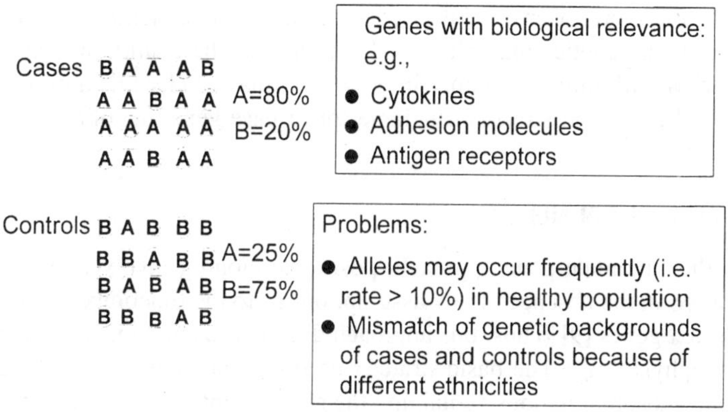

Cases B A A A B

    A A B A A A=80%

    A A A A A B=20%

    A A B A A

> Genes with biological relevance: e.g.,
> - Cytokines
> - Adhesion molecules
> - Antigen receptors

Controls B A B B B

    B B A B B A=25%

    B A B A B B=75%

    B B B A B

> Problems:
> - Alleles may occur frequently (i.e. rate > 10%) in healthy population
> - Mismatch of genetic backgrounds of cases and controls because of different ethnicities

FIGURE 3 Candidate genes which "make sense" in terms of their relevance to disease pathophysiology (e.g., for an inflammatory disorder, cytokine or adhesion molecule genes may be selected) are identified and an association study is performed to determine whether a particular allele (in this example, alleles A and B) is likely to be found more frequently in affected individuals (cases) than in a matched, healthy population (controls). Positive results can be verified by analysis of allele transmission from heterozygous parents to affected and unaffected children. In this example, the frequencies of both the A and B alleles are very different in the case compared to the control populations, which may be indicative of an association between this gene variant and the disease under study.

ease phenotype characterization, analysis of isolated populations or subgroups for which a mutation/variation is not generally applicable, and other sources of type I error, may all account for the many instances in which genetic association data cannot be replicated in independent studies. In this context, a set of guidelines delineating standards expected for rigorous genetic association studies has now been derived [15]. Criteria included in these guidelines are: large sample sizes on the order of 1000 (preferably unrelated) cases and at least as many controls; the requirement for low P values (10^{-6} to 10^{-8}) with high odds ratios; "biological sense" for the demonstrated association—that is, the disease-associated allele(s) should affect the gene product in a physiologically meaningful way; and inclusion of a replication study performed on an independently ascertained population. However, even when these criteria are fulfilled, data from an association study may prove nonreproducible and accordingly the potential for genetic association studies to elucidate the etiology of complex genetic disease is not clear at present. However, with the increasing availability of tools such as single-nucleotide polymorphisms (SNPs) and high-density SNP maps, advances in genotyping automation, more extensive knowledge of the human genome sequence, and improvements in genetic epidemiological approaches, the quality of genetic association studies will almost certainly improve and may render this approach the most practical and rapid strategy available for disease gene identification.

3 POSITIONAL CLONING

In contrast to the candidate gene approach, positional cloning involves disease gene identification in the absence of any assumptions as to the functional properties of the relevant genes [9]. Thus, this approach does not require understanding of disease pathophysiology. The basic strategy used in positional cloning is the definition of chromosomal regions containing the genes of interest and the subsequent analysis of the genes within this region for disease-associated mutations (Fig. 4). The enormity of this task, which involves screening the ~ 3 billion base pairs in the haploid human genome for as minor a change as a single base pair alteration, can be likened to the challenge posed in locating a specific individual on this planet with no clues as to his/her address. However, despite the magnitude of the challenge, many genes associated with single gene disorders have been successfully identified by positional cloning (Table 1). These successes have validated positional cloning as a highly valuable strategy for disease gene isolation

---

FIGURE 4 (a) Multicase family collections are required to achieve the disease gene localization integral to positional cloning. Genotyping is performed on each individual using ~300 microsatellite markers that span the entire genome (3300 cM) at 10 cM or 10 million bp intervals (genomewide scan). Marker-disease cosegregation can then be assessed so as to elucidate loci linked with disease expression. (b) Linkage analysis allows disease genes to be mapped to broad (>5 cM) chromosomal regions that must then be refined to allow disease gene identification. Such refinement is achieved by genotyping with a more dense marker set that provides at least 1 cM coverage of the region of interest. Improved localization of the gene of interest may also be obtained using additional statistical approaches such as the TDT, a test in which trios (one affected child and both parents) are evaluated for evidence of marker linkage disequilibrium (i.e., transmision of a particular marker allele to affected offspring more frequently than expected by chance). (c) Once a chromosomal region has been sufficiently refined to make gene identification feasible (<1 cM), the DNA sequence across the region is aligned and various techniques (e.g., gene prediction programs, comparison with EST databases) are employed to identify the genes within the region. The sequences and expression of these genes are then studied in patients and controls so as to identify the disease-causing gene.

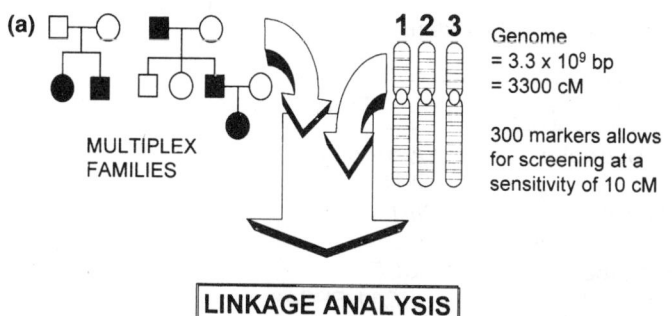

(a)

MULTIPLEX FAMILIES

1 2 3

Genome
= 3.3 x 10^9 bp
= 3300 cM

300 markers allows
for screening at a
sensitivity of 10 cM

LINKAGE ANALYSIS

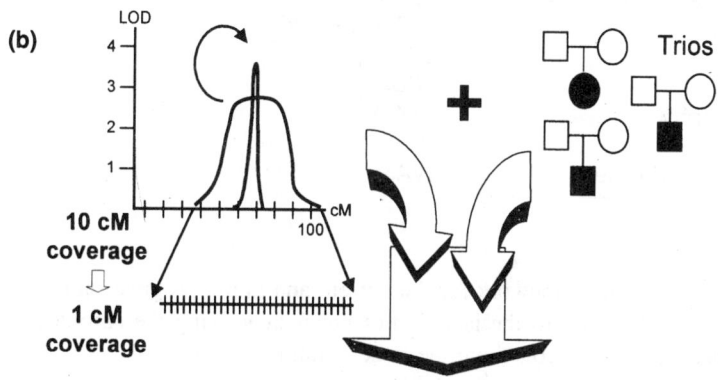

(b)

LOD

10 cM coverage
⇩
1 cM coverage

cM

Trios

LINKAGE DISEQUILIBRIUM ANALYSIS

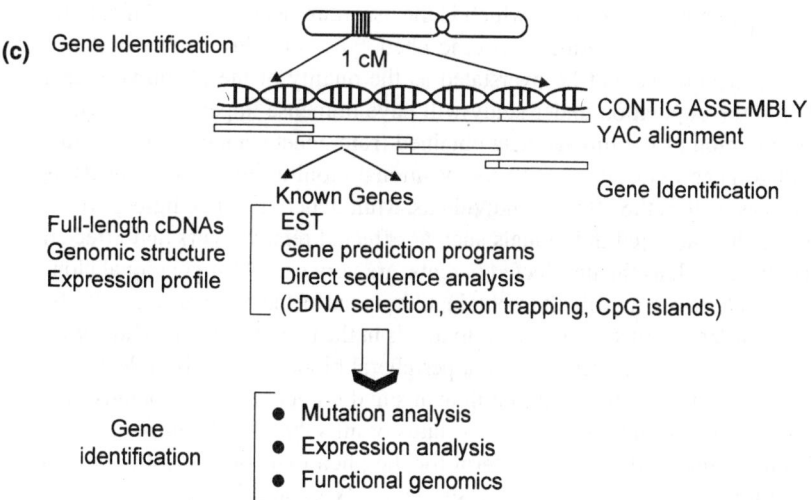

(c) Gene Identification

1 cM

CONTIG ASSEMBLY
YAC alignment

Gene Identification

Full-length cDNAs
Genomic structure
Expression profile

Known Genes
EST
Gene prediction programs
Direct sequence analysis
(cDNA selection, exon trapping, CpG islands)

Gene
identification

• Mutation analysis
• Expression analysis
• Functional genomics

TABLE 1 Examples of Disease Genes Identified by Positional Cloning

Disease	Gene
Duchenne muscular dystrophy	*Dystrophin*
Cystic fibrosis	*CFTR*
Neurofibromatosis type 1	*NF1*
Familial adenomatous polyposis	*APC*
Treacher Collins syndrome	*TCOF1*
Hereditary breast cancer	*BRCA1/BRCA2*
Branchio-oto-renal syndrome	*EYA1*
Alzheimer's disease, early onset	*PSEN1, APP*
Fanconi anemia	*FANCA, FANCC*
Lafora disease	*EPM2A*
Friedreich ataxia	*FRDA1*
Myotonic dystrophy	*DMPK*
Wilson disease	*ATP7B*
Wiskott-Aldrich syndrome	*WAS*

and have thus provided the framework for the current and future progression of positional cloning studies toward the isolation of genes underlying the chronic multifactorial disorders which constitute the bulk of human disease [16].

3.1 Clinical Material

Positional cloning generally involves a series of somewhat discrete steps, the earliest and often rate-limiting of which is the ascertainment and clinical characterization of patients exhibiting a specific phenotype (Fig. 4a). The importance of patient collection cannot be overstated as the quality of the phenotypic data collected in the population under study will have immense impact on the results and interpretation of the linkage data obtained from genetic analysis. In contrast to candidate gene association analysis, positional cloning involves the analysis of families as well as the affected individuals. Multigenerational pedigrees which include multiple affected individuals such as affected relative pairs and affected sibling pairs as well as the unaffected parents, are very useful for positional cloning studies but are often difficult to obtain. Other unaffected relatives may also be included in order to ''link'' affected individuals in the pedigree. Genetic material, usually genomic DNA extracted from a peripheral blood sample, is collected on the affected and unaffected study participants and clinical records obtained and reviewed so as to ensure the affectation status of all subjects. The importance of establishing stringent diagnostic criteria for the phenotype of interest is crucial as the failure to do so may obfuscate subsequently obtained linkage data [17].

These clinical data should in turn be formatted and stored in electronic databases in a fashion that facilitates easy retrieval to conduct multivariate analyses and stratification of the study population based on clinical and/or laboratory features.

After family collection is completed, linkage analysis can then be performed to facilitate disease gene localization. Linkage refers to the fact that loci which map in close proximity on the same chromosome tend to segregate together, whereas loci which map to different chromosomes or far apart on the same chromosome will segregate independently in conjunction with meiotic recombination. The greater the distance between two loci on a given chromosome, the higher the likelihood that these loci will be separated by meiotic crossover events and show a greater interloci recombination fraction (proportion of recombinants between the two loci). By contrast, loci mapping close to one another on a given chromosome are unlikely to be separated by recombination and as such, are referred to as "linked." Importantly, "linkage" implies a physical relationship between genetic loci and needs to be distinguished from the concept of gene "association," the latter of which refers to the coincident presence of a specific marker allele and a given disease phenotype, but which does not imply physical proximity between the disease gene and the marker locus [18–20].

3.2 Genetic Markers for Linkage Analysis

In recognition of the potential for linkage to localize and ultimately reveal novel disease susceptibility genes, an enormous research effort has been directed at identifying genetic markers that are sufficiently polymorphic to be of value in linkage studies. The search for polymorphic markers initially led to the identification of restriction fragment length polymorphisms (RFLPs), that is, biallelic polymorphisms which map within, and thus alter, restriction enzyme cleavage sites, and which can be detected by Southern analysis of restricted genomic DNA. Low levels of informativeness, however, reduced the utility of many RFLP markers, a problem partially resolved by the identification of variable number tandem repeats (VNTRs), that is, sites of highly repetitive DNA referred to as minisatellites. However, even with the addition of VNTRs, coverage of the genome for linkage studies remained a significant problem until the identification of microsatellite loci. These loci represent regions of the genome which contain tandem repeats of about two to seven nucleotides and which occur frequently throughout the genome. Microsatellite regions are highly polymorphic and can be easily detected by PCR amplification using primer pairs from the conserved flanking sequences. These properties have rendered microsatellites a very valuable tool for disease gene mapping and now represent a core reagent for most genomewide scans used in disease gene localization. Most microsatellite marker-based genome scans involve the use of ~ 300 di-, tri-, or tetranucleotide repeat markers spaced at about 10-centimorgan (cM) intervals so as to provide coverage of the approximately 3300 cM genome with a map density of 10 cM (~10% recombination per meiosis between adjacent markers) (Fig. 4a) [8].

While microsatellite markers have proven highly useful for disease gene mapping in single-gene disorders, it is currently unclear whether the level of resolution provided by these markers (at best ~ 1 cM or ~ 1 million base pairs in physical distance) is sufficient to allow for the mapping of genes responsible for complex genetic disease. It is in this context that attention has turned to SNPs, a form of sequence variation which represents the most common source of genome variation [21]. SNPs represent sites in which single base pair variation occurs from person to person and in which the least frequent allele has a frequency of 1% or greater. SNPs have several advantages over microsatellites in terms of both genomewide scanning or candidate gene analysis. SNPs, for example, occur at a frequency of about 1 per 1000 base pairs and, in contrast to microsatellites, are mutationally stable. In addition, many SNPs occur within genes, and accordingly, some SNPs will represent variations which alter gene function and as such, may represent the genetic lesion of interest. By contrast, the utility of SNPs is reduced by the fact that ~ 2.5 biallelic SNPs are required to derive the same amount of information as a simple, more polymorphic microsatellite marker. Thus, to provide whole genome coverage comparable to that of a standard microsatellite genomewide scan incorporating 300 markers, a SNP-based genome scan requires at least 1000 markers. In fact, recent estimates of the numbers of SNPs required for genomewide genetic association studies have been as high as 0.5 million to 1.0 million [22]. Notwithstanding this problem, new technologies such as the use of mass spectrometry and array technologies should render high-throughput SNP genotyping increasingly feasible and, in conjunction with the efforts of SNP consortia to identify novel SNPs, should provide the framework for the whole-genome association studies that may be required for disease gene mapping in complex genetic diseases [16].

3.3   Use of Families for Positional Cloning

In conjunction with polymorphic markers spanning the genome, family collections represent the cornerstone of gene mapping studies. The choice of family structures to be used in positional cloning is very much influenced by the disease under study. For example, large pedigrees including multiple affected individuals are of enormous value in mapping single-gene disorders in which the pattern of inheritance is known and parametric linkage methods are thus easily applied. By contrast, in instances in which the mode of inheritance is unknown, as is usually the case in complex genetic disorders, a preferable family structure is the affected sibling pair which can be studied by nonparametric methods that assess sharing of chromosomal regions by the affected individuals. Affected sib pair analysis is predicated upon the fact that siblings are expected to share 0, 1, or 2 parental alleles at frequencies of 0.25, 0.5, and 0.25, respectively, if the alleles segregate at random. However, siblings affected by a given disease would predictably share the chromosomal region containing the disease relevant loci as revealed by their sharing of an allele or group of alleles at frequencies greater than those predicted by chance. Sib pair analysis has proven very valuable in the search for complex disease gene loci; however, there are drawbacks to this approach including, for example, the fact that sib pairs may share many chromosomal segments by chance and the analysis may therefore easily yield false-positive results.

Once genotypes have been derived from genome-wide scans, the data must be analyzed so as to identify whether any markers cosegregate with the disease (or phenotype). Segregation of alleles is evaluated using linkage analysis and is generally quantitated using a lod (logarithm of the odds) score (Z) which depicts the likelihood of linkage (recombination frequency between two loci < 0.5) versus the null hypothesis of no linkage. For single-gene disorders and two-point linkage analysis, a lod score of 3.0 (5% chance of a false-positive error) has been considered definitive evidence of linkage; under these conditions, linkage is rejected if $Z < -2.0$ while values between -2.0 and $+3.0$ are considered inconclusive. However, these standards do not hold in the context of multiple testing in genome-wide scans, wherein the simultaneous analysis of 300 rather than one or two individual loci markedly increases the chance for false-positive results. Accordingly, for linkage analysis in which genomewide scans are used to identify single-gene disease loci, the threshold for genomewide significance for linkage is considered to be 3.3 [8].

For complex genetic diseases, defining the level of significance in a genomewide study is crucial to determining which loci are linked to true disease susceptibility loci. The difficulties inherent to this issue arise in part from the incorporation of the multiple markers tested. While it is generally agreed that genomewide scans require a threshold P value more stringent than that required for two-point analyses ($P < .05$), some controversy has existed as to what this value should be. However, a set of criteria for interpreting linkage data proposed by Lander and Kruglyak [23] have now been generally accepted. Based on these criteria, a lod score of 3.6 ($P < 2 \times 10^{-5}$) is now considered the threshold for significant linkage while a lod score of > 2.2 or $P < 7 \times 10^{-4}$ is considered to be suggestive of linkage in affected sibling pair-based analyses. Replication of previously reported significant linkage data required a P value $< .01$. In view of the increasing complexity and density of genotype data derived from genomewide scans, a number of sophisticated computer programs have been developed to facilitate linkage analyses. These include, for example, LINKMAP and GENEHUNTER, programs which generate linkage curves showing lod or nonparametric linkage (NPL) scores obtained using multiple sets of microsatellite markers [20,24].

As evidenced by the extensive variation in the recent linkage data derived from independent groups in relation to several complex genetic disorders, linkage analysis in multifactorial disease is not straightforward. While some of the disparities may reflect easily correctable errors such as misread gels, switched samples, incorrect scoring of family relationships and misdiagnosis or misclassification of phenotype, other problems such as incomplete penetrance and genetic heterogeneity are more difficult to address (Table 2). An additional problem is the relatively low resolution of microsatellite marker-based scans, and the consequent necessity for analysis of very large numbers of families so as to delineate a target region amenable to gene identification (i.e., <2 cM). At present, much of the linkage data emanating from microsatellite marker scans has revealed target regions that are far too large (e.g., 10–40 Mb) to attempt disease gene isolation. Accordingly, genomewide scanning needs to be complemented by additional strategies so as to refine the regions of interest to sizes amenable to physical mapping and candidate gene analysis.

3.4 Refinement of Chromosomal Localizations

While the disease gene localizations provided by microsatellite marker, genomewide scans are usually broad, the regions of interest can be refined by using several additional genetic strategies. One commonly used approach is to test for associations between the disease locus and markers in the candidate region. To accomplish this, additional microsatellite markers which increase the density of coverage across the region from 10 cM to 1 cM are required in order to search for disease-associated linkage disequilibrium (LD). The term LD is used if there is association in the presence of linkage, as opposed to the case where association is found without linkage as a result of other factors such as population stratification. When LD is present, the cosegregation of two or more alleles across many generations with the consequent transmission of a "haplotype" of shared alleles can be demonstrated [25]. The utility of LD analysis in disease gene localization is predicted upon cumulative data showing given disease gene alleles to segregate in association (i.e., in linkage disequilibrium) with a set of flanking alleles that comprise an ancestral haplotype derived from the individual (founder) who origi-

TABLE 2 Reasons for Failure to Replicate Linkage in Complex Diseases

Genetic heterogeneity
False-positive and false-negative results
Inadequate population size
Characteristics of patient population:
    Differences in admixture of disease phenotype
    Errors in phenotyping (misdiagnosis/misclassification)
    Differences in ethnic/geographic origin of population

nally introduced the disease gene allele into the population (Fig. 5). These affected individuals within a population may share a set of contiguous alleles within a chromosomal region that comprise a disease-associated haplotype encompassing the disease-related allele. Such linkage disequilibrium can facilitate refinement of candidate regions elucidated from linkage data (Fig. 4b). The transmission disequilibrium test (TDT) was initially introduced as a test for linkage in the presence of association, but it can also be used as a test of association in the presence of linkage (i.e., linkage disequilibrium) if the data consist of nuclear families with a single affected child [26]. This test involves a comparison of the number of times a specific allele is transmitted versus nontransmitted to the affected individual. As TDT is carried out on "trios" (affected individual and two parents), it is often possible to perform this evaluation on many more families than could be ascertained for a sib pair analysis. Increasing the size of the study population in conjunction with an increased density of microsatellite markers lays the groundwork for LD analysis and the definition of a marker haplotype that allows for substantive refinement of the chromosomal region under study. Along similar lines, SNPs also provide a valuable resource for high saturation coverage and refinement of a region of interest to a size (< 2 Mb) amenable to candidate gene identification and analysis.

The potential for SNP-based genomewide association studies to identify disease genes in complex conditions has been revealed by data from several re-

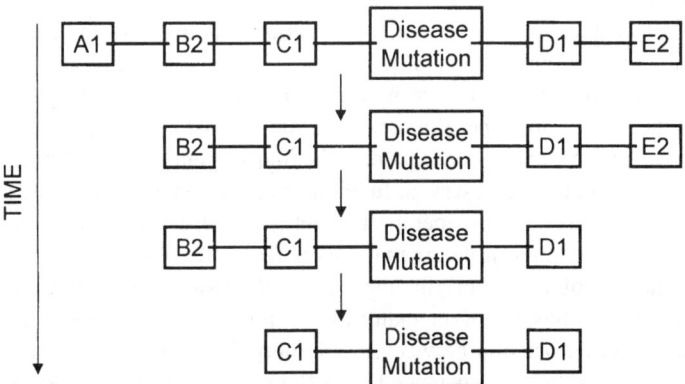

FIGURE 5 Particular alleles of genetic markers (haplotypes) in close proximity to a disease-causing mutation are often associated with the disease. A1, B2, C1, D1, and E2 are alleles initially associated with a disease-relevant allele/mutation. Over time, meiotic recombination disrupts most of these allelic associations. However, the C1 and D1 alleles remain associated with the disease mutation, thus constituting a disease-relevant ancestral haplotype.

cent studies addressing the extent of linkage disequilibrium between known disease susceptibility genes and specific SNP markers that flank such genes [27]. For example, an analysis of the *ApoE* gene, a gene implicated in late-onset Alzheimer's disease, has revealed that of 10 SNPs lying on 800 kb on either side of the gene, only 3 SNPs 10, 12–30, and 440 kb from *ApoE* showed significant LD with *ApoE* and strong association with Alzheimer's disease [28]; by contrast, SNPs located as little as 60–80 kb from the gene showed no evidence of LD or association. These findings highlight the difficulty in elucidating candidate genes based only on the detection of LD between these genes and nearby SNPs. The data suggest that this type of association study will require comprehensive SNP analyses incorporating all SNPs in proximity to the candidate genes of interest.

3.5   Utility of Isolated Populations

Isolated inbred populations have been used successfully in the identification of disease loci, including putative susceptibility loci for complex traits such as type 1 and 2 diabetes mellitus [29,30], multiple sclerosis [31], hyperlipidemia [32], and Hirschsprung's disease [33,34]. In such populations, inbreeding and genetic isolation result in differences in disease alleles and their frequencies and often a reduction in genetic heterogeneity compared with panmictic populations. Also, since homozygotes are more likely to share functional alleles identical by descent in this setting than in outbred populations, the number of alleles contributing to a complex trait is likely to be lower and recessive genetic effects on phenotypes more easily identified. Previous data from association studies have in fact revealed the ability to detect small genetic effects on a quantitative trait to be enhanced in consanguineous populations [35]; similarly, inbreeding coefficients of ~0.01 have been shown to be associated with increased power in detecting the effect of a candidate gene [36]. These observations are at least in part related to shared genetic background and a consequent reduction in genetic variation on which these recessive alleles are observed. In addition to consanguinity, isolated societies often contain large, multigenerational families with multiple affected individuals, a desirable pedigree structure that greatly facilitates linkage analysis. In founder populations of recent origin, the extent of linkage disequilibrium across a genetic interval may be larger than in older populations and therefore the ability to detect an association between a polymorphic marker and disease trait extends over a greater genetic distance [37–39]. Finally, population isolates may also have common traditions and lifestyles contributing to a shared environment which probably lessens the confounding effects of background environment heterogeneity.

Despite these advantages, there are a number of caveats to the analysis of genetic data garnered from inbred populations. For example, in isolated populations wherein allelic heterogeneity is predictably reduced, distinguishing a mutant allele from a rare polymorphism unique to the population may be very difficult

[40]. Furthermore, consanguinity may increase the type 1 error rate in sibling pair linkage analysis, leading to falsely positive linkage results [36]. Lastly, alleles identified as being disease causative variants in isolated populations may be rare alleles that are not relevant to disease etiology in more diverse populations and the clinical utility of such information may therefore be rather limited.

4 PHYSICAL MAPPING

The strategy of positional cloning [41,42] in which a disease gene is identified by virtue of its position within the genome rather than by functional characterization has been used in the mapping and identification of >100 disease loci [43]. The success of the strategy is very much dependent on the accuracy and resolution of the map to which the disease locus is assigned. Genome maps have historically been constructed from different resources and have varying scales of resolution which include, in order of least to highest resolution: genetic maps, radiation hybrid maps, ordered library contigs, and ultimately the genomic sequence. These maps can be further complimented by chromosomal or cytogenetic maps, which have improved dramatically due to advances in fluorescence in situ hybridization (FISH) analysis. Recent advances in delineating the full human genome sequence are radically altering strategies of disease gene mapping. A description of these and other advances in physical mapping is provided below, but it is important to note that the approach to disease gene mapping is in rapid evolution in conjunction with the culmination of the human genome project and associated changes in genomic technologies.

4.1 Genetic Maps

The utility of the genetic map is in its application as a tool to position disease gene loci on a framework of genetic markers. The report of a restriction fragment length polymorphism (RFLP) genomewide genetic linkage map in 1980 by Botstein and colleagues [44] marked the beginning of a new era in genetic map construction. The informativeness of the genomewide linkage maps was markedly improved by the introduction of multiallelic short tandem repeat polymorphisms (microsatellites) as a substitute for the relatively less informative di-allelic polymorphic markers [45,46]. The success of linkage studies and hence positional cloning studies relies on the accuracy and density of these reference genetic linkage maps. The Généthon linkage map is one such map derived by genotyping eight CEPH reference families for 5264 short tandem repeat polymorphic markers and then ordering 2032 of these markers on the map with an acceptable level of accuracy. The map spans a sex-averaged distance of 3699 cM and the average interval size between markers is 1.6 cM [47]. There now exist an enormous number of genetic maps which provide the framework for the gene mapping studies described above.

4.2 Radiation Hybrid Mapping

Radiation hybrid (RH) panels are generated from human/hamster somatic cell hybrids containing radiation-induced fragments of human chromosomes that have integrated into hamster chromosomes and undergone stable mitotic segregation. Panels of these cells containing selected human chromosomal fragments can be used as mapping reagents for ordering markers and determining distances between them. The frequency of radiation-induced breakage between two markers is used as a measure of distance, the marker order being determined in much the same manner as in meiotic linkage mapping [48]. Unlike genetic maps in which markers have to be polymorphic, any unique PCR amplicon can be used in RH mapping. Radiation hybrid maps have been constructed from three whole-genome RH panels, including the GB4 panel [49] and the G3 panel [50], which contain fragments of ~25 and 2.4 Mb, respectively. The G3 RH panel and a third panel, the TNG RH panel [51], can be used to order markers at 500 and 50-kb resolution, respectively. Using the RH method, a human gene map was established by integrating 30,181 gene-based markers onto a background set of microsatellite markers. This gene map is an important resource for the study of complex genetic disease, positional cloning, cross-referencing mammalian genomes, and validating and identifying human transcribed sequences [52].

4.3 Ordered Library Contigs

At the next level of mapping resolution are ordered library contigs which may be derived from yeast artificial chromosomes (YACs), bacterial artificial chromosomes (BACs), P1 artificial chromosomes (PACs), cosmids, or a combination of clones, each of which contain inserts of human genomic DNA. Maps covering regions or entire chromosomes can be generated by identifying overlapping clones and ordering these clones based on their marker content. YACs were initially envisioned as the cloning system of choice for genesis of contigs, as this vector can accommodate inserts on the order of 1 Mb. Two whole-genome YAC-based physical maps have been reported [53,54] and there are a number of chromosome-specific YAC-based maps of selected human chromosomes, for example, chromosomes Y [55], 21 [56], 3 [57], 12 [58], 16 [59], 22 [60], X [61], and 7 [62,63]. All of this mapping data is currently available on the respective, chromosome-specific internet sites. These YAC-based maps have enormously facilitated positional cloning studies, allowing for coverage of the very large genomic regions, which may represent the best refinement of a disease-relevant chromosomal region identifiable by linkage analysis. However, the high rate of YAC chimerism (incorporation of insert fragments from more than one genomic location within a single YAC), YAC instability, and difficulties inherent to YAC manipulation and purification render these cloning vectors unsuitable as reagents for human genome sequencing efforts. YACs are very useful as an intermediary vehicle in the ordering of "sequence ready" physical maps of the smaller and more stable PACs and BACs [64]. These latter bacterial cloning vectors, which can accommodate inserts sizes ranging from 100 to 200 kb, can be ordered into contigs using restriction enzyme fingerprinting analysis and marker content mapping, and can be used for subcloning and DNA sequencing. The generation of the entire genome sequence within bacterial contigs has laid the groundwork for development of the most comprehensive physical map with the highest resolution—that is, the complete human sequence [65].

The above mapping strategies can be complemented by cytogenetic mapping using FISH analysis. Genomic clones, labeled with fluorescent tags can be positioned on cytogenetic maps and used to verify contig construction and other mapping information. The resolution of FISH mapping is improving, being 1–5 Mb on condensed metaphase chromosomes, but 50–100 kb on interphase chromosomes [66]. Resolution is also increasing in the context of newer FISH techniques which employ various methods of stretching a single DNA molecule over a supporting matrix [67]. Positional cloning studies can be greatly accelerated by FISH analysis if the disease under study is associated with chromosomal rearrangements.

Importantly, the capacity to physically map chromosomal regions of interest has been greatly enhanced in the context of advances wrought by Human Genome Project research and the concomitant technological and bioinformatic advances. Thus, for example, once a disease gene-containing chromosomal region has been sufficiently refined, it is now possible to identify, through public databases, YAC contigs which include STS markers at 100- to 200-kb intervals across the region of interest. The STS markers can be utilized as primers or probes for screening BAC or cosmid libraries and BAC/cosmid contigs spanning the critical region thus generated. These clones can be subcloned, sequenced, and then queried against databases such as dbEST and Genbank in order to identify coding segments within the critical region. From these latter segments, candidates can be selected and full-length cDNAs then isolated and screened for mutations that cosegregate with disease. Currently, the generation of BAC tiling paths (minimal overlapping clones within a region) is expedited through the use of public databases including the BAC end library sequence database [68] as well as the human BAC fingerprinting database [69]. Mining of these two databases can markedly expedite chromosome walking and greatly reduce cost and labour. However, as outlined below, these technologies are rapidly changing and the availability of the human genome sequence may render obsolete much of the "physical mapping" facet of positional cloning.

5 POSITIONAL CLONING USING COMPUTATIONAL ALGORITHMS AND DATABASE MINING

At the time of this writing, 0.65 billion bp of finished sequence and 2.3 billion bp of unfinished (draft) sequence representing a total of ~90% of the human genome are available in public databases [70]. This resource has and will continue to dramatically change the positional cloning process. As the human genome sequence unfolds, for example, it is becoming increasingly possible to map disease genes to regions for which the entire sequence has been elucidated and many of the genes already delineated. This sequence can be analyzed by computational methods to identify additional candidate genes and mutation analysis then performed to immediately identify the etiologic disease gene. Clearly, under such conditions, disease gene discovery will be enormously expedited.

Analysis of given chromosomal regions for disease gene candidates has traditionally involved such strategies as exon trapping, CpG island identification, and cDNA selection. While some of these technologies may still be required to identify all genes encoded within a given region, the need to involve these labour intensive strategies is rapidly diminishing in conjunction with the extensive sequence data derived from the human genome project and the tremendous explosion in gene identification and mapping data. By contrast, gene identification within a given chromosomal region is increasingly performed using gene prediction programs and EST (expressed sequence tags) databases (Fig. 6).

A number of programs incorporating algorithms for gene or exon prediction are now available on the Internet. Examples of such programs include RepeatMasker [71] and Censor [72]. These programs integrate a so-called "masking" function, which mask repetitive sequences and hence reduce the amount of false positive prediction. This process is not perfect, however, as some genes, such as genes derived from transposable elements and many ESTs, may contain interspersed repeats in the 3′ UTR that can be inadvertently masked and thus not identified. Once masked, the test sequence is subjected to gene and exon prediction programs such as GRAIL2 [73], GENSCAN [74], FGENESH [75] and MZEF [76]. The algorithms incorporated in these programs have varying sensitivity and specificity for exon/gene identification and a robust analysis therefore requires the use of several of these programs. The region of interest can also be scanned for other indications of coding sequence such as transcription start sites, potential splice sites, polyadenylation signals, and CpG islands [77,78]. In addition, the sequence of interest can be submitted to an EST database (dbEST) so as to identify previously known ESTs within the region. ESTs that occur in clusters, align to genomic sequence, are predicted by exon/gene prediction algorithms and exhibit intron-exon structure, are highly likely to represent fragments of genuine genes and warrant further investigation. This can be accomplished, for example, by retrieval of the full-length cDNA and mRNA tissue expression.

Once the full complement of genes within a region of interest has been elucidated, the disease-relevant gene can then be investigated. Identification of the sought after gene may be facilitated by prior knowledge of gene product functions, the hope being to identify a gene encoding a protein with predicted relevance to the disease under study. Genes can then be prioritized based on this

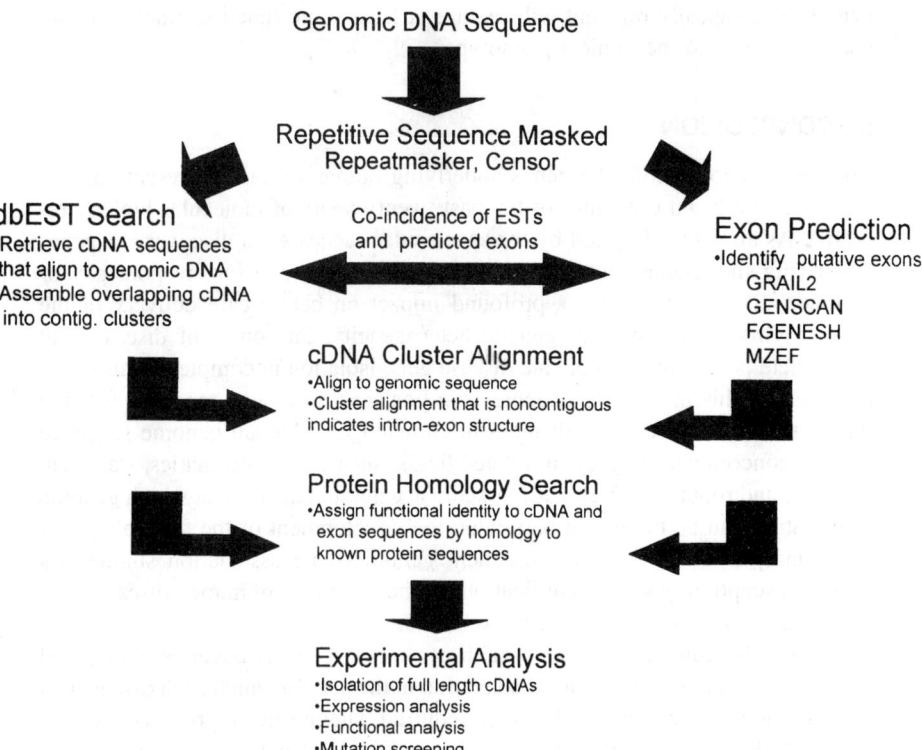

Genomic DNA Sequence

Repetitive Sequence Masked
Repeatmasker, Censor

dbEST Search
•Retrieve cDNA sequences
that align to genomic DNA
•Assemble overlapping cDNA
into contig. clusters

Co-incidence of ESTs
and predicted exons

Exon Prediction
•Identify putative exons
  GRAIL2
  GENSCAN
  FGENESH
  MZEF

cDNA Cluster Alignment
•Align to genomic sequence
•Cluster alignment that is noncontiguous
indicates intron-exon structure

Protein Homology Search
•Assign functional identity to cDNA and
exon sequences by homology to
known protein sequences

Experimental Analysis
•Isolation of full length cDNAs
•Expression analysis
•Functional analysis
•Mutation screening

FIGURE 6 With the availability in the near future of the complete human genome reference sequence, computational methods will play an increasingly prominent role in disease gene identification. Current algorithms exist that will analyze masked genomic sequence and identify by BLASTN alignment those ESTs that map to the sequence. Exons and genes can be predicted using available gene finding programs. Further information can be gleaned by performing protein homology searches on any putative gene. Ultimately, the expression of predicted genes needs to be proven, for example, by identifying the full-length cDNA and performing expression and functional analyses.

type of information and studied by direct sequence analysis for nucleotide changes which distinguishes patients from healthy controls. As the genetic lesions responsible for complex genetic disease are likely to be more subtle (i.e., SNPs) than those found in single-gene disease and will not be entirely correlated with the presence or absence of disease, it is likely that the verification of a candidate gene as etiologically relevant will require at least some functional data relating the gene defect to the clinical phenotype.

6 CONCLUSION

The capacity to identify the genes underlying human disease represents one of the most significant outcomes of the past twenty years of molecular biology research. As already evidenced by the spectacular successes in discovery of genes underlying single-gene diseases, definition of the genetic lesions responsible for common diseases will have a profound impact on health care delivery of the future. While issues such as genetic heterogeneity, late onset of disease, and incomplete penetrance complicate disease gene isolation in complex, multifactorial disease, this previously unachievable goal has now been rendered feasible thanks to the extraordinary advances in knowledge of human genome sequence and the concomitant progress in related fields, such as bioinformatics, statistical genetics, and robotics, which has markedly accelerated the pace at which genome information can be mined. In particular, the development of the technology for rapid analysis of SNPs and consequent genome-scale association studies has moved susceptibility gene identification for the full range of human disease from the spectrum of possibility to real likelihood.

To fully capitalize on the wealth of disease gene discoveries anticipated over these next few decades, an acceleration in the pace at which such discoveries are translated to the clinic will also be required. Diagnostics represents one area in which disease gene discovery can be easily translated to medical practice, but brings to the field many attendant complications including complex ethical, sociological, and legal issues that will need to be addressed as genetics is increasingly integrated into the practice of adult medical care. Therapeutics will likely be the next major area to be substantively modified by disease gene discovery with genetic information providing new avenues for gene therapy, definition of disease-specific targets for pharmacological intervention, and pharmacogenetics. Finally, disease gene discovery creates a framework for the large-scale population studies directed at definition of the environmental-gene interactions which underlie disease and the elucidation of molecular markers that can be used to stratify patient populations so as to predict severity, prognosis, and drug responsiveness. Ultimately, knowledge of the genes which cause and modulate disease will shift the paradigm of medical care to "individualized" care wherein risk for disease can be identified and mitigated in healthy individuals and treatment for those affected by disease can be tailored so as to minimize toxicity and optimize efficacy of selected therapies. The era of genomic medicine has begun and the challenge in this new millennium will be to both delineate the genetic basis of all human disease and to translate this extraordinary achievement to radical improvements in the quality of health care delivery.

ACKNOWLEDGMENTS

Compilation of this chapter was made possible by grants from the Medical Research Council of Canada, the Arthritis Society of Canada, and the Crohn's and Colitis Foundation of Canada. M.S. is a research fellow supported by the Canadian Association of Gastroenterology, the Medical Research Council of Canada, and Axcan Pharma, Inc. A.B. is a reseach fellow supported by the Medical Research Council of Canada. K.A.S. is a Research Scientist of the Arthritis Society of Canada.

REFERENCES

1. FS Collins, A Patrinos, E Jordan A Chakravarti, R Gesteland, L Walters. New goals for the US Human Genome Project:1998–2003. Science 282:682–689, 1998.
2. TJ Hudson. The Human Genome Project: tools for the identification of disease genes. Clin Invest Med 21:267–276, 1998.
3. J Gitschier, WI Wood, TM Goralka, KL Wion, EY Chen, DH Eaton, GA Vehar, DJ Capon, RM Lawn. Characterization of the human factor VIII gene. Nature 312: 326–330, 1984.
4. MD Koob, ML Moseley, LJ Schut, KA Benzow, TD Bird, JW Day, LP Ranum. An untranslated CTG expansion causes a novel form of spinocerebellar ataxia (SCA8). Nat Genet 21:379–384, 1999.
5. KJH Robson, T Chandra, RTA MacGillivray, SLC Woo. Polysome immunoprecipitation of phenylalanine hydroxylase mRNA from rat liver and cloning of its cDNA. Proc Natl Acad Sci USA 79:4701–4705, 1982.
6. M Schalling, TJ Hudson, KH Buetow, DE Houseman. Direct detection of novel expanded trinucleotide repeats in the human genome. Nat Genet 4:135–139, 1993.
7. DJ Weatheral. The thalassemias. In: G Stamatoyannopoulos, AW Nienhuis, PH Majerus, H Varmus, eds. The Molecular Basis of Blood Diseases. Philadelphia: W.B. Saunders, 1994, pp 157–205.
8. ES Lander, N Schork. Genetic dissection of complex traits. Science 265:2037–2048, 1994.
9. FS Collins. Of needles and haystacks: finding human disease genes by positional cloning. Clin Res 39:615–634, 1991.
10. B Lee, M Godfrey, E Vitale, H Hori, MG Mattei, M Sarfarazi, P Tsipouras, F Ramirez, DW Hollister. Linkage of Marfan syndrome and a phenotypically related disorder to two different fibrillin genes [see comments]. Nature 352:330–334, 1991.
11. HC Dietz, GR Cutting, RE Pyeritz, CL Maslen, LY Sakai, GM Corson, EG Puffenberger, A Hamosh, EJ Nanthakumar, SM Curristin et al. Marfan syndrome caused by a recurrent de novo missense mutation in the fibrillin gene. Nature 352:337–339, 1991.
12. L Fugger, R Tisch, R Libau, P van Endert, HO McDevitt. The role of human major histocompatibility complex (HLA) genes in disease. In: CR Scriver, AL Beaudet, W Sly, D Valle, eds. The Metabolic and Molecular Basis of Inherited Disease. Toronto: McGraw-Hill, 1995, pp 555–585.

13. AD Long, CH Langley. The power of association studies to detect the contribution of candidate genetic loci to variation in complex traits. Genome Res 9:720–731, 1999.

14. Editor. Freely associating. Nat Genet 22:1–2, 1999.

15. JA Todd. Interpretation of results from genetic studies of multifactorial diseases. Lancet 354(suppl 1):15–16, 1999.

16. N Risch, K Merikangas. The future of genetic studies of complex human diseases. Science 273:1516–1517, 1996.

17. MC King. Leaving Kansas . . . finding genes in 1997 [news]. Nat Genet 15:8–10, 1997.

18. DE Weeks, K Lange. A multilocus extension of the affected pedigree member method of linkage analysis. Am J Hum Genet 50:859–868, 1992.

19. L Kruglyak, ES Lander. Complete multipoint sib-pair analysis of qualitative and quantitative traits. Am J Hum Genet 57:439–454, 1995.

20. L Kruglyak, MJ Daly, MP Reeve-Daly, ES Lander. Parametric and nonparametric linkage analysis: a unified multipoint approach. Am J Hum Genet 58:1347–1363, 1996.

21. DA Nickerson, C Whitehurst, C Boysen, P Charmley, R Kaiser, L Hood. Identification of clusters of biallelic polymorphic sequence-tagged sites (pSTSs) that generate highly informative and automatable markers for genetic linkage mapping. Genomics 12:377–387, 1992.

22. L Kruglyak. The use of a genetic map of biallelic markers in linkage studies. Nat Genet 17:1–4, 1997.

23. ES Lander, L Kruglyak. Genetic dissection of complex traits: guidelines for interpreting and reporting linkage results. Nat Genet 11:241–247, 1995.

24. A Kong, NJ Cox. Allele sharing models: LOD scores and accurate linkage tests. Am J Hum Genet 61:1179–1188, 1997.

25. M Xiong, S-W Guo. Fine-scale genetic mapping based on linkage disequilbrium: theory and applications. Am J Hum Genet 60:1513–1531, 1997.

26. RS Spielman, RE McGinnis, WJ Ewens. Transmission test for linkage disequilibrium: the insulin gene region and insulin-dependent diabetes mellitus (IDDM). Am J Hum Genet 52:506–516, 1993.

27. ER Martin, JR Gilbert, EH Lai, J Riley, AR Rogala, BD Slotterbeck, CA Sipe, JM Grubber, LL Warren, PM Conneally, AM Saunders, DE Schmechel, I Purvis, MA Pericak-Vance, AD Roses, JM Vance. Analysis of association at single nucleotide polymorphisms in the APOE region. Genomics 63:7–12, 2000.

28. AD Roses, MA Pericak-Vance. Alzheimer's disease and other dementias. In: DL Rimoin, ed. Emery and Rimoin's Principles and Practice of Medical Genetics. New York: Churchill-Livingston, 1997, pp 1807–1825.

29. JL Davies, Y Kawaguchi, ST Bennett, JB Copeman, HJ Cordell, LE Pritchard, PW Reed, SC Gough, SC Jenkins, SM Palmer. A genome-wide search for human type 1 diabetes susceptibility genes [see comments]. Nature 371:130–136, 1994.

30. CL Hanis, E Boerwinkle, R Chakraborty, DL Ellsworth, P Concannon, B Stirling, VA Morrison, B Wapelhorst, RS Spielman, KJ Gogolin-Ewens, JM Shepard, SR Williams, N Risch, D Hinds, N Iwasaki, M Ogata, Y Omori, C Petzold, H Rietzch, HE Schroder, J Schulze, NJ Cox, S Menzel, VV Boriraj, X Chen. A genome-wide

search for human non-insulin-dependent (type 2) diabetes genes reveals a major susceptibility locus on chromosome 2 [see comments]. Nat Genet 13:161–166, 1996.

31. S Kuokkanen, M Sundvall, JD Terwilliger, PJ Tienari, J Wikstrom, R Holmdahl, U Pettersson, L Peltonen. A putative vulnerability locus to multiple sclerosis maps to 5p14–p12 in a region syntenic to the murine locus Eae2 [see comments]. Nat Genet 13:477–480, 1996.

32. P Pajukanta, I Nuotio, JD Terwilliger, KV Porkka, K Ylitalo, J Pihlajamaki, AJ Suomalainen, AC Syvanen, T Lehtimaki, JS Viikari, M Laakso, MR Taskinen, C Ehnholm, L Peltonen. Linkage of familial combined hyperlipidaemia to chromosome 1q21–q23. Nat Genet 18:369–373, 1998.

33. EG Puffenberger, ER Kauffman, S Bolk, TC Matise, SS Washington, M Angrist, J Weissenbach, KL Garver, M Mascari, R Ladda. Identity-by-descent and association mapping of a recessive gene for Hirschsprung disease on human chromosome 13q22. Hum Mol Genet 3:1217–1225, 1994.

34. EG Puffenberger, K Hosoda, SS Washington, K Nakao, D deWit, M Yanagisawa, A Chakravarti. A missense mutation of the endothelin-B receptor gene in multigenic Hirschsprung's disease. Cell 79:1257–1266, 1994.

35. E Genin, F Clerget-Darpoux. Association studies in consanguineous populations. Am J Hum Genet 58:861–866, 1996.

36. E Genin, F Clerget-Darpoux. Consanguinity and the sib-pair method: an approach using identity by descent between and within individuals. Am J Hum Genet 59:1149–1162, 1996.

37. TM Fujiwara, K Morgan, RH Schwartz, RA Doherty, SR Miller, K Klinger, P Stanislovitis, N Stuart, PC Watkins. Genealogical analysis of cystic fibrosis families and chromosome 7q RFLP haplotypes in the Hutterite Brethren. Am J Hum Genet 44:327–337, 1989.

38. L Peltonen, A Uusitalo. Rare disease genes—lessons and challenges. Genome Res 7:765–767, 1997.

39. B Glaser, KC Chiu, L Liu, R Anker, A Nestorowicz, NJ Cox, H Landau, N Kaiser, PS Thornton, CA Stanley. Recombinant mapping of the familial hyperinsulinism gene to an 0.8 cM region on chromosome 11p15.1 and demonstration of a founder effect in Ashkenazi Jews [published erratum appears in Hum Mol Genet 4:2187–2188, 1995]. Hum Mol Genet 4:879–886, 1995.

40. VC Sheffield, EM Stone, R Carmi. Use of isolated inbred human populations for identification of disease genes. Trends Genet 14:391–396, 1998.

41. FS Collins. Positional cloning: let's not call it reverse anymore [news]. Nat Genet 1:3–6, 1992.

42. A Ballabio. The rise and fall of positional cloning? [news]. Nat Genet 3:277–279, 1993.

43. FS Collins, MS Guyer, A Charkravarti. Variations on a theme: cataloging human DNA sequence variation. Science 278:1580–1581, 1997.

44. D Botstein, RL White, M Skolnick, RW Davis. Construction of a genetic linkage map in man using restriction fragment length polymorphisms. Am J Hum Genet 32:314–331, 1980.

45. JL Weber, PE May. Abundant class of human DNA polymorphisms which can be typed using the polymerase chain reaction. Am J Hum Genet 44:388–396, 1989.

46. H Donis-Keller, P Green, C Helms, S Cartinhour, B Weiffenbach, K Stephens, TP Keith, DW Bowden, DR Smith, ES Lander. A genetic linkage map of the human genome. Cell 51:319–337, 1987.

47. C Dib, S Faure, C Fizames, D Samson, N Drouot, A Vignal, P Millasseau, S Marc, J Hazan, E Seboun, M Lathrop, G Gyapay, J Morissette, J Weissenbach. A comprehensive genetic map of the human genome based on 5,264 microsatellites [see comments]. Nature 380:152–154, 1996.

48. DR Cox, M Burmeister, ER Price, S Kim, RM Myers. Radiation hybrid mapping: a somatic cell genetic method for constructing high-resolution maps of mammalian chromosomes. Science 250:245–250, 1990.

49. G Gyapay, K Schmitt, C Fizames, H Jones, N Vega-Czarny, D Spillett, D Muselet, JF Prud'Homme, C Dib, C Auffray, J Morissette, J Weissenbach, PN Goodfellow. A radiation hybrid map of the human genome. Hum Mol Genet 5:339–346, 1996.

50. EA Stewart, KB McKusick, A Aggarwal, E Bajorek, S Brady, A Chu, N Fang, D Hadley, M Harris, S Hussain, R Lee, A Maratukulam, K O'Connor, S Perkins, M Piercy, F Qin, T Reif, C Sanders, X She, WL Sun, P Tabar, S Voyticky, S Cowles, JB Fan, DR Cox. An STS-based radiation hybrid map of the human genome. Genome Res 7:422–433, 1997.

51. KL Lunetta, M Boehnke, K Lange, DR Cox. Selected locus and multiple panel models for radiation hybrid mapping. Am J Hum Genet 59:717–725, 1996.

52. P Deloukas, GD Schuler, G Gyapay, EM Beasley, C Soderlund, P Rodriguez-Tome, L Hui, TC Matise, KB McKusick, JS Beckmann, S Bentolila, M Bihoreau, BB Birren, J Browne, A Butler, AB Castle, N Chiannilkulchai, C Clee, PJ Day, A Dehejia, T Dibling, N Drouot, S Duprat, C Fizames, DR Bentley. A physical map of 30,000 human genes. Science 282:744–746, 1998.

53. TJ Hudson, LD Stein, SS Gerety, J Ma, AB Castle, J Silva, DK Slonim, R Baptista, L Kruglyak, SH Xu. An STS-based map of the human genome [see comments]. Science 270:1945–1954, 1995.

54. IM Chumakov, P Rigault, I Le Gall, C Bellanne-Chantelot, A Billault, S Guillou, P Soularue, G Guasconi, E Poullier, I Gros. A YAC contig map of the human genome. Nature 377:175–297, 1995.

55. S Foote, D Vollrath, A Hilton, DC Page. The human Y chromosome: overlapping DNA clones spanning the euchromatic region. Science 258:60–66, 1992.

56. I Chumakov, P Rigault, S Guillou, P Ougen, A Billaut, G Guasconi, P Gervy, I LeGall, P Soularue, L Grinas. Continuum of overlapping clones spanning the entire human chromosome 21q [see comments]. Nature 359:380–387, 1992.

57 RM Gemmill, I Chumakov, P Scott, B Waggoner, P Rigault, J Cypser, Q Chen, J Weissenbach, K Gardiner, H Wang. A second-generation YAC contig map of human chromosome 3. Nature 377:299–319, 1995.

58. K Krauter, K Montgomery, SJ Yoon, J LeBlanc-Straceski, B Renault, I Marondel, V Herdman, L Cupelli, A Banks, J Lieman. A second-generation YAC contig map of human chromosome 12. Nature 377:321–333, 1995.

59. NA Doggett, LA Goodwin, JG Tesmer, LJ Meincke, DC Bruce, LM Clark, MR Altherr, AA Ford, HC Chi, BL Marrone. An integrated physical map of human chromosome 16. Nature 377:335–365, 1995.

60. JE Collins, CG Cole, LJ Smink, CL Garrett, MA Leversha, CA Soderlund, GL Mas-

len, LA Everett, KM Rice, AJ Coffey. A high-density YAC contig map of human chromosome 22. Nature 377:367–379, 1995.

61. R Nagaraja, S MacMillan, J Kere, C Jones, S Griffin, M Schmatz, J Terrell, M Shomaker, C Jermak, C Hott, M Masisi, S Mumm, A Srivastava, G Pilia, T Featherstone, R Mazzarella, S Kesterson, B McCauley, B Railey, F Burough, V Nowotny, M D'Urso, D States, B Brownstein, D Schlessinger. X chromosome map at 75-kb STS resolution, revealing extremes of recombination and GC content. Genome Res 7:210–222, 1997.

62. http://www.genet.sickkids.on.ca/chromosome7

63. GG Bouffard, JR Idol, VV Braden, LM Iyer, AF Cunningham, LA Weintraub, JW Touchman, RM Mohr-Tidwell, DC Peluso, RS Fulton, MS Ueltzen, J Weissenbach, CL Magness, ED Green. A physical map of human chromosome 7: an integrated YAC contig map with average STS spacing of 79 kb. Genome Res 7:673–692, 1997.

64. MA Marra, TA Kucaba, NL Dietrich, ED Green, B Brownstein, RK Wilson, KM McDonald, LW Hillier, JD McPherson, RH Waterston. High throughput fingerprint analysis of large-insert clones. Genome Res 7:1072–1084, 1997.

65. L Goodman. The Human Genome Project aims for 2003. Genome Res 8:997–999, 1998.

66. BJ Trask, S Allen, H Massa, A Fertitta, R Sachs, G van den Engh, M Wu. Studies of metaphase and interphase chromosomes using fluorescence in situ hybridization. Cold Spring Harb Symp Quant Biol 58:7677, 1993.

67. J Herrick, A Bensimon. Imaging of single DNA molecule: applications to high-resolution genomic studies. Chromosome Res 7:409–423, 1999.

68. http://www.tigr.org/tdb/humgen/bac_end_search/bac_end_intro.html

69. http://genome.wustl.edu/gsc/human/human_database.shtml

70. http//www.ebi.ac.uk/~sterk/genome-MOT

71. http://ftp.genome.washington.edu/cgi-bin/RepeatMasker

72. http://charon.girinst.org/Censor_Server_Data_Entry_Forms.html

73. Y Xu, JR Einstein, RJ Mural, M Shah, EC Uberbacher. An improved system for exon recognition and gene modeling in human DNA sequence. Ismb 2:376–384, 1994.

74. C Burge, S Karlin. Prediction of complete gene structures in human genomic DNA. J Mol Biol 268:78–94, 1997.

75. VV Solovyev, AA Salamov, CB Lawrence. Predicting internal exons by oligonucleotide composition and discriminant analysis of spliceable open reading frames. Nucleic Acids Res 22:5156–5163, 1994.

76. MQ Zhang. Identification of protein coding regions in the human genome by quadratic discriminant analysis [published erratum appears in Proc Natl Acad Sci USA 94:5495, 1997]. Proc Natl Acad Sci USA 94:565–568, 1997.

77. L Milanesi, I Rogozin. Prediction of human gene structure. In: M Bishop, ed. Guide to Human Genome Computing. Cambridge: Academic Press, 1998, pp 215–259.

78. http://www3.oup.co.uk/nar/Volume_28/Issue 01/html/gkd115_gml.html

19

General Conclusions and Future Directions

Werner Kalow
University of Toronto, Toronto, Ontario, Canada

Arno G. Motulsky
University of Washington, Seattle, Washington

1 OVERVIEW

We hope that the different chapters of this book will convey to anyone interested in pharmacogenomics some idea of the various themes and areas of specialized knowledge that will have to come together to convert expectations to reality. The expectations which have been aroused by pharmacogenomics are substantial and involve the gradual development of personalized medicine or therapeutics, leaving behind the present statistically based medicine. There are variable estimates of the time which these processes may require; perhaps it will take 15–20 years. Eventually, however, pharmacogenomics is hoped to be a major payoff for society from the scientific and technical revolution called ''genomics.''

There is no doubt that some of the specialized techniques described in individual chapters are useful at the present time but may be outdated relatively fast as time goes on. This is always a danger for technical descriptions. In addition, the book covers many principles and problems which will remain with us for a long time to come. The main hope of the editors is that all who see and decide to read the book (or to read in the book) will feel to have gained new insights or new knowledge.

Pharmacogenetics and pharmacogenomics will have their impact on medicine, the biomedical sciences, and drug development in several ways. Variable responses to drugs and adverse events have always been observed. Modern genetic approaches have the promise of uncovering the genetic and molecular basis of such variability thereby identifying individuals who are at risk for harmful drug reactions. Appropriate testing before a drug is used will often be possible and the potentially offending drug can be avoided. For some drugs, pretesting may help in defining an appropriate dosage regimen that is effective and avoids toxicity. Drug development will be aided by finding effective medications whose design is based on disease-specific genomic and phenomic alterations. These scientific developments may lead to the elaboration of ''pharmacogenetic efficiency profiles'' for a given drug and more individualized therapy for the patient.

Clinical trials of new drugs will more frequently include only those individuals who on pharmacogenetic and pharmacogenomic grounds have a greater chance of favorably responding to the new drug. Adverse drug reactions are usually difficult to predict but better understanding of drug metabolism, drug response, and more data on genetic polymorphisms will provide occasional opportunities to screen out those at risk for currently unsuspected adverse events.

The best-understood pharmacogenetic examples relate to processes or reactions mediated by a single gene where a mutation grossly interferes with a crucial step in drug metabolism or drug response [1]. However, while more such examples will be discovered, the more frequent role of genetics and genomics will involve multifactorial phenomena where multiple different genes affecting drug metabolism and drug action interact with the environment and with each other. The resultant bell-shaped curve (i.e., number of individuals plotted against a biologic endpoint such as drug half-life) is unlike the bimodal curve classically seen with monogenic drug reactions where ''normals'' and ''abnormals'' represent different populations. As knowledge augments, it will be increasingly possible to define the specific role of each of the various components of polygenic variation by genetic, molecular, and biochemical approaches with careful attention to fixed biologic characteristics (such as age and gender) as well as to various environmental factors.

Pharmacogenetics is not a new science. The role of genes in drug response had been known for over 40 years [2,3] but recognition of a broader applicability of these concepts for drug therapy and drug development only occurred more recently, particularly as molecular techniques for in vitro studies became available and the need to administer a drug to healthy individuals and their family members no longer existed in pharmacogenetic studies. An additional reason for delay in the development of pharmacogenetics was the existence of only a few examples of pharmacogenetic variation that were not considered relevant for drug action in general. The demonstration that metabolism for many drugs as assessed by drug half-life differed among individuals but was very similar in identical twins as compared to nonidentical twins [4] pointed to an important role of genetic factors to explain variation of drug metabolism. Identical twins share all their genes while nonidentical twins have only half of their genes in common.

Major emphasis in pharmacogenetics has remained on monogenic variation which can be studied readily with a variety of modern techniques. In this regard, pharmacogenetics mirrors progress in medical genetics in general. While superb advances continue in unraveling the role of single-gene mutations in genetic diseases, success in isolating and elucidating the role of specific genes in the common multifactorial conditions has been much slower, even though considerable effort has been devoted to various approaches to find these genes [5]. Chromosomal localizations of possibly involved genes have often been suggested. However, repeat studies have tended to be unsuccessful in confirming initial results. Few genes except those represented by the less common monogenic subtypes of a given common disease (such as the autosomal dominant breast and colon cancer genes) have been identified. Identification of the genes that contribute to ''polygenic pharmacogenetics'' may be simpler to achieve since the number of genes involved in drug disposal and drug response are likely to be fewer than in multifactorial diseases. The identification of genes in pharmacogenetics may therefore be less difficult.

A consortium of the pharmaceutical industry together with the Wellcome Trust and several academic institutions are now carrying out a search for common DNA variants known as single-nucleotide polymorphisms (SNPs) across the whole human genome in the hope that such DNA variants can be used as markers to signal the presence of very closely linked genes involved in pharmacogenetic processes [6]. The likelihood of ultimate success in this endeavor is difficult to predict [5,7]. If cSNPs and other DNA changes are detected and related to drug responses, one still has to (1) apply the classical techniques of cloning and identifying the entire gene, (2) express its protein products, and (3) study its function under physiological conditions. The population history, the evolutionary age, and possible selective factors of different SNPs as well as recombination rates between a SNP and the linked gene of interest will vary among populations. The total number of SNPs needed and the number of individuals requiring testing for identifying a relevant gene therefore will often vary between different genes and different populations. Use of genetically more homogeneous populations such as Icelanders in such studies may not necessarily be more helpful [but see 8]. However, data of successful narrowing the genetic region carrying the apo E4 allele (of interest in Alzheimer's disease) have been published by using the SNP approach [9].

2 SOCIETAL PROBLEMS

Fundamental research that led to potential practical applications of pharmacogenetics has usually been carried out in academic institutions. Together with a shift of more biomedical research to pharmaceutical and biotechnology companies, pharmacogenetic and pharmacogenomic approaches now occupy an important place in the research portfolio of such companies. With this shift and an interest of academic institutions to derive income from research discoveries, more patents are being applied for. Efforts have already been made to patent newly discovered human genes without any knowledge of their function. It appears now that the U.S. Patent Office is unlikely to issue such patents unless they describe a novel function or application that has utility such as the commercialization of a discovery. Since introduction of a new drug has become very expensive, granting of patents will make novel drugs more expensive still, increasing the cost of medical care, a major problem in much of the world.

The total impact of pharmacogenetics and pharmacogenomics on the pharmaceutical industry in the long run is hazardous to predict. However, even though some analysts on the business side of the pharmaceutical industry are concerned about reducing market size by targeting smaller segments of the population, most companies have placed large investments in genetic and genomic applications in the belief that these approaches will lead to ultimate success and profitability. The impact of pharmacogenetics and pharmacogenomics on the practice of medicine as compared with the development of new drugs should be considered separately. New drug development is of key interest to industry but of less importance to practicing physicians until a new drug becomes available for use. Genomic concepts and techniques together with the application of proteomics are likely to point out new targets for drug therapy based on better understanding of the biologic mechanism of disease. A more rational therapy is therefore likely to evolve. Effectiveness of a given drug in only some patients is currently common. Occasionally, the reason may be simple and relates to differences in drug metabolism such as "rapid inactivators" who require larger doses to maintain effective blood levels of a given drug. Studies of other kinds of genetic variation such as drug targets may reveal novel genetic mechanisms responsible for differential responses.

Pharmaceutical companies often want orphan drug status given to a new drug. Under current FDA rules, drugs for rare conditions affecting fewer than 200,000 people in the United States receive tax breaks on clinical trials, and 7 years of marketing exclusivity. Drugs that currently have a larger market but that following pharmacogenetic testing would be predictably effective in <200,000 people might qualify under current rules. Will more drugs therefore be given orphan status? Developments in this area will be followed with much interest.

3 ETHICAL PROBLEMS

Not covered in this book are ethical issues which may be harder to solve than some technical problems. Considering ethical issues, it is useful to start by contemplating the Hippocratic Code: The patient, after having agreed to be treated by a physician, trusts the physician to act in the patient's best interest; no other ethical problem arises. This is an entirely different situation from one in which the physician's interest is not only the patient's well-being but the promotion of knowledge—in other words, the promotion of research.

Protection of a patient's interest who participates in a research project has led to many statements and laws. A major start was the Nuremberg Code [10]. In the United States, the Office of Protection from Research Risks (OPRR) has issued regulations known as the "Common Rule." Almost everywhere are institutional review boards, safeguarding the rights of the individuals.

The point to be considered in the present context is that with the aim to create personalized medicine, most investigations will be designed to benefit the patient as well as to promote general knowledge. The logical consequence for the formulation of protective laws should be to combine the new rules with the spirit of the Hippocratic Code. It remains to be seen to which extent this will be possible.

If the medical choice of drug or drug dosage depends on a patient's genes, the prescriber has to know the genes of the patient which may affect these choices; this requires a look into the patient's genetic privacy. However, it also requires the prescriber to know from a study of pharmacogenetics or pharmacogenomics which genotypes are compatible with which drug, necessitating a restructuring of medical education within the framework of the many other problems posed by developments in genetic and genomic medicine.

Many ethical and societal issues of pharmacogenetics and pharmacogenomics are not unique and raise issues similar to those brought up by the recent advances. While different human populations regardless of geographic origin of their ancestors share the vast majority of their genes, considerable genetic variation remains which renders everyone genetically unique. There is considerably more genetic variation within a given population (or "race") than among populations [11]. The concept of race is based on external resemblances only and therefore makes little genetic sense. Nevertheless, the frequencies of pharmacogenetic traits usually differ in populations from various parts of the world (see Chapter 6) due to different selective factors but often for unknown reasons. Since such differences may cause adverse drug reactions or variable drug responses, knowledge of a patient's ethnic origin will often be useful to select appropriate pharmacogenetic tests for clinical trials or in medical practice. If a given allele (or set of alleles) that leads to differential drug metabolism or variable drug response differs between ethnic groups, selection of the appropriate PCR reactions (or similar test) characteristic for a given population can be made. However, it may often be difficult logistically to assign ethnic origin and ethnic mixture is increasingly common as well. All alleles of a given pharmacogenetic system rather than a population specific set may therefore need to be included in the test system. Utilization of biochemical tests such as measurement of enzyme activity may sometimes be more appropriate since it could detect low enzyme activity regardless of which one of multiple DNA alleles that reduce enzyme activity is involved. Molecular diagnosis, however, is currently simpler and more accurate, and can be more readily automated. The technical and population problems encountered will vary for different biochemical and molecular measurements of a given pharmacogenetic trait.

DNA testing has raised public worries regarding privacy, and legislative initiatives have been proposed to restrict DNA testing in medical settings. Such trends often relate to failure of differentiating forensic DNA tests from DNA tests designed to diagnose various diseases or disease susceptibilities. Genetic testing in medicine raises problems of informed consent, privacy, confidentiality, stigmatization, and discrimination (health insurance and occupation), and requires appropriate guidelines and oversight [12]. Roses has pointed out, however, that pharmacogenetic testing which aims to detect genes and SNP profiles involved in drug metabolism and drug action is different by only searching for a "pharmacogenetic efficiency" or "medicine response" profile [13]. He states that such a goal carries no special ethical or social problems and therefore should be considered differently than other kinds of genetic testing. Attempting to find the most appropriate drug for a patient is therefore considered similar to other diagnostic tests in medicine. However, an abnormal result is also relevant for drug therapy of relatives. As long as DNA specimens are only used for pharmacogenetic tests related to adverse events and effective drug responses, a good case can be made for treating such tests somewhat differently from more sensitive genetic tests with more serious implications.

Clinical trials on patients with a disease pose additional problems. Here, patients with variable disease mechanisms and often with a different natural history of their disease may require different treatments. Detailed descriptions of dietary habits, smoking, and other environmental exposures (depending on the condition under study) in addition to age, sex, and ethnic origin will be necessary in clinical trials to elucidate the interaction of environmental and genetic factors. Anonymity that strips a specimen of a name but retains demographic, genetic, and environmental information is one solution and allows additional investigation when new laboratory methodology and additional genetic and environmental markers for studies of the same disease become available. Retention of ethnic identity may be important for the reasons already mentioned. To prevent future abuses, it has been suggested to destroy DNA specimens after testing has been completed. Much valuable information in research studies would be lost under these circumstances, particularly if novel tests become available for the study of the same disease, thus causing problems in locating study subjects. Anonymity with retention of specimens therefore appears most appropriate but has the disadvantage that even a trial participant will not have access to his or her own specimen in the future.

Other problems arise. The intellectual property rights related to specimens from clinical trials are not always clear. Do the study participants whose SNPs lead to new drugs and more appropriate therapy own their DNA, or do all potential benefits go to the investigator or company who collect these specimens? Under what conditions could organizations that collect DNA for either clinical trials or other purposes sell this information to third parties?

REFERENCES

1. W Weber. Pharmacogenetics. New York: Oxford University Press. 1997.
2. A Motulsky. Drug reactions, enzymes and biochemical genetics. JAMA 165:835–837, 1957.
3. W Kalow. Pharmacogenetics—Heredity and the Responses to Drugs. Philadelphia: W.B. Saunders, 1962.
4. ES Vesell. Pharmacogenetic perspectives gained from twin and family studies. Pharmacol Ther 41:535–552, 1989.
5. NJ Risch. Searching for genetic determinants in the new millennium. Nature 405:847–856, 2000.
6. JJ McCarthy, R Hilfiker. The use of single-nucleotide polymorphism maps in pharmacogenomics. Nat Biotechnol 18:505–508, 2000.
7. L Kruglyak. Prospects for whole-genome linkage disequilibrium mapping of common disease genes. Nat Genet 22:139–144, 1999.
8. A Collins, C Lonjou, NE Morton. Genetic epidemiology of single-nucleotide polymorphisms. Proc Natl Acad Sci USA 96: 15173–15177, 1999.
9. ER Martin, EH Lai, JR Gilbert, AR Rogala, AJ Afshari, J Riley, KL Finch, JF Stevens, KJ Livak, BD Slotterbeck, SH Slifer, LL Warren, PM Conneally, DE Schmechel, I Purvis, MA Pericak-Vance, AD Roses, JM Vance. SNPing away at complex diseases: analysis of single-nucleotide polymorphism around APOE in alzheimer disease. Am J Hum Genet 67:383–394, 2000.
10. ME Sobel. Ethical issues in molecular pathology: paradigms in flux. Arch Pathol Lab Med 123:1076–1078, 1999.
11. LL Cavalli-Sforza. Genes, Peoples, and Languages. New York: North Point Press, 2000.
12. NA Holtzman. Promoting safe and effective genetic tests in the United States: work of the task force on genetic testing. Clin Chem 45:732–738, 1999.
13. AD Roses. Pharmacogenetics and the practice of medicine. Nature 405:857–865, 2000.

Index

ABC transporters, 83
Acetaldehyde, 123
Adenomatous polyposis coli, 240
β-Adrenergic receptor, 68, 140, 147
β-Adrenoreceptor, 16
Adverse drug reactions (ADRs), 45
Affymetrix, 184
Africa, 110, 113
AH receptors (*see* Arylhydrocarbon
    hydroxylase receptors)
AIDS, 70
AIDS resistance, 1
Albuterol, 147
Alcohol dehydrogenase, 3, 122
Aldehyde dehydrogenase, 122, 124
Allele-specific amplification assay,
    173
Allele-specific oligonucleotide
    assay, 172
ALOX5 promoter, 16

Alzheimer's disease, 337
Amerind, 110
Aminoglutethimide, 192
Amobarbital, 4
Androgen, 55, 58, 59
Angiotensin converting enzyme
    (ACE), 146, 337
Antidepressants, 12, 191
Antigen processing, 84
Antisense design, 333
Apolipoprotein E gene (APOE), 337
Applied bioinformatics, 311
Array-based systems, 161
Arrhythmias, 18
Arylhydrocarbon hydroxylase recep-
    tors, 63, 64
Asians, 110
Asthma, 17, 68, 366
Atherogenesis, 241
Australian, 110

AutoLoad plate, 196
Azathioprine, 42, 43, 145

Bandwidth, 308
Basic Local Alignment Search Tool
    (BLAST), 326
Baylor College of Medicine's
    MBCR, 302
BCRP (see Breast cancer resistance
    protein)
Bile salt export pump, 13, 90
Bioinformatics, 308
Biomarkers, 13
Breast cancer resistance protein, 94
Browsers, 308
Brute force variant identification,
    153
Butyrylcholinesterase, 2

Cancer, 17, 145
Candidate gene approaches, 365
Candidate gene strategy, 339
Capillary electrophoresis, 198
Capillary isoelectric focusing
    (CIEF), 278
Cardiac ion channels, 147
Cardiff Mutation Database, 302
Cardiovascular drugs, 192
Catalase, 120
Caucasians, 4
CCR5 receptor, 70
Cell surface receptors, 64, 67
CFTR, 94
Charge modification index (CMI),
    264
Chemical mismatch identification,
    159
Cheminformatics, 334
Chemokine receptor CCR5 gene
    (CMKBR5), 337
China, 35, 113
Chinese, 4

3-[(3-cholamidopropyl)dimethyl-
    ammonio]-1-propanesulfate
    (CHAPS), 258
Chromosome, 6, 22, 36, 44
Citalopram, 118, 144
Classification, 53
Climate, 114
Clomipramine, 118
CLUSTAL W, 329
Clustered genes, 333
Codeine, 5, 142, 145
Collision-induced dissociation
    (CID), 271
Common gateway interface (CGI),
    308
Complex (or multifactorial) dis-
    eases, 337, 338
Concatenation, 225
Coomassie blue staining, 261
Coomassie Brilliant Blue (CBB),
    262
Crohn's disease, 42
Cyclosporin A, 146
CYP1A1 activity, 63, 64
CYP2C19, 16, 115, 117, 137
CYP2C9, 135, 145
CYP2D6, 3, 115, 135, 138, 191,
    194
CYP2D6 polymorphism, 34, 42
Cytochromes P450, 112

Dapsone, 119
Data mining, 332
ddF, 156
Debrisoquine, 3, 4, 34, 144, 113,
    115, 117, 144
Decreased enzyme activity, 36
Depression, 17
Dextromethorphan, 144
DGGE, 157
dHPLC, 158
Diabetes, 17

Diagnostic assays, 22
Diazepam, 118
Dideoxy DNA sequencing, 186
Digoxin, 146
Dihydropyrimidine dehydrogenase
 (DPD), 137, 145
Dioxin, 63
Discovery, 34
Disease, molecular characterization,
 15
Dithiotreitol (DTT), 258
DNA chip microarrays, 139
DNA chip technology, 176
DNA Database of Japan (DDBJ),
 293, 297
DNA ligases, 192
DNA polymerases, 192
DNA polymorphisms, 340
Drugable targets, 11
Drug–drug interactions, 44
Drug safety vs. efficacy, 7
Drug substrates, 40
Duodenal ulcer, 17

Ecogenetics, terminology, 6
ED50, 5
Edge effect, 6
Electrospray ionization mass spec-
 trometry (ESI-MS), 270
EM (see Extensive metabolizers)
Endotoxic shock, 71
Enzymatic mismatch identification,
 159
Enzyme-based DNA sequencing, 186
Esterases, 112
Estrogen, 56, 59, 60
Ethanol, 122
Ethnic differences, 35, 37, 44
Ethnicity, 110
Ethylmorphine, 145
European Bioinformatics Institute
 (EBI), 293, 296

European Molecular Biology Labora-
 tory (EMBL), 293, 296
Europeans, 110
Exonuclease I, 203
Extensive metabolizers (EM), 138

Factor VIII gene, 366
FASTA, 305
FASTA formatted record, 318
Fatal adverse drug reactions, 135
Fenoxifenadin, 146
Fibrillin, 366
Fluoxetine, 144
Fluvoxamin, 144
Foods, adverse effects of, 1
Functional cloning, 339
Functional genomics, 34, 253

Gel shift assays, 154
Genatlas, 303
GenBank divisions, 313
GenBank Flat File Format (GBFF),
 315, 320
Gene deletion, 36
Gene duplication, 39, 117
Gene expressions, 3, 223
Gene scanning, 154
Généthon, 298
Genome Database (GDB), 298
Genomewide linkage scans, 345
Genotyping, 142
Geography, 110
Gilbert syndrome, 122
Glipicide, 145
Glucocorticoid, 55, 58
Glucocorticoid receptor, 304
Glucose-6-phosphate dehydrogenase
 (G-6-PD), 2, 120
Glucuronyltransferase, 122
Glutathione (GSH), 120
Glycoproteins, 272
G Protein Coupled Receptor, 304

HA, 158
Haloperidol, 42
Haplotype, 341
Hemophilia A, 366
Hepatocyte, 88
Hepatotoxicity, 18
Hexose monophosphate, 120
Hippocratic Code, 392
Histamine H_2 blocker, 12
HIV, 337
HLA-associated diseases, 349
HLA region, 339
HLA subtypes, 16
Homology analysis, 324
HOVERGEN, 323
Human Genome Nomenclature Com-
    mittee, 4
Human Genome Project, conse-
    quences of, 26
Huntington's disease, 338
Hybridization-based sequencing,
    185
Hydralazine, 119, 192
Hyperlipidemia, 17
Hypertension, 17

IgE, 68
Illumina, 184
Imipramine, 44, 118
Immobilized pH gradient electropho-
    resis (IPG), 259
Immunogenetics, 304
Immunosuppression, 42
Incomplete penetrance, 338
Insulin response, 65
Interethnic, 109, 134
Intrasubject variation (drug repeti-
    tion), 6
Ion channel receptors, 64, 65
Irinotecan, 145
Isoelectric focusing (IEF), 254, 256,
    259

Isoniazid, 2, 119
Isoniazid acetylation, 192
Isotope-coded affinity tags (ICATs),
    278

Japanese, 110, 124
Jervell Lange-Nielsen syndrome, 65

Koreans, 110

Leucopenia, 145
Leukocyte antigens (HLA), 366
Levomepromazine, 44
Library contigs, 378
Linkage analyses, 342, 371
Linkage disequilibrium, 341
Linkage disequilibrium analysis,
    369
Linkage disequilibrium mapping,
    346
5-Lipoxygenase inhibitor, 16
Long-QT syndrome (LQTS), 65
Luminex, 184

Major histocompatibility complex,
    339
Malaria, 120
MALDI-TOF MS, 202
Malnutrition, 114
Marfan's syndrome, 366
Mass MDR-1, 146
Matrix-assisted laser desorption/ion-
    ization (MALDI), 267
Matrix selection, 328
Maturity-onset diabetes of the
    young (MODY), 343
MDR1 (*see* P-glycoprotein)
MDR3, 12
MDRs (*see* Multidrug resistance pro-
    teins)
Mechanism of action, 14
Membrane transporters, 83, 146

Mephenytoin, 117
Mercaptopurine, 145
6-Mercaptopurine, 43
MFS (major facilitator superfamily),
    3
Microsatellites, 340, 343
Migraine, 17
Minisequencing, 191
Mismatch identification, 159
Mitochondrial Genome Database,
    304
MOA (*see* Mechanism of action)
Modifiergenes, 338
Molecular diagnostics, 169
Monogenic vs. multigenic varia-
    tions, 5
Morphine, 5, 142
MRP1, 16
MRP2/cMOAT, 17
MRP3, 6, 8
MRP subfamily C, 14, 15
MultAlin, 329
Multidrug resistance–associated pro-
    teins (MRP), 90–94
Multidrug resistance proteins, 84
Multifactorial variation, 6
Multiple sclerosis, 366
Multiplex fluorescent minisequenc-
    ing, 193
Multiplex genotyping, 208, 217
Multiplex genotyping mass spec-
    trometry, 201
Multispecific OCTs, 27
Myelosuppression, 43, 145
Myocardial infarction, 337

N-acetyltransferase, 137, 119
Nanogen, 184
NAT1, 119
NAT2, 119, 194
National Center for Biotechnology
    Information (NCBI), 293

Neonatal jaundice, 121
Neuroleptics, 191
Neurological disturbances, 119
Non-array-based systems, 163
Nonequilibrium pH gradient electro-
    phoresis (NEPHGE), 260
Nonresponders, 17
Nortriptyline, 40, 41, 140
Nuclear receptors, 55, 57

OATP (*see* Organic anion trans-
    porter) 21, 24
OATP-A, 22
OATP-B, 22
OATP-C, 24
OCT (*see* Organic cation trans-
    porter)
Office of Protection from Research
    Risks (OPRR), 393
Oligonucleotide ligation assay,
    174
Oligonucleotide primer, 206
Oligonucleotide probe, 333
Omeprazol, 118
Open reading frame, 330
Opioids, 145
Organic anion transporter (OATP),
    21, 24, 95, 97
Organic cation transporter (OCT),
    25, 97, 99
Orphan drug, 392
Osteoporosis, 62, 63
Osteo/rheumatoid arthritis, 17
Oxidases, 112

P-aminosalicylic acid (PAS), 119
Paroxetine, 144
PCR restriction enzyme assay, 172
Personalized medicine, 14, 24
P-glycoprotein (MDR1), 5, 12, 85,
    89, 146
Pharmaceutical proteomics, 279

Pharmacogenetics, history of, 1, 4, 135,
Pharmacogenomics:
  definition, 23
  terminology, 6, 7
Phase II and III trials, 18, 19
Phenotyping, 7
Phenytoin, 145
Physical mapping, 377
Physiology, 10
Plasma cholinesterase, 2
Plasma pseudocholinesterase, 137
Plasmodium falciparum, 120
Polydactyly, 338
Polymerase chain reaction (PCR), 36
Polynesian, 114
Polyvinylidene fluoride (PVDF), 267
Poor metabolizer (PM), 34, 139
Porphyria, 2
Positional cloning, 339, 363, 365, 368, 372
Positron emmission tomography (PET), 138
Previously identified gene variants, 161
Primaquine hemolysis, 2, 120
Primer extension assay, 175
Prizidilol, 192
Procainamide, 119
Procaine, 2
Proguanil, 118
Propanolol, 118
Protein deficiency, 114
Proteomes, 223
Proteomics, 253, 254
Pseudocholinesterase, 2
Pseudogenes, 192
Psoriasis, 366
Pyrosequencing, 186

QTc, 18

Receptor history, 51, 54
Receptor variants, 52
Reductases, 112
REF, 155
Renal toxicity, 18
Restriction length polymorphism (RFLP), 36
Retinoid acid, 57, 60, 61
Rheumatoid arthritis, 16
Rickets, 61, 62
Romano-Ward syndrome, 65

S-adenosine methionine, 42
SAGE, 224, 231, 233, 235
Salt intake, 1
Schizophrenia, 17
Selective serotonin reuptake inhibitors (SSRIs), 12
Sequence file formats, 314
Sequin, 294
Serial analysis of gene expression (SAGE), 223
Serious adverse experience (SAE), 12, 16
Serotonin reuptake inhibitors, 191
Sertraline, 144
Sickle cell anemia, 121, 338, 366
Similarity searches, 325
Single-nucleotide polymorphisms (SNPs), 3, 13, 183
Societal problems, 391
Sodium dodecyl sulfate electrophoresis, 254
Sodium dodecyl sulfate–polyacrylamide gel electrophoresis (SDS-PAGE), 356
Spain, 113
Sparteine, 3, 34, 117, 144
Spectrometry, 202

SSCP, 155
Stanford Human Genome Center, 301
Starvation, 1, 114
Strepatavidin, 193
Subfamilies, 84
Substrates, 43
Succinylcholine, 2
Sulfonamides, 119, 192
Sulfonylurea receptors, 19, 65, 94, 147
Sweden, 35, 113
SWISS-PROT, 297, 322

Tardive dyskinesia, 135
Target validation, 24
Taxonomy database, 323
TCDD (2,3,7,8-tetrachlorodibenzo-p-dioxin), 63
Terfenadine, 146, 147
TGGE, 158
Thalassemia, 121, 366
Thermal cycling, 207
ThermoSequence DNA polymerase, 196
Thioguanine, 145
Thiopurine methyltransferase (TPMT), 34, 137, 145
Thyroid hormone receptors, 304
Tolbutamide, 145, 147
Tolterodine, 44
Torsades de pointes (TdP), 16
TPMT, 34, 42, 44

Transcriptomes, 223, 224, 242, 254
TRANSFAC Database, 323
Transferases, 112
Transporter associated antigen processing, 84
Tributylphosphine, 258
Tuberculosis, 119
Tuberculosis resistance, 1
Twin studies, 2, 6
Two-dimensional gel electrophoresis, 254, 255
Type 1 diabetes, 343–345, 366

Ubiquitin, 245
UDP-glucuronosyltransferase (UGT1A1), 137
Ultrarapid metabolizer (UM), 139
Unigene databases, 317

Vanuatu, 118
Variant frequency, 111
Verapamil, 146
Vitamin D, 57

Warfarin, 145
Washington University Genome Sequencing Center, 301
Weizmann Institute of Science Genome Center, 300
Whitehead/MIT Center for Genome Research, 300
WWW resources, 291–310